# Statistics and the Language of Global Health

Yi-Tang Lin presents the historical process by which statistics became the language of global health for local and international health organizations. Drawing on archival material from three continents, this study investigates efforts by public health schools, philanthropic foundations, and international organizations to turn numbers into an international language for public health. Lin shows how these initiatives produced an international network of public health experts who, across various socioeconomic and political contexts, opted for different strategies when it came to setting global standards and translating local realities into numbers. Focusing on China and Taiwan between 1917 and 1960, Lin examines the reception, adaptation, and appropriation of international health statistics. She presents the dynamic interplay between numbers, experts, and policy-making in international health organizations and administrations in China and Taiwan. This title is also available as Open Access on Cambridge Core.

Yi-Tang Lin is a Swiss National Science Foundation postdoctoral fellow at the University of Geneva and a visiting scholar at the Harvard Fairbank Center for Chinese Studies for 2021–22.

*Global Health Histories*

*Series editor:*

Sanjoy Bhattacharya, University of York

*Global Health Histories* aims to publish outstanding and innovative scholarship on the history of public health, medicine and science worldwide. By studying the many ways in which the impact of ideas of health and well-being on society were measured and described in different global, international, regional, national and local contexts, books in the series reconceptualise the nature of empire, the nation state, extra-state actors and different forms of globalisation. The series showcases new approaches to writing about the connected histories of health and medicine, humanitarianism, and global economic and social development.

# Statistics and the Language of Global Health

*Institutions and Experts in China, Taiwan, and the World, 1917–1960*

Yi-Tang Lin

*University of Geneva*

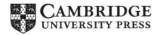

CAMBRIDGE UNIVERSITY PRESS

# CAMBRIDGE
## UNIVERSITY PRESS

University Printing House, Cambridge CB2 8BS, United Kingdom

One Liberty Plaza, 20th Floor, New York, NY 10006, USA

477 Williamstown Road, Port Melbourne, VIC 3207, Australia

314–321, 3rd Floor, Plot 3, Splendor Forum, Jasola District Centre, New Delhi – 110025, India

103 Penang Road, #05–06/07, Visioncrest Commercial, Singapore 238467

Cambridge University Press is part of the University of Cambridge.

It furthers the University's mission by disseminating knowledge in the pursuit of education, learning, and research at the highest international levels of excellence.

www.cambridge.org
Information on this title: www.cambridge.org/9781108845922
DOI: 10.1017/9781108991339

First published 2022

*A catalogue record for this publication is available from the British Library.*

ISBN 978-1-108-84592-2 Hardback

For my parents,
Chen Ying and Lin Kuo-Ching

# Contents

# Figures

# Tables

# Acknowledgments

This book tells the stories of people who traveled and learned. In my own travels and learning, I have relied on the help of many people.

For his support during the doctoral research on which this book is based, I would like to express my sincere gratitude to my dissertation advisor, Thomas David, for his scrupulous and critical reading, which pushed me to refine every part of my argument amid a sea of archival sources. My co-advisor, Davide Rodogno, was the first person to read my preliminary chapters and advised me to write more like a historian, a skill that I am still learning. Their mentorship, patience, and passion for research guided me throughout my doctoral work. The dissertation would not have been what it is without the comments and criticisms of my thesis committee, and for that I am profoundly indebted to Anne-Emanuelle Birn, Pierre Singaravélou, and Yohan Ariffin.

This book has greatly benefited from myriad discussions and critical comments, and the testing out of my arguments over the years. I want to address my gratitude to the members of the Swiss National Science Foundation's Sinergia research network "Patterns of Transnational Regulation" – Sandrine Kott, Martin Lengwiler, Roberto Sala, Matthieu Leimgruber, Jean-Christophe Graz, Milena Guthörl, and Nils Moussu – for stimulating discussions and comments on my drafts. I have enjoyed and learned so much from our meetings. I would also like to thank Lion Murard, Patricia Rosenfield, Dan Fox, Sean Hsiang-Lin Lei, Chang Li, Kawashima Shin, Dora Vargha, and the late Socrates Litsios for the inspiring discussions and encouragement.

The Swiss National Science Foundation provided important financial support for this book: the open access version of this book was funded by the Swiss National Science Foundation, and I would not have had access to such extensive archival materials without the financial support of the Foundation's Sinergia research network. I would also like to thank Reynald Erard of the World Health Organization Archives, Jacques Oberson of the League of Nations Archives, and Margaret Hogan, Monica Blank, and the late Tom Rosenbaum of the Rockefeller Archive Center:

not only did they share their knowledge, they slaked my thirst for sources by providing leads to more material. A chat with Tom provided leads for Chapter 2. My sincere thanks to Zhang Daqing, Liu Shiyung, and Zhang Yung-An for helping me to access Chinese archives. It was not easy to gain access to Chinese material from Switzerland; I am grateful to Chen Ju-Han, Kao Tzu-Yi, and Lin Yi-Hsuan for helping me access online databases, which saved me much trouble. I would also like to thank the Beijing Municipal Archives, the Peking Union Medical College Archives, the Archives of the Chinese Ministry of Foreign Affairs, the National Library of China, Shanghai Library, Academia Historica, the Institute of Modern History of the Academia Sinica, Taiwan Historica, the Alan Mason Chesney Medical Archives of the Johns Hopkins Medical Institutions, the American Philosophical Society, the Columbia University Libraries, the National Archives and Records Administration (College Park), the United Nations Archives and Records Management Section, the William H. Welch Medical Library, and Yale University Library.

I have given lectures based on parts of this book at the Peking University Department of History of Science, Technology and Medicine, the Chinese Academy of Science Institute for the History of Natural Science, and the Global Asia Research Center at National Taiwan University. I would like to thank Zhang Li, Zhang Daqing, Wu Chia-Lin, Lan Pei-Chia, and the participants at those lectures for the thought-provoking discussions and encouragement. Sanjoy Bhattacharya, Lucy Rhymer, and anonymous readers have helped this book become what it is today and live up to its potential. Rachel Blaifeder bore with my rookie editing questions. Margaret Besser copyedited the manuscript; her meticulous editing and knowledge of Chinese helped me overcome linguistic barriers and saved me from many embarrassing typos. Jess Farr-Cox, Stephanie Carter, Aaron Glasserman and Mathilde Sigalas provided precious advice at the final stretch of editing. Ludovic Tournès, Pierre-Yves Saunier, Lan Pei-Chia, Davide Rodogno, Harry Wu shared their experience of writing books and prepared me for this otherwise unimaginable ride.

Rewrites were completed during my postdoctoral research on the Swiss National Science Foundation Heralds of Globalization project. My teammates Ahmad Fahoum, Mathilde Sigalas, Hannah Tyler, and I are now sailing in an even larger sea of experts who have traveled and learned.

My friends and colleagues Sabina Widmer, Johanna Schnabel, Virginie Fracheboud, Andrea Pilotti, Caroline Bertron, Chuang Ya-Han, Lee Shih-Rong, and Michael Hutter were precious allies during the long thesis-writing process. Yi-Chien Chu, Chia-Fen Liao, De-Wei Chen,

Shu-Wen Tang, and Chang-Jr Lin helped me make it through the difficult period when I was unable to go home by "airdropping" Taiwanese food. Po-Jung Yang and Pei-Yin Chien always remind me of my deadlines and make sure I am making progress. Albert Hsu, Yung-wei Song, and Ray Ho were always welcoming during my trips to the New York archives – at a time when traveling was simpler.

Finally, special thanks to my family. My parents are always supportive of my odd life choices. My sister has been my reserve commander, supplying me with food. My partner, Dominique, has been amazingly supportive in so many ways – from taking photos in the archives while on vacation to taking care of household chores and enduring my monologues-disguised-as-questions with a delightfully weird sense of humor.

# Note on Language

This book uses the pinyin romanization system. The historical romanizations used in original sources are provided upon first mention in each chapter. Alternative forms are used for the following: (1) historical figures who are widely known under a different romanization (e.g. Sun Yat-Sen, Chiang Kai-Shek); (2) Taiwanese places; and (3) contemporary scholars, whose names are romanized according to their preference.

## Cited Works

Historical publications in Chinese are romanized using pinyin. Author names for English-language publications are cited in their original forms. Journals in Chinese are cited in pinyin alongside their official translations.

A glossary of Chinese individuals and organizations is provided at the end of this book.

# Abbreviations

| | |
|---|---|
| AICP | Association for Improving the Condition of the Poor |
| APHA | American Public Health Association |
| BCG | Bacillus Calmette–Guérin (vaccine) |
| CCMC | Committee on the Costs of Medical Care |
| CFHS | Central Field Health Station |
| DALY | Disability-Adjusted Life Year |
| GMEP | Global Malaria Eradication Program |
| ICA | International Cooperation Administration |
| ICD | International List of Causes of Death/International Classification of Diseases |
| IHB | International Health Board |
| IHD | International Health Division |
| ISI | International Statistical Institute |
| JCRR | Joint Commission on Rural Reconstruction |
| JHSPH | Johns Hopkins School of Public Health |
| LNHO | League of Nations Health Organization |
| MEM | Mass Education Movement |
| NHA | National Health Administration |
| OIHP | Office international d'hygiène publique |
| PAHO | Pan American Health Organization |
| PFHS | Peking First Health Station |
| PRC | People's Republic of China |
| PUMC | Peking Union Medical College |
| ROC | Republic of China |
| TMRI | Taiwan Malaria Research Institute |
| UNICEF | United Nations Children's Fund |
| UNRRA | United Nations Relief and Rehabilitation Administration |
| USPHS | United States Public Health Service |
| WHO | World Health Organization |
| WHOIC | World Health Organization Interim Commission |

# Introduction

World data ... are essential for international organizations assisting countries to organize their health services, as well as for institutions and individuals undertaking research into epidemiological and statistical matters of world or regional concern.[1]

In a World Health Organization (WHO) document entitled "International Work in Health Statistics, 1948–1958," WHO founding statisticians Yves Biraud (also known as Yves-Marie Biraud) and Satya Swaroop, along with a former consultant, Harry Sutherland Gear, set out their aspirations for global health data. The document was published in 1961, decades before the catchwords "evidence-based medicine" and "big data" came to epitomize the predominance of quantitative data in global health policy-making. The trio underscored the importance of incorporating statistics into research and policy-making, presenting a vision in which researchers and public health officers across the world would use statistics to advance understanding of epidemiological situations and devise policies aimed at improving people's health. The quotation above also encapsulates the main purpose of this book. Whereas policy publications tend to present numerical analysis as an innovative – if not exactly new – panacea for global health research and governance, this book aims to portray the historical process and sociopolitical contexts through which statistical practices circulated and eventually became a legitimate means of communication between international health organizations and national and local administrations. I also examine the strategies public health institutions and experts used to collect and disseminate statistics vis-à-vis international health organizations.

It is no accident that this book starts with the 1910s, when a wide array of transnational organizations, public and private, aspired to serve several countries at once and used statistics as a language to facilitate international collaboration. Governments, in Western Europe in particular,

---

[1] Harry Sutherland Gear, Yves Biraud, and Satya Swaroop, *International Work in Health Statistics, 1948–1958* (Geneva: WHO, 1961), 56.

had of course already been collecting numbers to better manage the health conditions of their populations in various ways.[2] Although historians have provided accounts of early (and often failed) European-led attempts to collect statistics at the international level ever since the first International Sanitary Conference of 1851,[3] little is known about how countries outside of Western Europe (including their colonies) and North America used similar statistical practices to tackle public health crises. As this book will demonstrate, it was only in the twentieth century that American philanthropic organizations began to provide resources and expertise to help administrations and research organizations on other continents to quantify their public health affairs. These programs, which aimed to improve the well-being of humanity across the globe through public health actions, spread the consensus on the usefulness of statistics for public health beyond Europe and North America, persuading research institutes and health administrations in a number of countries to learn the language of numbers.

It should be stressed that the statistical initiatives presented in this book were a continuation of nineteenth-century European initiatives that sought to standardize vital and health statistics at the international scale. Specifically, nineteenth-century Europe underwent a series of administrative changes – public health movements, the increased use of statistics by national administrations, and growing intergovernmental collaboration – which led to the collection and exchange of vital and health statistics at the international level. Existing historiographies chronicle how, during the first half of the nineteenth century, an increasing number of experts in Europe began to rely on numbers to tackle public health crises.[4] For instance, British experts Edwin Chadwick (1800–1890) and John Snow (1813–1858), along with their French counterparts Louis René Villermé (1782–1863) and Pierre-Charles Alexandre Louis (1787–1872), all used cross-tabulated birth and

---

[2] See, e.g.: Michael Donnelly, "William Farr and Quantification in Nineteenth-Century English Public Health," in *Body Counts: Medical Quantification in Historical and Sociological Perspectives/La Quantification Médicale, Perspectives Historiques et Sociologiques*, eds. George Weisz et al. (Montreal: McGill-Queens, 2005), 251–65; Mervyn Susser and Zena Stein, *Eras in Epidemiology: The Evolution of Ideas* (Oxford and New York: Oxford University Press, 2009).

[3] Valeska Huber, "The Unification of the Globe by Disease? The International Sanitary Conferences on Cholera, 1851–1894," *The Historical Journal* 49, no. 2 (2006): 453–76; Céline Paillette, "Épidémies, santé et ordre mondial. Le rôle des organisations sanitaires internationales, 1903–1923," *Monde(s)*, no. 2 (2012): 235–56.

[4] For more on public health experts' use of statistics in their work see, e.g.: Alfredo Morabia, *A History of Epidemiologic Methods and Concepts* (Basel: Birkhäuser, 2004); Susser and Stein, *Eras in Epidemiology*.

death statistics by district (or other criteria) to infer the origins of communicable diseases. At the same time, European public administrations were beginning to recruit specialists to collect and compile statistics. The best-known case was that of Louis' two pupils, William Farr (1807–1883) and Marc d'Espine (1806–1860), both of whom became official compilers of vital and health statistics (Farr in England and Wales, and d'Espine in Geneva). Farr and d'Espine further took on leading roles when the number of international conferences and congresses mushroomed in the 1850s, and the two men endeavored to standardize the collection of vital and health statistics across countries. Specifically, the International Statistical Congresses and the International Sanitary Conferences each produced a set of reporting standards for health statistics that are still maintained and revised by international health organizations: an international nomenclature of causes of death (the precursor to the International Classification of Diseases), which Farr and d'Espine were the first to draft, and the International Sanitary Regulations (now known as the International Health Regulations). Despite their differing priorities, the participants in the conferences managed to devise these standards in the hope of harmonizing vital and health statistical collection and reporting across countries. The goal was for statistics to be comparable and be used to alert the world to future epidemics. Reaching a consensus proved extremely difficult during both series of gatherings, as there was disagreement as to the etiology of communicable diseases for most of the nineteenth century. The International Sanitary Regulations also became embroiled in diplomatic disputes and international trade issues.[5]

If the main development in the nineteenth century was the birth of these sets of standards, the core achievement in the twentieth was the crystallization and implementation of statistics-led health administration procedures in different corners of the world through the work of various organizations, with financial support from American philanthropic

---

[5] For detailed historical accounts of these international gatherings and the standards they produced, see, e.g.: Norman Howard-Jones, *The Scientific Background of the International Sanitary Conferences, 1851–1938* (Geneva: World Health Organization, 1974); Éric Brian, "Statistique administrative et internationalisme statistique pendant la seconde moitié du XIXe siècle," *Histoire & Mesure* 4, no. 3 (1989): 201–24; Huber, "The Unification of the Globe by Disease? The International Sanitary Conferences on Cholera, 1851–1894"; Anne Rasmussen, "L'hygiène en congrès (1852–1912): circulation et configuration internationales," in *Les Hygiénistes: Enjeux, modèles et pratiques, (XVIIIe-XXe Siècles)*, ed. Patrice Bourdelais (Paris: Belin, 2011), 213–39; Sylvia Chiffoleau, *Genèse de la santé publique internationale: de la peste d'Orient à l'OMS* (Rennes: Presses universitaires de Rennes, 2012); Mark Harrison, *Contagion: How Commerce Has Spread Disease* (New Haven, CT: Yale University Press, 2013).

foundations. In 1917, the Johns Hopkins School of Public Health (JHSPH), financed by the Rockefeller Foundation, established the very first statistics department within a public health school, thus launching the legitimatization of statistical practices within public health academia. The establishment of the JHSPH dovetailed with the end of World War I, when the establishment of the League of Nations institutionalized a form of internationalism that promoted collaboration between nation-states.[6] In the decades that followed, health statisticians trained at the JHSPH went on to be employed by the League of Nations and health organizations around the globe. The Rockefeller Foundation also backed the Epidemiological Intelligence and Public Health Statistics Service of the League of Nations Health Organization (LNHO, 1922–1946), which aimed to standardize and legitimatize the statistical practices of national health authorities. The Service went further than its predecessors by developing knowledge and programs to help member countries integrate statistical collection into their health systems. The impact of the JHSPH and the LNHO statistical service at the international and local levels endured after World War II and left its mark on the United Nations Relief and Rehabilitation Administration (UNRRA, 1943–1947) and the vital and health statistics system of the WHO.

Some alumni of the JHSPH would become leading figures in China and Taiwan before or after the political upheavals of the mid-twentieth century. These statisticians brought their interwar and wartime experience to the postwar context, during which the WHO strove for an all-encompassing global statistical system, and Cold War rivalries came to be a critical factor in international organizations' work,[7] as well as in the attitudes of the two Chinese regimes vis-à-vis the organizations.

Over the course of seven chapters covering statistical initiatives in the interwar, wartime, and postwar periods, and their implementation in China and Taiwan, this book focuses first and foremost on investigating the circulation of statistical practices from the North Atlantic sphere to other parts of the world – that is, how health organizations at different levels came to use statistics in their work (for some, this also included devising a network to integrate standardized practices into other organizations). I also examine how various stakeholders – whether experts from

---

[6] This feature of interwar internationalism is discussed in Glenda Sluga, *Internationalism in the Age of Nationalism* (Philadelphia, PA: University of Pennsylvania Press, 2013).

[7] Scholars have argued that distinct countries and their experts had different ways of making use of the Cold War rivalry for their respective public health programs. See: e.g. Anne-Emanuelle Birn and Raùl Necochea López, *Peripheral Nerve: Health and Medicine in Cold War Latin America* (Durham, NC: Duke University Press, 2020).

international organizations or officers within national or local administrations – used statistics to evaluate health conditions on the ground and communicate (and argue) with one another.

Ultimately, this book asks the question: To what extent did statistics influence global health policy-making?

## Quantification, its Socio-Historical Context, and Politics

In this book, people and their statistical practices are kept center stage through the application of socio-historical research on the rise of statistical thinking.[8] (I use the term "statistical practices" to refer to all statistical work, including the collection, dissemination, and use of statistics to formulate arguments.) I postulate that statistics are closely intertwined with the people who produce them: the following chapters therefore present and analyze the visions and actions of individuals – researchers and administrators for the most part – in producing quantified data, and how their work impacted public health programs. Experts employed by research institutes and health organizations at the international, national, and local levels made use of a large variety of statistics to support their arguments.

In investigating how quantification fits into its socio-historical context, I do not seek to repeat or add to existing accounts on the intellectual genealogy of renowned statisticians and epidemiologists such as Karl Pearson or Major Greenwood;[9] nor do I intend to structure my narrative around the history of each type of statistics. Generally speaking, the statistics used for public health are divided into the following categories: demographic statistics, which aim to present the composition and changes in a given population in terms of age, sex, and marital status;[10] vital and health statistics,

[8] See, e.g.: Ian Hacking, *The Taming of Chance* (Cambridge: Cambridge University Press, 1990); Alain Desrosières, *La politique des grands nombres: histoire de la raison statistique* (Paris: Éd. La Découverte, 1993); Theodore M. Porter, *Trust in Numbers: In Pursuit of Objectivity in Science and Public Life* (Princeton, NJ: Princeton University Press, 1995).

[9] See, e.g.: J. Rosser Matthews, *Quantification and the Quest for Medical Certainty* (Princeton, NJ: Princeton University Press, 1995); Eileen Magnello and Anne Hardy, ed., *The Road to Medical Statistics* (Amsterdam; New York: Rodopi, 2002); Anne Hardy and M. Eileen Magnello, "Statistical Methods in Epidemiology: Karl Pearson, Ronald Ross, Major Greenwood and Austin Bradford Hill, 1900–1945," *Sozial- und Präventivmedizin* 47, no. 2 (2002): 80–9; Susser and Stein, *Eras in Epidemiology*.

[10] See, e.g.: Simon Szreter, "The Idea of Demographic Transition and the Study of Fertility Change: A Critical Intellectual History," *Population and Development Review* 19, no. 4 (1993): 659–701; Keith Breckenridge and Simon Szreter, *Registration and Recognition: Documenting the Person in World History* (Oxford: Oxford University Press/British Academy, 2012).

which record the health conditions of a given population, including morbidity, mortality, cases of disease, etc.;[11] and health economic statistics, which are based on the first two categories but which add in the cost of health services and disease prevention.[12] As all three categories were gradually combined within the collection and dissemination work coordinated by international organizations during the period under study, to examine them separately would be to lose sight of how statistical practices as a whole were integrated into the global health domain.

Instead, I do as many historians, philosophers, and sociologists of quantification have done and outline the relationship between quantification work and its socio-historical context. Researchers rooted in the disciplines of philosophy and history, such as Theodore Porter, Ian Hacking, and Alain Desrosières, have studied how socio-political contexts give rise to different ways of quantifying a phenomenon, and how numbers in turn shape knowledge about the phenomenon in question.[13] Taking case studies from North Atlantic countries, these scholars bridge the gap between historiographies that focus on the statisticians themselves and those that focus purely on the political context. Sociologists, inspired by such work, have adopted a similar approach to study quantification and its social effects in the contemporary world, such as in global rankings of universities and policing statistics.[14] Even closer to the themes discussed here, a book edited by anthropologist Vincanne Adams' edited volume presents a variety of case studies on the use of quantified data in public

---

[11]  See, e.g.: Iris Borowy, "Counting Death and Disease: Classification of Death and Disease in the Interwar Years, 1919–1939," *Continuity and Change* 18, no. 3 (2003): 457–81; Iwao Moriyama et al., *History of the Statistical Classification of Diseases and Causes of Death* (Hyattsville, MD: National Center of Health Statistics, 2011).

[12]  See, e.g.: Dan Bouk, *How Our Days Became Numbered: Risk and the Rise of the Statistical Individual* (Chicago, IL: University of Chicago Press, 2015); Michelle Murphy, *The Economization of Life* (Durham, NC: Duke University Press, 2017).

[13]  See, e.g.: Theodore M. Porter, *The Rise of Statistical Thinking: 1820–1900* (Princeton, NJ: Princeton University Press, 1986); Porter, *Trust in Numbers*; Hacking, *The Taming of Chance*; Desrosières, *La politique des grands nombres*; Alain Desrosières, *Gouverner par les nombres*.

[14]  Wendy Nelson Espeland and Mitchell L. Stevens, "Commensuration as a Social Process," *Annual Review of Sociology* 24, no. 1 (1998): 313–43; Wendy Nelson Espeland and Mitchell L. Stevens, "A Sociology of Quantification," *European Journal of Sociology* 49, no. 3 (2008): 401–36; Martha Lampland and Susan Leigh Star, *Standards and Their Stories: How Quantifying, Classifying, and Formalizing Practices Shape Everyday Life* (Ithaca, NY: Cornell University Press, 2009); Michael Sauder and Wendy Nelson Espeland, "The Discipline of Rankings: Tight Coupling and Organizational Change," *American Sociological Review* 74, no. 1 (2009): 63–82; Emmanuel Didier, "Globalization of Quantitative Policing: Between Management and Statactivism," *Annual Review of Sociology* 44, no. 1 (2018): 515–34; Andrea Mennicken and Wendy Nelson Espeland, "What's New with Numbers? Sociological Approaches to the Study of Quantification," *Annual Review of Sociology* 45, no. 1 (2019): 223–45.

health governance and resource allocation.[15] All of the above point to the salient role played by statistics in knowledge production and policy-making from the eighteenth century to today, as well as demonstrating the unintended consequences of quantification on the social world.

In addition to Adams, other emerging scholarly works also attempt to construct historical narratives on the use of health metrics at the international level. Research by Martin Gorsky and Christopher Sirrs compares metrics from statistical publications by international organizations in the interwar and postwar years, and draws a broad picture of the organizations' attempts to create records of their member countries' health systems: from mortality and morbidity to health expenditures and hospital numbers.[16] David Reubi's article starts by examining a contemporary program, the Bloomberg Initiative to Reduce Tobacco Use in Developing Countries, and traces the history of metrics and surveys back to the interwar years.[17] Both of these publications show that the pervasive reach of quantification in international organizations' health work has its origins in the interwar period. In this book, I will further argue that pervasive quantification began to radiate outside of the North Atlantic world well before the postwar years. Through multi-archival studies, I trace how the LNHO and WHO worked to include countries in regions with less administrative capacity, and how Chinese experts interacted with the organizations when it came to implementing and reporting statistics. In that sense, this book also complements the literature on how the use of customs statistics, social surveys, and national statistics came to be used in modern China.[18]

More specifically, the following quote from Desrosières encapsulates the approach employed here:

Quantification provides a specific language, with remarkable properties of transferability, the possibility for standardized manipulations by calculations, and of routinized interpretation systems. Thus, quantification provides social actors

---

[15] Vincanne Adams, ed., *Metrics: What Counts in Global Health* (Durham, NC: Duke University Press, 2016).

[16] Martin Gorsky and Christopher Sirrs, "World Health by Place: The Politics of International Health System Metrics, 1924–c. 2010," *Journal of Global History* 12, no. 3 (2017): 361–85.

[17] David Reubi, "A Genealogy of Epidemiological Reason: Saving Lives, Social Surveys and Global Population," *BioSocieties* 13, no. 1 (2017): 1–22.

[18] See, e.g.: Andrea Bréard, "Robert Hart and China's Statistical Revolution," *Modern Asian Studies* 40, no. 3 (2006): 605–29; Tong Lam, *A Passion for Facts: Social Surveys and the Construction of the Chinese Nation-State, 1900–1949* (Berkeley, CA: University of California Press, 2011); Arunabh Ghosh, "Accepting Difference, Seeking Common Ground: Sino-Indian Statistical Exchanges 1951–1959," *BJHS Themes* 1 (2016): 61–82; Arunabh Ghosh, *Making It Count: Statistics and Statecraft in the Early People's Republic of China* (Princeton, NJ: Princeton University Press, 2020).

and researchers with "objects that hold" [*des objets qui tiennent*] in the triple sense of their robustness (holding water in face of criticism), of their capacity to combine together, and finally, of the fact that they "hold people together" by encouraging them (or obliging them) to use this language with universalist aims, instead of others.[19]

Here, Desrosières provides a promising way of considering statistics within their socio-historical context. Instead of plunging into the classic debate as to whether statistics are a manipulated or faithful representation of a given phenomenon, studying statistics as a language that actors use to present their ideas and advance their agendas offers a fruitful third way to understand such practices without losing the nuances inherent to statistical collection and reporting. The language metaphor brings us back to the quotation that opened this book, and the implication by WHO statisticians that international organizations would one day use statistical data to communicate with public health research institutes and administrations at the national, regional, and international levels. In other words, statistics would act as a lingua franca. Numbers would eventually become a language into which public health conditions and fieldwork could be translated in order to provide that information to stakeholders in different localities or at different organizational levels.

In this sense, I hope to open a fresh chapter in the debate on the use of statistics for policy-making, which has been monopolized by political and social scientists for far too long. Inspired by Michel Foucault's accounts of biopolitics and governmentality, some researchers have presumed that actors trusted and lauded the capacities of statistics, and regarded statistical practices as a governing technique that organizations, whether national or international, used to influence the behavior of populations.[20] In general, these authors believe that the organizations

---

[19] Translated from: Alain Desrosières, *Pour une sociologie historique de la quantification* (Paris: Presses de l'Ecole des mines, 2008), 10. Original text: *"La quantification offre un langage spécifique, doté de propriétés remarquables de transférabilité, de possibilités de manipulations standardisées par le calcul, et de systèmes d'interprétations routinisées. Ainsi, elle met à la disposition des acteurs sociaux ou des chercheurs « des objets qui tiennent », au triple sens de leur robustesse propre (résistance à la critique), de leur capacité à se combiner entre eux, et enfin de ce qu'ils « tiennent les hommes entre eux » en les incitant (ou parfois en les contraignant) à user de ce langage à visée universaliste, plutôt que d'un autre."*

[20] For an analysis at the national level, see, e.g.: Graham Burchell, Colin Gorden, and Peter Miller, eds., *The Foucault Effect: Studies in Governmentality* (Chicago, IL: University of Chicago Press, 1991); Andrew Barry, Thomas Osborne, and Nikolas Rose, eds., *Foucault and Political Reason: Liberalism, Neo-Liberalism and the Rationalities of Government* (Chicago, IL: Chicago University Press, 1996). On the application of Foucauldian analysis to international organizations, see e.g.: Arturo Escobar, *Encountering Development: The Making and Unmaking of the Third World* (Princeton, NJ: Princeton University Press, 1995); Tania Murray Li, *The Will to*

trained experts to evaluate the status quo and make political decisions in a certain way (using statistical analysis, for example) and that the experts and their governing techniques served as intermediaries that translated local situations into a given analysis, based upon which certain policies were applied. Drawing on multi-archival sources, this book will put such conjectures into historical context by revealing the mechanisms that led public health experts to turn to statistics in their work and the standardized techniques used in health organizations at different levels. I will also illustrate how statistical practices – and the extent to which they were trusted as a basis of reasoning – evolved depending on the global sociopolitical context.

My focus is on the making of an international health statistics system through the transfer of statistical practices from public health schools, intergovernmental health organizations, and philanthropic public health programs to their counterparts in China and Taiwan. What makes this research unique in quantification studies is the extensive span of time and space covered. The relatively long time period serves to show the continuities and changes in international health statistics and to follow actors' endeavors to create a consolidated international statistical system for public health. The sections focusing on the LNHO (Chapter 3) and its postwar successors, UNRRA and the WHO (Chapter 5), juxtapose the underlying differences within the international health statistical network managed in Geneva. Theodore Porter posits that statistics build trust in groups of experts in need of authority,[21] and the history of the international health statistical network further shows that the collection of statistics also hinges upon the leading organization's authority.[22] Trust in numbers and in organizations can thus be symbiotic.

The broad geographic span under analysis here also signals the heterogeneity of quantification practices. Public health experts in different localities, in both the interwar and postwar periods, played different roles in the life cycle of making and circulating health statistics. The LNHO,

*Improve: Governmentality, Development, and the Practice of Politics* (Durham, NC: Duke University Press Books, 2007); Jeremy Youde, *Biopolitical Surveillance and Public Health in International Politics* (New York: Palgrave Macmillan, 2010); Jonathan Joseph, *The Social in the Global: Social Theory, Governmentality and Global Politics* (Cambridge: Cambridge University Press, 2012); Nicholas J. Kiersey and Doug Stokes, eds., *Foucault and International Relations: New Critical Engagements* (London: Routledge, 2011).

[21] Porter, *Trust in Numbers*. For a concrete example of experts resorting to mechanical objectivity, see Porter's fifth chapter, in which he discusses the case of accountants and actuaries.

[22] Porter also briefly touches upon the organizational basis for trust in numbers. See: Porter, *Trust in Numbers*, 213–14.

as discussed in Chapter 3, formed separate circles of experts when creating a global health statistics exchange system: North Atlantic statisticians sat in expert meetings, whereas others merely participated in training sessions. In the postwar period, statisticians from regions outside of the North Atlantic world were invited to join WHO expert committees, and the organization's experts tailored standards to localities with different levels of administrative capacity (see Chapter 5).

Throughout this book, I also investigate the diachronic implementation of public health initiatives, including statistical practices. During the interwar and postwar years, experts and researchers used statistical data to formulate their arguments, yet gave themselves leeway to select the statistics that supported their ongoing policies. During the interwar health demonstrations in both the United States and China, experts implicitly or explicitly designed their programs in line with controlled laboratory principles, which led them to include statistical collection in the hope of demonstrating the programs' effectiveness (see Chapters 2 and 4). However, when numbers were lacking, interwar program designers mostly resorted to their authority as experts to promote the program in question and simply dismissed the statistics. Thus, during this period, statistics did not always serve as an effective language for communication between organizations. Statistics became more embedded in argumentation for policy decisions after World War II, as the WHO centralized its various types of statistical data and devised statistical practices that connected fieldwork administration, research, and policy-making. Public health experts both within and outside the WHO were pushed to select statistics more meticulously to support their arguments.

## The Globalization of Health Administrations

This is, by its very nature, a history that transcends national borders: a study of how statistical practices and data were transferred between international health organizations and local agencies. Phenomena that span borders have been a heated subject in historical studies. The number of such studies has peaked in the last two decades with the publication of a number of introductory books on how to conduct research on different kinds of border-crossing phenomena.[23]

---

[23] Pierre-Yves Saunier, "Circulations, connexions et espaces transnationaux," *Genèses* 57, no. 4 (2004): 110–26; Madeleine Herren, Martin Rüesch, and Christiane Sibille, *Transcultural History: Theories, Methods, Sources* (Berlin: Springer, 2012); Pierre-Yves Saunier, *Transnational History* (New York: Palgrave Macmillan, 2013); Akira Iriye, *Global and Transnational History: The Past, Present, and Future* (New York: Palgrave

Though all share a common interest in moving beyond the nation-state as the traditional unit of historical writing, these studies have given rise to different methodologies: "transcultural history," "transnational history," and "global history." Advocates of trans*cultural* history emphasize the intercultural encounter; trans*national* historians make a meticulous study of a wide array of connections; and scholars of global history emphasize the structural contexts that allow those connections to be made. All three methodologies study connections by placing emphasis on either the micro level (cultural encounters), the meso level (trans-boundary formations), or the macro level (global context). All three approaches center on the study of mobility, connection, exchange, and the circulation of people, ideas, practices, and institutions across politics and societies.[24] Nonetheless, it is worth noting that the three are not mutually exclusive – authors from one camp do not deny the importance of the others' angles of emphasis.

Rather than subscribing to one of these methodologies in particular, my approach is to emphasize the interaction between institutions and experts at different levels, putting my work in dialogue with that of researchers who explicitly underscore the importance of "playing with levels" (*jeux d'echelles*), an approach through which historians investigate the interaction of events or phenomena that took place at the local, national, and global levels.[25] By focusing on people, ideas, practices, and data that circulated between local/national administrations and organizations (usually based in the United States or Western Europe) tackling public health affairs at the international level, this book tells the story of international health experts and their visions, paying equal attention to how those visions were put into practice on the ground by experts working in national or local organizations. This research details how statistical practices in public health became globalized by investigating the historical formation of quantification mechanisms within health organizations at different levels – mechanisms that public health experts played a decisive role in implementing. And by taking different levels into account, this

Macmillan, 2013); Akira Iriye and Pierre-Yves Saunier, *The Palgrave Dictionary of Transnational History: From the Mid-19th Century to the Present Day* (New York: Palgrave Macmillan, 2009); Sebastian Conrad, *What Is Global History?* (Princeton, NJ: Princeton University Press, 2016).

24  Herren, Rüesch, and Sibille, *Transcultural History*, vi, 11; Saunier, *Transnational History*, 3, 8; Iriye and Saunier, *The Palgrave Dictionary of Transnational History*, xix; Iriye, *Global and Transnational History*, 11; Conrad, *What Is Global History?*, 5.

25  Jacques Revel, ed., *Jeux d'échelles. La micro-analyse à l'expérience* (Paris: Seuil, 1996); Caroline Douki and Philippe Minard, "Histoire globale, histoires connectées: un changement d'échelle historiographique?," *Revue d'histoire moderne et contemporaine* 54–4, no. 5 (2007): 7–21; Saunier, *Transnational History*, 122.

method provides a nuanced reading that shows the extent to which political interests were incorporated into the international health statistical system.

This book builds on a wealth of scholarly research on international health organizations, from the LNHO to the WHO.[26] In digging under the surface of global health governance, it joins abundant historical accounts of international health programs, most of which nonetheless focus on one specific public health program (such as malaria control, mass Bacillus Calmette–Guérin vaccination campaigns, or the development of public health work in a specific territory).[27] By focusing on statistical practices, I seek to explain how public health officials communicated outside of official policy communiqués and how their standardized programs were implemented both in the governing centers of the North Atlantic world and in national administrations and fieldwork. This book recounts the reality of international health governance on the ground, showing why and how experts designed a statistical reporting network, how their standard practices were transferred, and how their colleagues at the national and local levels – who believed in the power of public health programs but were hindered by small government budgets – used statistical data to maximize foreign funding of their work. Having been trained in public health schools established by international health organizations, these workers were familiar with the rationale used to award funding and the statistical language necessary for presenting a convincing project. The production of health statistical data was thus

---

[26] For general accounts on these two organizations and more, see, e.g.: Iris Borowy, *Coming to Terms with World Health: The League of Nations Health Organisation 1921–1946* (Bern: Peter Lang, 2009); Randall M. Packard, *A History of Global Health: Interventions into the Lives of Other Peoples* (Baltimore, MD: Johns Hopkins University Press, 2016); Anne-Emanuelle Birn, Yogan Pillay, and Timothy H. Holtz, *Textbook of Global Health* (Oxford: Oxford University Press, 2017); Marcos Cueto, Theodore M. Brown, and Elizabeth Fee, *The World Health Organization: A History* (Cambridge: Cambridge University Press, 2019).

[27] See, e.g.: Marcos Cueto, *Cold War, Deadly Fevers: Malaria Eradication in Mexico, 1955–1975* (Washington, DC: Woodrow Wilson Center Press, 2007); Randall M. Packard, *The Making of a Tropical Disease: A Short History of Malaria* (Baltimore, MD: Johns Hopkins University Press, 2007); Sanjoy Bhattacharya, "International Health and the Limits of its Global Influence: Bhutan and the Worldwide Smallpox Eradication Programme," *Medical History* 57, no. 4 (2013): 461–86; Christian W. McMillen, *Discovering Tuberculosis – A Global History, 1900 to the Present* (New Haven, CT: Yale University Press, 2015); Harry Yi-Jui Wu, "World Citizenship and the Emergence of the Social Psychiatry Project of the World Health Organization, 1948–c.1965," *History of Psychiatry* 26, no. 2 (2015): 166–81; Dóra Vargha, *Polio Across the Iron Curtain: Hungary's Cold War with an Epidemic* (Cambridge: Cambridge University Press, 2018).

co-constructed by officers working in health organizations with different scopes.[28]

## China: An Ideal Site for Studying the Transfer and Implementation of International Health Statistics

China provides the perfect setting for answering this book's core question regarding the process by which national and local experts came to use statistical standards to communicate with international organizations. The country was the object of significant interest from international health organizations – including the LNHO, the Rockefeller Foundation, UNRRA, and the WHO – all of which designed and implemented programs in China and provided technical support starting between the 1910s and 1960 (in 1949, that support shifted to Taiwan). China thus provides a rich case for comparing the local implementation of those initiatives and studying the continuities among them over different periods.

This research thus joins existing historiographies that study the relationship between colonial medicine and international health.[29] Though never a colony, China was a battlefield in which imperial powers competed for political and economic domination from the mid-nineteenth century. Until 1943, there were a total of fifty-four treaty ports in the country.[30] And because foreign powers controlled parts of China's territory, Chinese soil was itself intergovernmental, offering spaces and opportunities for intergovernmental organizations

---

[28] On the idea of co-construction, see, e.g.: Kapil Raj, "Colonial Encounters and the Forging of Knowledge and National Identities: Great Britain and India, 1760–1850," in *Social History of Science in Colonial India*, eds. S. Irfan Habib and Dhruv Raina (Oxford: Oxford University Press, 2007), 83–101.

[29] See, e.g.: David Arnold, *Colonizing the Body: State Medicine and Epidemic Disease in Nineteenth-Century India* (Berkeley, CA: University of California Press, 1993); Warwick Anderson, *Colonial Pathologies: American Tropical Medicine, Race, and Hygiene in the Philippines* (Durham, NC: Duke University Press, 2006); Packard, *A History of Global Health*; Jessica Lynne Pearson, *The Colonial Politics of Global Health: France and the United Nations in Postwar Africa* (Cambridge, MA: Harvard University Press, 2018).

[30] The first treaty ports were established in China in 1842 following the country's defeat by the United Kingdom in the First Opium War. To guarantee its commercial interests in China, the British government included an article in an unequal treaty with the Qing government (1644–1911) requiring it to provide the British government with extraterritorial rights over five Chinese ports. Other imperial powers later signed similar treaties with the Qing government, increasing the number of treaty ports in China (Robert Nield, *China's Foreign Places: The Foreign Presence in China in the Treaty Port Era, 1840–1943* [Hong Kong: Hong Kong University Press, 2015]).

to intervene.[31] International health organizations were no exception: they had been providing health programs and considerable funding to the country since the early years of the Republic of China (ROC). Moreover, at the time, China was often depicted as a great civilization in decline, and providing aid to the country was in line with the guiding philosophy of philanthropic foundations. In the 1910s, the Rockefeller Foundation launched its most expensive medical and public health projects in China, establishing the elite Peking Union Medical College (PUMC).[32] In the late 1920s, China also became one of three countries to receive LNHO support in devising their national health systems.[33] The collaboration between the ROC and the LNHO came at a time when the Nationalist government regained control of most of the mainland following the Northern Expedition.[34] Recovering sovereignty was a diplomatic priority for the Nationalists, who were increasingly involved in international negotiations with the primary aim of reclaiming authority over customs controls.[35] Collaboration with the LNHO on quarantine reform was a win-win proposition for the LNHO and China. The LNHO could include Chinese ports in

[31] Foreign powers also established an intergovernmental organization in Tianjin during their occupation of the city in the aftermath of the Boxer Rebellion (Pierre Singaravélou, *Tianjin Cosmopolis. Une histoire de la mondialisation en 1900* [Paris: Le Seuil, 2017]).

[32] On Rockefeller-funded medical philanthropy in China, see, e.g.: Mary Brown Bullock, *An American Transplant: The Rockefeller Foundation and Peking Union Medical College* (Berkeley, CA: University of California Press, 1980); Mary Brown Bullock and Bridie Andrews, eds., *Medical Transitions in Twentieth-Century China* (Bloomington, IN: Indiana University Press, 2014).

[33] The other two countries were Greece and Bolivia. For more information on the League of Nations' collaboration with the ROC during the interwar years, see, e.g.: Chang Li, *Guoji hezuo zai Zhongguo: Guoji Lianmeng jiaose de kaocha [International Collaboration in China: A Study of the Role of the League of Nations (1919–1946)]* (Taipei: Academia Sinica, 1999); Margherita Zanasi, "Exporting Development: The League of Nations and Republican China," *Comparative Studies in Society and History* 49, no. 1 (2007): 143–69.

[34] In 1926, the Nationalist government in Guangdong launched the Northern Expedition, a military campaign aimed at reunifying China, which was divided by warlords, including the Beiyang government, which occupied the ROC's then capital, Beijing. The Northern Expedition concluded in 1928, with the Nationalist government regaining most of the mainland, ending the Warlord Era.

[35] These efforts were considered successful, as several treaties were revised between 1928 and 1931, before the outbreak of the Manchurian Crisis (William C. Kirby, "The Internationalization of China: Foreign Relations at Home and Abroad in the Republican Era," *The China Quarterly*, no. 150 [1997]: 443). On the late Qing and the ROC's efforts to be included in the international system before 1949, see e.g.: Chang Li, *Guoji hezuo zai Zhongguo*; Guoqi Xu, *China and the Great War: China's Pursuit of a New National Identity and Internationalization* (Cambridge: Cambridge University Press, 2005).

its statistical information network, and China could use the LNHO's impartial standing and expertise to recover quarantine authority.

Foreign health organizations did not shift their attention away from China with the outbreak of the Second Sino-Japanese War (1937–1945). Rather, the country's plight attracted the sympathy of the LNHO and other foreign associations, which provided funding for various wartime relief activities.[36] As the center of a World War II arena, and later as a permanent member of the United Nations Security Council, China received a large share of aid from international health organizations such as UNRRA and the WHO.[37]

In 1949, the Chinese Communist Party took control of the mainland, establishing the People's Republic of China (PRC), and the ROC government was exiled to Taiwan. The two Chinese regimes' contrasting relationships with the international health organizations offers an intriguing parallel in terms of international health statistics against the backdrop of the Cold War. As most socialist countries were absent from the WHO in the 1940s and for a large part of the 1950s, the Cold War divided WHO-led international epidemiological intelligence into separate circuits. During their absence from the WHO, socialist countries exchanged epidemiological information among themselves. The PRC was one of the countries most hostile to the UN system, cutting off relations with the WHO until 1971. During this period, the PRC government devised its own international medical and health exchanges with individual countries, both socialist and non-socialist (see Chapter 7). The ROC, on the other hand, was part of the WHO network. It hosted many WHO campaigns, as the Western bloc considered it to be a critical frontier of the "free world," and the WHO strove to reinforce its public health campaigns there. As I will demonstrate in Chapters 5–7, both the PRC and ROC continued to collect and report statistics for their own public health governance, despite the Cold War divide. The constant political upheaval in China during the period under study provides a rich field for analysis of the continuities and ruptures in the implementation

---

[36] Brazelton's book focusing on Yunnan proffers interesting accounts of wartime vaccination campaigns and relief programs by the ROC and the LNHO, as well as other relief organizations, and how they laid the basis for the postwar development of Chinese public health (Mary Augusta Brazelton, *Mass Vaccination: Citizens' Bodies and State Power in Modern China* [Ithaca, NY: Cornell University Press, 2019]). On medical relief programs by other foreign organizations in wartime China, see also: John R. Watt, *Saving Lives in Wartime China: How Medical Reformers Built Modern Healthcare Systems Amid War and Epidemics, 1928–1945* (Leiden: Brill, 2014).

[37] On the ROC's prominent role in the immediate postwar years, see: Rana Mitter, "Imperialism, Transnationalism, and the Reconstruction of Post-War China: UNRRA in China, 1944–7," *Past & Present* 218, no. suppl. 8 (2013): 51–69.

of statistical practices by international health organizations, in two distinctly different socio-political contexts.

This book surveys the statistical practices of Chinese and Taiwanese health officials from the interwar to the postwar years, and joins emerging historiographies of medicine and health in which China is studied as a knot of globalization of biomedicine; these historiographies offer accounts of how the Chinese government interacted with the outside world in terms of medical and public health service.[38] More specifically, this book enters into dialogue with research into the appropriation of a Western-style public health system by China in the nineteenth and twentieth centuries. Specifically, a number of historians have investigated public health actions implemented by foreign organizations in China from the perspective of cultural history.[39] Their work mainly focuses on the ROC before 1937 and examines the introduction of public health measures into Chinese daily life.[40] This book covers a larger

[38] See, e.g.: David Luesink, William H. Schneider, and Zhang Daqing, eds., *China and the Globalization of Biomedicine* (Rochester, NY: University of Rochester Press, 2019); Wayne Soon, *Global Medicine in China: A Diasporic History* (Stanford, CA: Stanford University Press, 2020). Other researchers, who have not put transnational networks at the center of their research, still offer pertinent accounts of China's interaction with the world in terms of medicine and public health. See, e.g.: Brazelton, *Mass Vaccination*; Xun Zhou, *The People's Health: Health Intervention and Delivery in Mao's China 1949–1983* (Montreal: McGill-Queen's University Press, 2020).

[39] Ruth Rogaski, *Hygienic Modernity: Meanings of Health and Disease in Treaty-Port China* (Berkeley, CA: University of California Press, 2004); Yang Nianqun, *Zaizao "bingren": Zhongxiyi chongtu xia de kongjian zhengzhi (1832–1985) [Remaking "Patients": Space Politics under the Conflict between Chinese and Western Medicine (1832–1985)]* (Beijing: China Renmin University Press, 2006); Sean Hsiang-Lin Lei, *Neither Donkey nor Horse: Medicine in the Struggle over China's Modernity* (Chicago, IL: University of Chicago Press, 2014).

[40] In a series of articles, for example, Yang Nianqun demonstrates how the new public health system altered the landscape of social life in cities; Hsiang-Lin Lei's two works respectively investigate the Chinese equivalent for the term "public health" – which translated literally means "guarding life" – and the implementation of tuberculosis control measures in China. See: Yang Nianqun, "'Lan Ansheng moshi' yu Minguo chunian Beijing shengsi kongzhi kongjian de zhuanhuan ['The John B. Grant Model' and the Transfer of Spaces of Birth and Death Control in the Early Years of the Republic of China]," *Shehuixue yanjiu [Sociological Studies]* , no. 4 (1999): 98–133; Yang Nianqun, "Beijing 'weisheng shifanqu' de jianli yu chengshi kongjian gongneng de zhuanhuan [The Establishment of Beijing Health Demonstration and the transformation of Urban Space Functions]," *Beijing dangan shiliao [Beijing Archives Series]*, no.1 (2000): 205–31; Hsiang-Lin Lei, "Weisheng weihe bushi baowei shengming? Minguo shiqi linglei de weisheng, ziwo, yu jibing [Why Weisheng Is Not About Guarding Life? Alternative Conceptions of Hygiene, Self, and Illness in the Republican China]," *Taiwan shehui yanjiu jikan [Taiwan: A Radical Quarterly in Social Studies]*, no. 54 (2004): 17–59; Sean Hsiang-Lin Lei, "Habituating Individuality: The Framing of Tuberculosis and its Material Solutions in Republican China," *Bulletin of the History of Medicine* 84, no. 2 (2010): 248–79.

time period (up to the Cold War), thus complementing a corpus of historiographies that offers accounts of the establishment and transformations of the ROC Ministry of Health (which later became the National Health Administration), from the interwar to the postwar years.[41] Specifically, I chart the continuities and ruptures during a long period of constant political change and provide accounts of the on-the-ground implementation of the national health systems in China and Taiwan. The last chapter, in which I focus on the PRC's vital and health statistics, also complements research on PRC-era public health campaigns.[42]

A detailed analysis of the process of statistical communication at the local, national, and international levels reveals that Chinese public health officers had a tendency to curate the statistics used in their arguments to their sponsor organizations. Once on the ground, experts had to reconcile their vision with the suspicion and mistrust of local inhabitants regarding government collection of their personal data. Given the limited local administrative capacity, statistical practices for health tended to be reduced to routinized work, and public health experts recorded statistics that they did not actually believe in or make use of when taking decisions in the field.[43] On other occasions, despite differences in their statistical practices, these experts used statistical data to present their programs as conforming to the standards set out by international organizations, or as a potential showcase for universal implementation of the organizations' ongoing policies, in the hope of receiving financial and technical support.

## Playing with Levels: Research Methods

To establish an accurate picture of the globalization of statistical practices, I have drawn on archival sources as well as publications in both English and Mandarin Chinese. By comparing the worldviews of public health experts in different languages and different health organizations, I am able to show how some experts adapted their discourse when writing in a different language. A *jeux d'echelles* analysis also offers a reading of how stakeholders at different levels, each with their own policy priorities,

---

[41] Book-length research works include: Lei, *Neither Donkey nor Horse*; Liping Bu and Ka-Che Yip, eds., *Public Health and National Reconstruction in Post-War Asia: International Influences, Local Transformations* (London: Routledge, 2015); Liping Bu, *Public Health and the Modernization of China, 1865–2015* (London: Routledge, 2017).

[42] Book-length research works include: Xiaoping Fang, *Barefoot Doctors and Western Medicine in China* (Rochester, NY: University of Rochester Press, 2012); Miriam Gross, *Farewell to the God of Plague: Chairman Mao's Campaign to Deworm China* (Berkeley, CA: University of California Press, 2016); Zhou, *The People's Health*.

[43] Similar testimonials can be found in Chapters 2, 4, and 5.

Table 0.1 *List of institutional archival holdings*

|  | International organizations | National and local organizations |
|---|---|---|
| Public | • LNHO<br>• UNRRA<br>• WHO<br>• United States federal aid agencies | • PRC Ministry of Foreign Affairs<br>• ROC Ministry of Health<br>• ROC Ministry of Foreign Affairs<br>• City of Beijing<br>• City of Shanghai |
| Private | • Rockefeller Foundation<br>• Milbank Memorial Fund<br>• JHSPH<br>• American Bureau for Medical Aid to China<br>• PUMC | |

interacted and negotiated with regard to vital and health statistical practices. To carry out this analysis, I drew on the institutional archives of fourteen organizations at different levels and localities (see Table 0.1).

To carry out a *jeux d'echelles* analysis, the different levels are first categorized (see Table 0.1) in order to clarify how statistical practices and data were transferred between levels. I classify as "international" any organization with international ambitions that implemented programs in countries outside of that in which it was headquartered. I also divide organizations at the international level into public and private. The public organizations at the international level are the LNHO, UNRRA, and the WHO. These organizations devised standardized programs that spanned national borders, with national governments contributing as member states. All American federal aid agencies are categorized at the international level, as the United States government conceived programs to be implemented in territories outside its borders, thus acting in a similar spirit to the international organizations. Private organizations whose programs shared the same traits include American philanthropic foundations based in New York (the Rockefeller Foundation and the Milbank Memorial Fund), schools that received funding from the Rockefeller Foundation to train public health experts from different countries (the JHSPH and the PUMC), and a New York-based private organization that supported medical work in China (the American Bureau for Medical Aid to China). Unlike the public international organizations, these private entities did/do not represent national governments, despite the fact that they often collaborated closely with public administrations.

In the national/local context, my research draws on the institutional archives of Chinese public organizations at distinct administrative levels, which leaves one category empty: local, private organizations. This is for two interrelated reasons. During the period under study, Chinese civil society was rather fragile. To ensure their statistical practices were properly implemented, some international organizations established their own dependent organizations in China (such as the PUMC); all partnered with the national government. Local and private organizations were thus relegated to the margins. The only exception was the Chinese Mass Education Movement (see Chapter 4), which also received funds from international organizations. Nevertheless, the Movement was relatively unstable in terms of organization and depended largely on support from the public authorities. This brings us to another reason for its absence in the table above: it did not conserve independent archival holdings that illustrate its institutional vision about statistical practices or were of any relevance to this research.

Organizations at different levels were intertwined in several ways. Organizations and individuals collaborated by providing funding, technical consulting, and staff, or simply kept in contact about their work on the ground. The relationship between health organizations at different levels was complex and changed over time. Indeed, as I will demonstrate, the transfer of statistical practices was not implemented in an orderly fashion: from public international organizations to the national administration, and then on to the local authorities. Instead, some private actors (e.g. the Milbank Memorial Fund) were able to connect directly with partners in China, skipping (or receiving minimal assistance from) intergovernmental and national agencies. Inversely, some international organizations, both public and private (e.g. the LNHO and the Rockefeller Foundation), had to coordinate with the ROC's national or local administrations before they could implement their initiatives in interwar China. By mobilizing archival sources from health organizations at different levels, I seek to demonstrate the complexity of the configuration of the different levels and show how every connection played a crucial role in quantifying health – in international health organizations, China, and postwar Taiwan.

## Book Structure

By examining the work of organizations in four different localities (the United States, Western Europe, mainland China, and Taiwan), I faced the challenging prospect of writing a history in which the main players were active at the same time but in different places. Moreover, the four territories in which this historical account takes place were interlinked in complex ways.

I do not wish to give the impression of an orderly lineage between the statistical practices of international health organizations and their implementation on the ground. When examining the full range of statistical practices, the divergences are impossible to ignore and indeed are vital for understanding the implementation process. True to the complex relationship between the various organizations, each chapter – excepting Chapter 1 (which sets the stage) and Chapter 7 (on the early PRC) – recounts a different circuit through which key statistical knowledge and practices were transferred between international organizations and their Chinese partners. With an emphasis on cross-continental transfers, I pay equal attention to international health organizations and national and local health administrations. In each chapter, I first present how statistical initiatives were devised and implemented in the West, then how they intermingled and metamorphosed in China or Taiwan once confronted with the local context and the visions of health officials there. I then explore how experts made their arguments using the data they collected. It should be noted that although each chapter presents a self-contained circuit, all the circuits were connected in one way or another. By narrating each circuit and the connections between them, this book paints a picture of how statistical knowledge and practices circulated between places with very different administrative cultures.

Chapter 1 presents the historical context and the key players who called for the collection of statistics for public health programs in the interwar period. I then examine those programs in detail in Chapters 2, 3, and 4. Striving to promote the health of "others" – poor rural communities, or a foreign country – using scientific methods, the Rockefeller Foundation and the Milbank Memorial Fund provided support to these statistical initiatives, with the help of bacteriologists trained in laboratory methods who aimed to extend those principles to the social world as well, as other experts with knowledge of Chinese culture and/or public health in China. It was these experts who made the public health programs, and the associated statistical practices, possible.

Chapter 2 details how Karl Pearson's mathematical statistics methods were integrated into public health education by focusing on the Rockefeller-funded statistics department at the JHSPH and its Chinese counterpart in Beijing. In this chapter, I illustrate how conceptions of the role of statistics in science differed at the two schools. Chapter 2 also contains an account of the JHSPH's transition from a biological focus, in Pearson's tradition, to a focus on public health and epidemiology. The

JHSPH's approach was transferred – up to a point – to the PUMC. The major intermediaries were a JHSPH alumnus and Rockefeller Foundation officer, John B. Grant, and his student Yuan Yijin (Yüan I-Chin, commonly known as I. C. Yuan). Grant promoted the idea that statistics should not be used for research (as they were at the JHSPH), but rather for adapting health programs to the Chinese context. Lastly, I provide case studies showing how graduates of the two schools used mathematical statistics in their fieldwork, in the course of which they encountered resistance from other field experts and locals. Nonetheless, statistical reporting took on an increasingly prominent role in public health work in New York, Geneva, and Beijing.

Chapter 3 focuses on the LNHO's Epidemiological Intelligence and Public Health Statistics Service and its relationship with the Chinese government. Using Rockefeller funding, the LNHO positioned itself as a center of statistics and strove to lead international health collaboration. The LNHO's statistical authority, however, was a patchwork, as the organization had to negotiate with existing stakeholders individually. I also explain how the Service devised separate circles for generating and diffusing statistical standards and data. A focus on the Chinese government's strategies of cooperation with the Service is illuminating as to the geopolitical context, which played a salient role in the epidemiological reporting network, given that the ROC was also collaborating with the LNHO with a view to recovering its customs controls from the imperial powers.

Chapter 4 recounts the rising prominence of public health demonstrations as a policy-making method. In such demonstrations, a zone was demarcated in which public health services were provided and financial needs calculated as a policy experiment. The Milbank Memorial Fund popularized the concept as a modus operandi through its demonstrations in New York State. Edgar Sydenstricker – formerly one of the founding statisticians at the LNHO – was hired by the Milbank Memorial Fund and worked with a cohort of the graduates of the PUMC to reproduce Milbank's demonstration in Ding Xian (Ting Hsien), a rural county some 200 kilometers southwest of Beijing. In both New York and Ding Xian, statistics were central to setting up the experiment but less so in terms of policy follow-up. The Ding Xian demonstration converged with European health programs in rural areas conducted through the LNHO and served as the prototype for China's Central Field Health Station, a national research institute where public health situations, whether social or bacteriological, were quantified. Yet again, however, this quantification did not feed directly into policy-making, as the experts in charge retained the authority to make sense of the numbers.

Chapters 5, 6, and 7 bring the storyline up to the end of World War II and its aftermath. Together, they paint a picture of the reconstruction and expansion of the international statistical system during the postwar years. An account of China and Taiwan's implementation of statistical programs during this period illustrates vividly how the Cold War political divide influenced how statistics were used at the national and local levels. Chapter 5 provides an account of efforts by UNRRA and the WHO to rebuild a health statistics reporting system from 1943, when UNRRA took over the LNHO's international epidemiological intelligence efforts, and continues into the postwar years. The WHO also developed an all-encompassing statistical system to gather statistics collected through research, administration, and policy-making via a network that took better account of local variation when making standards; the WHO's network for spreading its ideas was also broader than that of the LNHO. A case study on the ROC – which ruled the mainland in 1943 but was exiled to Taiwan as of 1949 – shows that UNRRA and the WHO's statistical reporting was often undermined by geopolitics and administrative constraints.

In Chapter 6, I investigate the WHO's malaria and tuberculosis control programs in the 1950s and 1960s, which made use of statistical collection and analysis. Numbers had become omnipresent in program design and implementation by this time, and experts both at the WHO and in the Taiwanese government used their knowledge to justify their selection of statistics. I also chronicle how WHO experts and Taiwanese health officers used numbers in advocating for their programs. In particular, experts curated their numbers to bolster their arguments in the context of ongoing policy disputes at the WHO. The WHO experts mobilized their knowledge on the diseases in question to justify their selection of certain statistics over others, and their Taiwanese colleagues also used numbers to present Taiwan as a viable testing ground for WHO's policies, with a view to obtaining financial and technical support.

Lastly, in Chapter 7, I explore the ways statistics were used to govern public health in the PRC in the 1960s, showcasing another way the language of statistics was spoken during the postwar years. The PRC was cut off from the WHO's network during this time, instead becoming part of an international health network made up of socialist countries. I detail the ebb and flow of socialist statistics within the PRC and the continuity running through public health researchers' methods, despite the central government's enforced implementation of socialist statistics in the 1950s, as well as a series of anti-intellectual campaigns aimed at challenging experts' authority. Chapter 7 presents a case in which statistical thinking continued to develop, at a time when this authority was being called into question.

By examining different areas of statistical application involving different organizations and actors, this book presents the complex cross-continental circulation of statistical practices and data between the United States, Europe, China, and Taiwan, revealing the strategies employed by public health institutions and experts when making and interacting with statistical reporting systems.

# 1 The Call for a Language of Public Health
## Philanthropic Foundations, Bacteriologists, and Health Administrators

Our age is marked by two tendencies, the democratic and the scientific. In Dr. Welch and his work we find an expression of the best in both tendencies. He not only represents the spirit of pure science but constantly sees and seizes opportunities to direct its results into the service of human kind.[1]

On April 8, 1930, United States President Herbert Hoover delivered a speech to 1,600 guests at the Memorial Continental Hall in Washington, DC, which had served as the venue for the Washington Naval Conference nine years previously. The occasion was the eightieth birthday celebration of the pathologist and founder of the Johns Hopkins University School of Public Health (JHSPH), William Welch. Hoover praised Welch for his contributions to science and democracy: the two guiding spirits of the time. Hoover's speech also conveyed the key principles of public health work in the interwar United States: public health experts were to advance science and apply their discoveries to achieving progress for all humanity.

Welch's birthday celebration vividly encapsulated the interwar, American public health milieu, which contributed to the standardization of statistics at the international level in three important ways. First, the event brought together key stakeholders in American public health work: government workers, representatives of philanthropic foundations, and public health researchers. Specifically, the United States government was represented at the event by Hoover and Hugh Cumming, the surgeon general of the United States Public Health Service (USPHS). Key players from philanthropic foundations were involved in organizing the celebration, including John D. Rockefeller, Jr., the patron of the Rockefellers' philanthropic enterprises; Simon Flexner, the first director of the Rockefeller Institute for Medical Research; and Albert Milbank, president of the Milbank

---

[1] "Committee on the Celebration of the Eightieth Birthday of Doctor William Henry Welch," *The Eightieth Birthday of William Henry Welch: The Addresses Delivered* (New York: Milbank Memorial Fund, 1930), 25.

Memorial Fund. The event's organizers also included important names in public health research: C. E. A. Winslow of Yale University and Sir Arthur Newsholme, the former principal officer of the United Kingdom Local Government Board and a visiting professor at the JHSPH, to name just two.[2] These three strands of power – the United States government, philanthropic foundations, and public health researchers – orchestrated American public health work during the interwar years and, as the following chapters will show, played a salient role in institutionalizing statistical practices in public health at the international level.

Second, the event featured a transnational network for public health. Welch's birthday celebration was not a purely American affair, despite the prominent role of American stakeholders in this network. Local events were held in health organizations and medical institutes across the world, including the League of Nations Health Organization (LNHO) in Geneva, the Pasteur Institute in Paris, the London School of Hygiene and Tropical Medicine, and the Peking Union Medical College (PUMC) in Beijing. In Tokyo, a meeting was even organized to listen to the live radio broadcast of the celebration.[3] Composed of different branches of public health work, the same transnational network laid the foundation for international standards in public health statistics and strove to implement initiatives to establish them.

Lastly, and perhaps most essentially, the main organizer and sponsor of the celebration was the Milbank Memorial Fund, a general-purpose philanthropic foundation specializing in social work and public health.[4] Just as the Milbank Memorial Fund played an essential role in turning Welch's birthday celebration into an international public health event, many public health initiatives both within and outside the United States became a reality through the financial support of American philanthropic foundations. These foundations underwrote public health campaigns and recruited experts who ended up spreading American-style public health work to other parts of the world.[5]

---

[2] Ibid., 39.

[3] Ibid., 19, 36.

[4] Researchers use the term "general-purpose philanthropic foundation" to refer to foundations able to amend their programs according to changing needs without being bound by a deceased donor's will. (See, e.g.: Daniel M. Fox, "Foundations and Health: Innovation, Marginalization, and Relevance since 1900," in *American Foundations: Roles and Contributions*, eds. Helmut K. Anheier and David C. Hammack [Washington, DC: Brookings Institution Press, 2010]; Olivier Zunz, *Philanthropy in America: A History* [Princeton, NJ: Princeton University Press, 2014].)

[5] On the transnational nature of philanthropic foundations, see, e.g.: Thomas David and Ludovic Tournès, "Introduction. Les philanthropies: un objet d'histoire transnationale," *Monde(s)*, no. 6.2 (2014): 7–22.

The aforementioned actors, and the partnerships they formed, paved the way for the international public health statistical practices that are this book's focus. Before delving into specific themes within those practices, this chapter provides a detailed overview of the zeitgeist and key actors that led to the dependence on statistics in public health. Rooted in the Progressive Era (1896–1916) in the United States, philanthropic foundations, bacteriologists, and Chinese-born experts trained in North America – with their respective priorities and capacities – came to contribute to promoting (and sometimes implementing) statistics in public health projects at the international level.

## The Progressive Era and Philanthropic Foundations

The golden age of general-purpose philanthropic foundations lasted from the 1890s to the early 1930s.[6] This started with the Progressive Era: the economic boom at the turn of the twentieth century had created a growing class of nouveau riche but had worsened living conditions for the poor. It was also a time when the United States federal government was slow to formulate social policies, and it was left to such foundations to fill the void by implementing innovative social and public health programs.[7]

As Olivier Zunz indicates, the golden age began in 1893 with the passing of a New York State law, known as the Tilden Act, permitting the establishment of general-purpose foundations in which trustees were allowed to redefine and alter donors' plans to meet current social needs. Soon after, general-purpose philanthropic foundations began to thrive in the United States.[8] They tackled issues ranging from public health to social work, competing with the faith-based organizations to which their founders had once entrusted the lion's share of their donations.[9] The foundations reached the height of their influence in 1922, when

---

[6] Despite minor disagreements regarding the end of the golden age of American philanthropic foundations due to interests in different programs, researchers specializing in the history of such foundations tend to start their accounts in the 1890s, with the 1930s marking the moment when the foundations largely retired from American socioeconomic policy-making. (See, e.g.: Steven Wheatley, "The Partnerships of Foundations and Research Universities," in *American Foundations: Roles and Contributions*, 74; Fox, "Foundations and Health," 121; Inderjeet Parmar, *Foundations of the American Century: The Ford, Carnegie, and Rockefeller Foundations in the Rise of American Power* [New York: Columbia University Press, 2012], 3.)

[7] Fox, "Foundations and Health." For general accounts on public health development during the Progressive Era, see, e.g.: Paul Starr, *The Social Transformation of American Medicine* (New York: Basic Books, 1982); George Rosen, *A History of Public Health* (Baltimore, MD: Johns Hopkins University Press, 2015).

[8] Zunz, *Philanthropy in America*, 16.

[9] Ian Tyrrell, *Reforming the World: The Creation of America's Moral Empire* (Princeton, NJ: Princeton University Press, 2010), 227–9.

Hoover – then secretary of commerce – implemented his "compound republic" policy, through which the United States federal government sought to systematically integrate philanthropic foundations' programs into the government's social policies.[10] Hoover's defeat in the 1932 presidential election put an end to the golden age of philanthropic foundations. The New Deal of his successor, Franklin D. Roosevelt, created a more powerful federal government that took charge of social policies in the aftermath of the Great Depression.[11] With the federal government taking on the central role in socioeconomic policy-making in areas ranging from social work to public health, philanthropic foundations gradually stopped directly implementing campaigns on American soil and instead intensified their activities in foreign countries.[12]

Before philanthropic foundations began to lose prominence, starting in 1930, their financial support had been the foundation of American public health activities and research. Specifically, the two main philanthropic foundations investing in public health – the Rockefeller Foundation and the Milbank Memorial Fund – carried out health campaigns while also providing support to local health authorities, universities, and research institutes. Not only did the philanthropic foundations provide financial resources to these entities, they also exchanged technical advice, fieldwork training, political backing, and data that reinforced each other's programs. Both the Rockefeller Foundation and the Milbank Memorial Fund extended this modus operandi to foreign countries. By working with foreign governments and establishing research institutes, universities, and public health campaigns, they influenced the methods that local authorities used in their public health programs.

The transnational network described above, comprised of public and private stakeholders and fueled by American philanthropic funding, led statistical practices gradually to filter into public health research and policies in various parts of the world. But how did these actors come to focus on numbers in their public health programs? The Rockefeller Foundation's ideas about and dependence on numbers can be traced back to its founding years and were visible in its management culture. Established in 1913 by John D. Rockefeller, the Foundation sought to "promote

---

[10] Zunz, *Philanthropy in America*, 104; Fox, "Foundations and Health," 121.
[11] In historiographies of American philanthropic foundations, researchers have shown how the foundations' roles changed before World War II. See, e.g.: Judith Sealander, *Private Wealth and Public Life: Foundation Philanthropy and the Reshaping of American Social Policy from the Progressive Era to the New Deal* (Baltimore, MD: Johns Hopkins University Press, 1997); Fox, "Foundations and Health"; Zunz, *Philanthropy in America*.
[12] Parmar, *Foundations of the American Century*, 3.

the well-being of mankind throughout the world."[13] Frederick Gates, Rockefeller's right-hand man in business affairs, was also his adviser on philanthropic matters. Besides Gates, many of Rockefeller's business partners were also involved in managing the Foundation. The fact that Rockefeller hired professional managers in the 1920s is yet another sign of the businesslike mindset that reigned within the Foundation.[14]

The Rockefeller Foundation's trust in statistics was also related to its emphasis on using science to improve the well-being of humanity. Science was central to decision-making from day one of the Foundation's public health work. Before the Foundation was even established, Rockefeller had donated to the hookworm control campaign in the American South in 1909, blazing the trail for the establishment of the Foundation's International Health Board (IHB). Rockefeller supported the hookworm campaign because of scientific advances that had made it possible to identify hookworm ova using a microscope and to invent new treatments.[15] From the early days of the IHB, the Foundation endorsed various ways of collecting and using statistics that were closely related to its commitment to science. In the 1910s, the Foundation underwrote the JHSPH, including its statistics department, to promote science-based public health. In the 1920s, under the direction of former United States army officer Frederick Russell, the IHB collected vital and health statistics linked to scientific research; the idea took hold not just at the IHB headquarters in New York but also in its public health fieldwork in Europe, the Americas, and Asia.[16] In 1926, the IHB recruited JHSPH-trained Persis Putnam to be its first statistician. Putnam assessed vital statistics from fieldwork reports using mathematical statistical analysis. Through Putnam, statistical analysis came to be integrated into the IHB's management.[17]

The Milbank Memorial Fund linked statistics to business management in a manner similar to the Rockefeller Foundation. Albert Milbank, the Fund's president from 1922, was also head of the Borden Company, the leading producer of condensed milk at the time. Milbank transformed the Fund from a purely grant-giving organization into one that carried out its own public health programs. He managed the Fund as he would a business: one prominent proof being that, on its twenty-fifth anniversary,

[13] The Rockefeller Foundation, "The Rockefeller Foundation Annual Report 1913–1914," 1914, 7, www.rockefellerfoundation.org/wp-content/uploads/Annual-Report-1913-1914-1.pdf.

[14] Anne-Emanuelle Birn, *Marriage of Convenience: Rockefeller International Health and Revolutionary Mexico* (Rochester, NY: University of Rochester Press, 2006), 22.

[15] Ibid., 17–18.

[16] On Frederick Russell's policies while working for the IHB (which became the International Health Division in 1927), see: John Farley, *To Cast Out Disease: A History of the International Health Division of the Rockefeller Foundation* (Oxford: Oxford University Press, 2004).

[17] I will elaborate on Persis Putnam's statistical practices in Chapter 2.

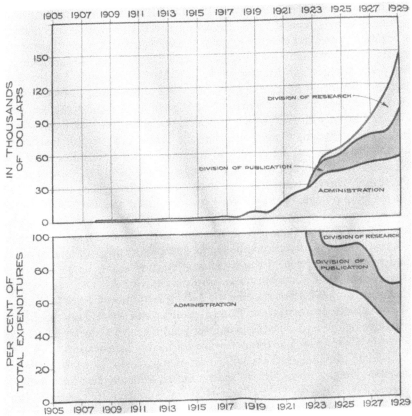

Figure 1.1 Comparative expenditures for administration, research, and publication (1905–1929).
Milbank Memorial Fund, "Twenty-Five Years of Philanthropy," 1930, 1–2, IV/32/2 Historical records, twenty-fifth anniversary: charts and tables, Milbank Memorial Fund Archives, University of Yale. Courtesy of Milbank Memorial Fund Records (MS 845). Manuscripts and Archives, Yale University Library.

the Fund published its finance and expenditure records dating back to 1905 (in full color), claiming the publication would be useful for other, younger organizations in administrating a general-purpose foundation.[18] Figure 1.1 is an example of how the expenditure report was presented, illustrating how the Fund's spending on administration grew along with the research and publication expenditure categories that emerged in 1923.

18 Milbank Memorial Fund, "Twenty-Five Years of Philanthropy," 1930, 1–2, IV/32/2 Historical records, twenty-fifth anniversary: charts and tables, Milbank Memorial Fund Archives, University of Yale.

The way the Milbank Memorial Fund collected statistics from its programs is closely related to the American social survey movement. John Kingsbury, the chief executive of the Fund from 1922, was a passionate collector of statistics in the early stage of his career. In 1911, when Kingsbury was the general director of the New York Association for Improving the Condition of the Poor (AICP),[19] he contributed statistical data on its beneficiaries to a report by the Russell Sage Foundation entitled "Wage Earner's Illness," which indicated that illness caused poverty and bolstered support for the campaign for compulsory health insurance, as advocated for by the American Association for Labor Legislation.[20] Kingsbury also worked with Paul Kellogg (1879–1958), the leader of the Pittsburgh Survey from 1910 to 1914, who drafted policy propositions on the living wage, hours of work, and so on for the 1912 Republican Convention.[21] Kellogg reformed the magazine *Charities and the Commons* and supplied information to American charity workers in the journal *Survey*, which underscored the importance of surveys in charity work and marked the peak of the social survey movement.[22] It is therefore unsurprising that Kingsbury, too, emphasized the role of surveys in public health work while overseeing the Milbank Memorial Fund. His ideas about surveys prompted the Fund to collect and share vital and health statistics before and after carrying out public health programs. As I will show in Chapter 4, Kingsbury endorsed health demonstration in New York State that included the collection of statistics on the cost of health services. He also hired Edgar Sydenstricker, a former health statistician at the LNHO and the USPHS, to oversee the collection of statistics from the Milbank health demonstrations.

Influenced by the traditions of scientific health research and social surveys, respectively, the leaderships of the Rockefeller Foundation and the Milbank Memorial Fund were convinced that numbers were a reliable medium for communicating public health conditions. It is worth noting that the two organizations were in constant contact at the highest level, as well as on the ground. John D. Rockefeller, Jr., and Albert Milbank

[19] "Kingsbury C.V.," n.d., II/24/15 Kingsbury, John A. Speeches 1937–1938, 1956, Milbank Memorial Fund Archives, University of Yale.
[20] The Russell Sage Foundation report compiled the AICP's data with that of the United Hebrew Charities. The report was never published, however. (Beatrix Hoffman, *The Wages of Sickness: The Politics of Health Insurance in Progressive America* [Chapel Hill, NC: University of North Carolina Press, 2001], 36–7, 191.)
[21] Shelton Stromquist, *Reinventing "The People": The Progressive Movement, the Class Problem, and the Origins of Modern Liberalism* (Urbana and Chicago, IL: University of Illinois Press, 2006), 100.
[22] Ibid., 100–1.

had been classmates at the Tony Cutler School.[23] When the Milbank Memorial Fund lacked funding for its health demonstration project in China owing to the economic depression, Rockefeller began funding the project at Milbank's request.[24] The Rockefeller Foundation's officers also sought advice from the Milbank Memorial Fund on a regular basis regarding nutrition and tuberculosis control.[25]

Both organizations worked in foreign terrain – be it geographically or socioeconomically – and depended on numbers to communicate local situations to their headquarters and the research institutes that they financed. Between the two of them, they funded three initiatives that improved the reliability of statistics and techniques for interpreting them. The Rockefeller Foundation financed a public health school (the JHSPH) and an intergovernmental organization (the LNHO's epidemiological intelligence service). The former legitimatized the use of mathematical statistics for analyzing vital and health statistics in academia, while the latter standardized vital and health statistics collection and dissemination among public administrations. The Milbank Memorial Fund, with its considerably smaller budget, devised health demonstrations in New York State through which it financed local public health administrations, in collaboration with local governments, to test their financial feasibility. The Milbank demonstrations established the essential role of statistical practices in health policy-making through a number of publications that described the results.

Although the above three initiatives had different priorities and were independent of one another, the experts who contributed to their design and implementation were in contact and had very similar career paths. Examining their profiles can help us grasp the context that led to the development of the international health statistical system.

### Bacteriologists and Their Ventures into Public Health

Both the Rockefeller Foundation and the Milbank Memorial Fund sought guidance from public health researchers when designing their initiatives. Three medical doctors, who had also trained in bacteriological

---

[23] Ron Chernow, *Titan: The Life of John D. Rockefeller, Sr.* (New York: Knopf Doubleday Publishing Group, 2007), 232.

[24] John D. Rockefeller Jr., "To Albert Milbank," November 30, 1932, Family/Cultural Interests/E/11/114, Rockefeller Archive Center.

[25] Paul Weindling, "American Foundations and the Internationalizing of Public Health," in *Shifting Boundaries of Public Health: Europe in the Twentieth Century*, eds. Susan Gross Solomon, Lion Murard, and Patrick Zylberman, Rochester Studies in Medical History (Rochester, NY: University of Rochester Press, 2008), 69–70.

laboratory research methods, acted as statesmen of science and were sought out by the philanthropic foundations in order to secure scientific credentials for their actions. These were William Welch (1850–1934), Hermann Biggs (1859–1923), and Ludwik Rajchman (1881–1965), who would become the principal advocates of the three statistical initiatives discussed in the following chapters.

Welch and Biggs had almost identical early career trajectories. Born in the mid-nineteenth century, they were part of the first generation of physicians to convert to germ theory and related laboratory methods when the theory began to gain traction at the end of the century. Welch and Biggs both began their medical careers at Bellevue Hospital Medical College in New York City, in the 1870s and 1880s, respectively. Welch then embarked on a two-year tour of Europe, during which he worked with Julius Cohnheim in Breslau (current-day Wrocław, Poland), and through him became acquainted with Robert Koch.[26] Afterwards, Welch returned to Bellevue to teach pathology and contributed to the establishing the United States' first pathology laboratory.

Welch's lectures were greatly admired by his students, including a young Hermann Biggs, and Welch's laboratory demonstration of Koch's experiment inspired Biggs' passion for bacteriology.[27] Just like his mentor, Biggs departed for Europe to apprentice under renowned bacteriologists, including Robert Koch in Berlin and Louis Pasteur in Paris. In 1884, a year after Biggs' departure for Europe, Welch himself took a second European tour in search of inspiration for his design of a medical college and laboratory at Johns Hopkins University. 1884 was also when Robert Koch isolated the pathogen responsible for cholera. Welch and Biggs' European experiences meant that they were steeped in bacteriological laboratory methods focused on isolating pathogens in pure culture in the era when that trend reached its climax.[28]

Upon returning home, Welch and Biggs imported European laboratory training into the American public health system. Welch became a professor of pathology at Johns Hopkins and the first pathologist-in-chief of its hospital five years later; Biggs took over the Carnegie Laboratory at Bellevue, and convinced the New York City government to enlarge its municipal diagnostic laboratory (which also produced vaccines) at the

[26] David Riesman, "William Henry Welch, Scientist and Humanist," *The Scientific Monthly* 41, no. 3 (1935): 253.
[27] Simon Flexner and James Thomas Flexner, *William Henry Welch and the Heroic Age of American Medicine* (New York: The Viking Press, 1941), 119; Richard Adler, *Robert Koch and American Bacteriology* (Jefferson, NC: McFarland, 2016), 145.
[28] For more detail on Welch's training during his second visit to Europe, see: Adler, *Robert Koch and American Bacteriology*, 145–9.

end of the nineteenth century, with Biggs at the helm.[29] Biggs spent the rest of his career in New York public health administrations: he served as the first general medical officer of the Health Department of the City of New York in 1902, and as the New York State Commissioner of Health in 1914.[30]

The final effort of both men's careers was the promotion of statistical practices in public health in the 1910s. Biggs was in his fifties and Welch in his sixties, and both were well established in research. Their emphasis on statistical collection can be understood as an effort to apply laboratory methods to the social world. Theodore Porter's work is useful for grasping Welch and Biggs' reasons for supporting statistics: Porter draws a parallel between laboratory science and quantification, pointing out that statistics put the messy reality of the social world into a purified form and represented social reality while being suited to laboratory-like manipulations.[31] As the collection and calculation of statistics had traits in common with laboratory research, it is not surprising that Welch and Biggs became strong advocates for statistical practices in public health, though neither of them would have considered himself a statistician.

Welch and Biggs' voices were amplified by their close relationship with the philanthropic foundations. Both were, in one way or another, associated with the Carnegie Laboratory at Bellevue, and both had served on the board of directors of the Rockefeller Institute for Medical Research since its establishment in 1901,[32] making them a natural choice for the foundations to consult when designing their programs. When Welch submitted his design for the Johns Hopkins School of Public Health and its statistics department, he was a professor of pathology at Johns Hopkins and was frequently called upon by the Foundation to advise its IHB and China Medical Board. He also visited China on a Rockefeller mission in 1915 and participated in designing the PUMC.[33] Biggs was the general medical officer of the New York Public Health Board, and had spearheaded a variety of public health activities in New York, including the Framingham health demonstration launched in 1916. With the Milbank Memorial Fund's financial support, the demonstration aimed to lower the number of tuberculosis cases in the Massachusetts town

[29] John Duffy, *The Sanitarians: A History of American Public Health* (Urbana, IL: University of Illinois Press, 1992), 195.
[30] "Hermann M. Biggs," *Science* 58, no. 1508 (1923): 413–14.
[31] Porter, *Trust in Numbers*, 16–21.
[32] Darwin H. Stapleton, *Creating a Tradition of Biomedical Research: Contributions to the History of the Rockefeller University* (New York: Rockefeller University Press, 2004), 20.
[33] Flexner and Flexner, *William Henry Welch*, 402.

of Framingham.[34] These prior collaborations gave Welch's and Biggs' suggestions on statistical initiatives considerable weight with the philanthropic foundations. Notably, Welch and Biggs were also associated with each other's initiatives via the philanthropic foundations that funded them. Welch sat on the advisory board of the Milbank Memorial Fund, which funded the New York State demonstrations supported by Biggs; and Biggs participated in the Rockefeller Foundation's conferences on designing a new school of public health, a conference that paved the way for Welch's proposed school at Johns Hopkins.[35]

On the other side of Atlantic, the bacteriologist Ludwik Rajchman – the main instigator of the LNHO's use of statistics – had a career that took a rather different trajectory. Rajchman was born, decades after Welch and Biggs, into a family of intellectuals in Russian-controlled Warsaw in 1881. When Rajchman began his medical education at the Jagiellonian University in Krakow, bacteriology was already well established across Europe. His teacher, Odo Bujwid, was a student of Louis Pasteur and Robert Koch. When Rajchman was released from prison after his involvement in the Polish Revolution of 1905, Bujwid organized his exile in Paris at the Pasteur Institute. Rajchman stayed in Paris until 1910, when he was hired as a bacteriologist by the Royal Institute of Public Health in London. When Poland gained independence in 1918, Rajchman returned to his home country and convinced the newly established government to establish an epidemiological institute, later known as the National Institute of Hygiene. Rajchman and his institute were instrumental in containing the typhus epidemic that was raging in Russia and Eastern Europe following World War I. He became known to the Rockefeller Foundation, which was active in the provision of medical relief in Eastern Europe. Rajchman's leading role in responding to that crisis eventually led him to be named the first director of the LNHO in 1921. His first mission for the League, before becoming director, was to form international partnerships to combat typhus in Eastern Europe.[36]

As the first director of the LNHO, Rajchman was in charge of designing the organization, and he created the statistical service with the express aim of gaining financial support from the Rockefeller IHB. Like Welch and Biggs, Rajchman was an established bacteriologist and no

[34] Donald B. Armstrong, "The Framingham Health Tuberculosis Demonstration," *American Journal of Public Health* 7, no. 3 (1917): 318–22.
[35] Rockefeller Foundation, "Conference on Training for Public Health Service by Rockefeller Foundation – Committee on Institute of Hygiene," October 16, 1914, RF/1.1/200/184/2214, Rockefeller Archive Center.
[36] Marta Aleksandra Balinska, "Ludwik Rajchman (1881–1965): Médecin polonais et citoyen du monde," *La Revue du Praticien* 55, no.4 (2005): 458–61.

stranger to the Rockefeller Foundation. What distinguished Rajchman from Welch and Biggs was his rhetoric regarding the role of statistics. Rajchman, working as he did at the helm of an international health organization, emphasized the fact that statistics could serve as the basis for international collaboration, rather than focusing on advancing scientific research.[37]

Welch, Biggs, and Rajchman were neither the first nor the only individuals to use statistics to tackle public health crises, but they planted the seeds for initiatives that eventually institutionalized statistical practices within public health at the international level. Apart from their generational and geographical differences, the three researchers' careers had several traits in common: Their apprenticeships were transnational; they all received bacteriological laboratory training; and they were all known to the philanthropic foundations for their medical research before they sought to integrate statistical practices into public health. Their prior experience motivated and empowered them – with the support of philanthropic foundations – to venture into statistical initiatives for public health, which would have a profound impact in several regions of the world over the following years.

### Missionaries' Sons, Born in China and Trained in North America

To achieve their ambition of carrying out public health work that transcended national borders, the philanthropic foundations and their bacteriologist partners relied on experts with knowledge of both public health and local contexts. In China, missionaries' sons who had been born and raised in the country fit perfectly into this highly niche profile. Edgar Sydenstricker (1881–1936) and John B. Grant (1890–1962) were two notable examples. Their childhoods in China gave them knowledge of the country, while their university training in North America (Sydenstricker in the United States, and Grant in Canada and the United States) meant that their public health expertise was aligned with the needs of the foundations and bacteriologists. They were thus entrusted to lead the Chinese end of the circuits through which statistical initiatives crossed continents. Specifically, Sydenstricker was recruited by the LNHO in Geneva to design the epidemiological intelligence service, with earmarked funding from the Rockefeller Foundation. Upon returning to the United States, he was then associated with the Milbank Memorial

---

[37] See Chapter 3 for more information on Rajchman's attempts to secure IHB funding.

Fund's New York and Ding Xian (Ting Hsien) health demonstrations.[38]
Grant, for his part, was sent to China by the Rockefeller Foundation to
serve as professor of pathology at the PUMC, where he would carry out
a series of activities that laid the foundation for public health statistics in
China.[39] As executive officers, Grant and Sydenstricker were both pioneers of health statistics collection in China, a country separated from
the North Atlantic sphere by vast cultural and political differences.

Though they were involved in different initiatives and worked with
different foundations, Sydenstricker and Grant's family backgrounds
were surprisingly similar. Sydenstricker's father, Absalom Sydenstricker,
was an American Presbyterian missionary stationed in Shanghai, where
Edgar Sydenstricker was born in 1881. Nine years later, John Grant was
born into a Canadian missionary family based in Ningbo, some 200 kilometers south of Shanghai. The men's family backgrounds explain their
long-standing interest in public health in China in two ways. First, having
grown up in missionary families, they were steeped in charitable culture,
which in part explains why both undertook studies and careers that had
a humanitarian dimension. In 1896, the fifteen-year-old Sydenstricker
went to West Virginia to study sociology and economics at Washington
and Lee University;[40] some fifteen years later, Grant began his studies
in Nova Scotia and later studied medicine at the University of Michi-
gan.[41] Their childhoods also inspired their professional interest in China
at different stages of their careers. As will be discussed in the following
chapters, Sydenstricker brought the Milbank Memorial Fund's attention
to China in the late 1920s. And Grant spent eighteen years in China
representing the Rockefeller Foundation in the construction of a public
health system there before the Foundation transferred him to India in
1937 due to the outbreak of the Second Sino-Japanese War.[42]

With specializations in the social sciences and medicine, respectively,
Sydenstricker and Grant were trained to approach public health issues
from different angles. Sydenstricker applied a social-science perspective:

[38] These two initiatives will be discussed in Chapters 3 and 4, respectively.
[39] Grant and his contribution to vital and health statistics in China will be presented in
greater detail in Chapter 2.
[40] Dorothy G. Wiehl, "Edgar Sydenstricker: A Memoir," in *The Challenge of Facts:
Selected Public Health Papers of Edgar Sydenstricker*, eds. Richard V. Kasius (New York:
Prodist, 1974), 4.
[41] Liping Bu and Elizabeth Fee, "John B. Grant International Statesman of Public
Health," *American Journal of Public Health* 98, no. 4 (2008): 628.
[42] Li Lu and Zhang Daqing, "Lan Ansheng de gongxian: Zhongguo gonggong weisheng
jingyan zai yindu de zhuanyi" [John Black Grant's Contribution: Chinese Public
Health Experiences' Transplant in India], *Yixue yu Zhexue [Medicine & Philosophy]*
36, no. 9A (2015): 81–4.

He began his career by conducting social surveys on the wages, working conditions, and standards of living of industrial workers for the United States Immigration Commission. His venture into public health started in 1915, when he joined the USPHS and was appointed assistant to surgeon Benjamin S. Warren for a study on health insurance administration in European countries. He was subsequently transferred to South Carolina to work with Joseph Goldberger, also of the USPHS, on his epidemiological study of pellagra, which sought to ascertain the relationship between dietary, economic, and sanitary factors.[43] In contrast to Sydenstricker, Grant received more orthodox training for a public health expert: though originally trained in medicine, he began his career in public health after being recruited by the Rockefeller IHB in 1918. The IHB first sent Grant to Puerto Rico to work on hookworm control and later paid for his studies in public health at Johns Hopkins University in the early 1920s. Grant's work in China reflected the nature of his training and focused on adapting public health research and administration to the Chinese context.

Unlike the bacteriologists mentioned above, Sydenstricker and Grant did not come to focus on statistical practices only at the end of their careers; rather, their entire careers were intertwined with public health statistics. In the early 1920s, both men were associated with statistical initiatives by philanthropic foundations and designed programs that led to the professionalization of public health statisticians.[44] As I will demonstrate in the following chapters, Sydenstricker's work with the LNHO – aimed at institutionalizing the role of statisticians within national health authorities – was launched in 1922 with Rockefeller funding. Grant's plan for a public health school at the PUMC – where special attention was given to the training of statisticians – was endorsed by the Rockefeller Foundation in 1924.

Both men's influence in public health statistics extended beyond 1925. Following his work at the LNHO, Sydenstricker returned to the United States and continued conducting statistical research for the USPHS and the Milbank Memorial Fund. The latter would send Sydenstricker to China to run a health demonstration. Sydenstricker also became the director of the statistical section of the American Public

---

[43] Willford I. King, "Edgar Sydenstricker," *Journal of the American Statistical Association* 31, no. 194 (1936): 411–14.

[44] Sydenstricker was an author of two articles describing the role of statisticians in public health administrations: E. W. Kopf et al., "Educational and Professional Standards for Vital Statisticians," *American Journal of Public Health* 15, no. 6 (1925): 518–20; Edgar Sydenstricker, "The Statistician's Place in Public Health Work," *Journal of the American Statistical Association* 23, no. 162 (1928b): 115.

Health Association, and throughout his career sought to demonstrate the correlation between health and social factors – such as economic status, income, and sanitary conditions – up until his premature death in 1936.[45] As for Grant, he became a public health administration guru in China, with his students occupying key positions within Chinese public health administrations and research institutes even after 1945. Grant's influence also extended to other parts of the world after World War II. He was associated with United States President Harry Truman's administration, advised the World Health Organization, and consulted with several national governments on their health administration design. He also taught public health at the University of Puerto Rico until his death in 1962.[46]

It should be noted that Sydenstricker and Grant knew each other and consulted one another while working on their respective programs. The most significant encounter came in the late 1920s, when Sydenstricker arrived in China as Milbank's representative in charge of designing the health statistical system for the rural reconstruction programs in Ding Xian. At Grant's advice, he placed the Ding Xian program in the hands of Grant's former students at the PUMC.[47]

The life stories of Sydenstricker and Grant support historian Ian Tyrrall's argument that continuities existed between missionary societies and philanthropic foundations.[48] Tyrrall asserts that philanthropic foundations gradually replaced missionary societies as the major players in the American moral empire, but Sydenstricker and Grant's trajectories show that this replacement happened not only at the organizational level but also at the individual level. The sons of missionaries with cultural knowledge and humanitarian concerns attributable to their childhood in China and higher education in North America, they became the executors of American philanthropic foundations' plans to promote public health statistics on an international scale.

## Confluence and Networks

The life trajectories of the bacteriologists and health administrators introduced above represent two directions of migration. On the one hand, starting in the 1870s, American bacteriologists traveled to Europe for laboratory training and then returned to the United States to develop

[45] Wiehl, "Edgar Sydenstricker: A Memoir."
[46] Bu and Fee, "John B. Grant International Statesman of Public Health."
[47] See Chapter 4.
[48] Tyrrell, *Reforming the World*, 228–9.

their own laboratories. On the other, the sons of North American missionaries grew up in China and returned to North America for higher education, where they became acquainted with, and were later hired by, philanthropic foundations. New York was the meeting point for these two trajectories: it was where affluent American philanthropic foundations were headquartered and where experts with various skill sets were recruited to carry out the foundations' plans to improve health conditions and further crystallize statistical collection for public health at the international level.

The experts involved in the three interwar circuits of transfer for statistical practices covered in this book were aware of one another's initiatives and even collaborated in some cases. For example, Raymond Pearl, the first biostatistics professor at the JHSPH, recommended that Edgar Sydenstricker become the first director of the LNHO's epidemiological intelligence service.[49] Pearl was also part of the LNHO's study groups. Sydenstricker and his associates at the LNHO provided statistical services to the Milbank health demonstrations upon returning to the United States, and Sydenstricker's Milbank-funded research on the impact of depression on morbidity and malnutrition was published in the LNHO's bulletin.[50] This off-and-on collaboration is demonstrative of how the circulation of a given statistical practice was not self-contained; rather, different circuits interacted with one another.

This loosely organized collaborative network was not without its opponents. Major Greenwood and Raymond Pearl, both pupils of Karl Pearson (a leading founder of mathematical statistics), privately shared bitter criticisms of initiatives aimed at inserting statistics into public health. Although Greenwood and Pearl also made salient contributions to those same initiatives on several occasions, the duo complained to each other that such initiatives were a waste of money and energy because they tackled only the superficial manipulation of statistical techniques, thus diverging from the mathematical statistical research in which Greenwood and Pearl had been trained under Pearson.[51] Such criticisms make it evident that the circulation of statistical practices was not always straightforward and was challenged at various points. The challenges are revelatory of the ways in which some types of statistical thinking and practices were "lost in translation" when transferred to China from the North Atlantic sphere of influence. As I will detail later, North Atlantic experts and their

---

[49] Wickliffe Rose, "To Rajchman," July 18, 1922, 12b/26117/21836/R839/1923, League of Nations Archives.

[50] Borowy, *Coming to Terms with World Health*, 367–8.

[51] Major Greenwood, "To Raymond Pearl," August 5, 1923, Greenwood, Major (2) 1923/i, Raymond Pearl Papers, American Philosophical Society. I will also detail their criticisms in Chapter 2.

Chinese partners had to adapt their priorities when confronted with the Chinese context.

In the following chapters, I will further detail how the call for a language of public health was responded to and implemented through my analysis of the circulation of statistical practices among a network of experts composed of philanthropists, researchers, and administrators. This network spanned continents and laid the foundation for an international health statistical system from the 1910s to the 1960s. The network grew as more specialists were recruited to carry out statistical work, and some early initiatives trained new cohorts of health experts in statistical practices.

> We, first inspired by [Francis] Galton and Karl Pearson, fought this
> long battle without the least help from the professional mathematician
> and against the violent opposition of nearly the whole medical profes-
> sion. Now that the battle is won, that biometry and statistics are aca-
> demically respectable …[1]

In a letter supporting his American colleague Raymond Pearl's candidacy
for a professorship at Harvard University, Major Greenwood, a professor
of epidemiology and vital statistics at the London School of Hygiene and
Tropical Medicine, who also acted as the head of the Medical Research
Council's Statistical Department,[2] reminisced on the struggle to make
biostatistics an academic branch of medical science. As students of Karl
Pearson (1857–1936), Greenwood and Pearl represented the first generation of recognized academic researchers to use statistical analysis to
explain human life, disease, and death. Their research culminated in the
systematic integration of statistical methods into public health research:
the only domain of medical statistics in which "the language of quantity [was] very successful," according to Theodore Porter.[3] Meanwhile,
statistical thinking was struggling to become systematically integrated
into medical research. Although some researchers and administrators
had already begun to use descriptive statistics to exhibit and compare
the vital and health conditions of populations in the nineteenth century,
medical doctors – arguably up until the 1950s – still insisted, under-
standably, on their patients' individuality and inability to be quantified.[4]

---

[1] Major Greenwood, "To President A. Lawrence Lowell, University of Harvard,"
 July 20, 1929, I/Greenwood, Major (8) 1929, Raymond Pearl Papers, American
 Philosophical Society.
[2] Vern Farewell and Tony Johnson, "Major Greenwood (1880–1949): A Biographical
 and Bibliographical Study," *Statistics in Medicine* 35, no. 5 (2016): 654.
[3] Porter, *Trust in Numbers*, 203.
[4] Desrosières, *La politique des grands nombres*, 104; Porter, *Trust in Numbers*, 203–4. For
 examples of statistical collection prior to Pearl and Greenwood, see, e.g.: Edward

Greenwood and Pearl's statistical practices can be traced back to the eugenicist Francis Galton (1822–1911) and his experiment on pea seeds. Galton, a cousin of Charles Darwin, based his research on observations of the size of peas; he noticed that the size of large peas would gradually revert to an average size over the course of generations.[5] He published his observations in a book, *Natural Inheritance* (1889), which is generally considered to be the origin of correlation and regression theories. Pearson translated Galton's inheritance theory into pure mathematical equations that explained variations, and devoted himself to extending the application of mathematical statistics from biological research to other disciplines.[6] Pearson established the biometric laboratory at University College London in 1911, where he trained Greenwood and Pearl, who went on to become the first professors of vital statistics on their respective sides of the Atlantic.[7]

This chapter explores the socio-historical context that served as the basis for the integration of Pearson's mathematical statistical method into public health research and its influence beyond the North Atlantic world. While Pearson's contribution to the integration of mathematical statistics into medical research is well known among historians of statistics,[8] it was unclear until now how Pearson's methods became implanted in public health schools outside of the United Kingdom, let alone how they were transferred to China. In this chapter, I show how the Johns Hopkins School of Public Health (JHSPH) and the Peking Union Medical College (PUMC) – two academic institutions that received the lion's share of funding from the Rockefeller Foundation – played an essential role in that process. The Rockefeller Foundation, looking to advance scientific research through support for a public health school, selected

Higgs, *The Information State in England: The Central Collection of Information on Citizens Since 1500* (New York: Palgrave Macmillan, 2004); Morabia, *A History of Epidemiologic Methods and Concepts*; Susser and Stein, *Eras in Epidemiology*.

[5] Galton's theory was the basis for the eugenics movement that rose in prominence during the twentieth century. See: Alison Bashford and Philippa Levine, eds., *The Oxford Handbook of the History of Eugenics* (Oxford: Oxford University Press, 2010).

[6] See, e.g.: Porter, *The Rise of Statistical Thinking*, 286–97; Theodore M. Porter, *Karl Pearson: The Scientific Life in a Statistical Age* (Princeton, NJ: Princeton University Press, 2004).

[7] The two men's titles, however, were not identical. Greenwood's official title at University College London was "Professor of Epidemiology and Vital Statistics," whereas Pearl's was "Professor of Biometry and Vital Statistics." The difference is indicative of the unstable boundary between disciplines at that time when it came to research that used statistics to explain trends in lives, diseases, and deaths.

[8] See, e.g.: Eileen Magnello, "The Introduction of Mathematical Statistics into Medical Research: The Roles of Karl Pearson, Major Greenwood and Austin Bradford Hill," in *The Road to Medical Statistics*, eds. Eileen Magnello and Anne Hardy (Amsterdam; New York: Rodopi, 2002), 95.

the Johns Hopkins University project led by William Welch.[9] Welch's proposal included a statistics department, which was put under Pearl's leadership in 1917. As the JHSPH was also responsible for training American and foreign public health workers of all grades, the school's statistical practices eventually spread across national borders. As early as the interwar years, some JHSPH alumni later became leading statisticians in their home institutions or at the League of Nations Health Organization (LNHO); some were later recruited by the World Health Organization (WHO) after World War II.

The JHSPH had the resources to spread its statistical practices to public health research institutions in other countries; the PUMC was where those practices were adapted through local innovations. The founder of the PUMC Department of Hygiene and Public Health, John B. Grant (a JHSPH alumnus) and his collaborators played a central role in that process. Not only did they design the Chinese version of the International List of Causes of Death (ICD) and a statistical reporting system for part of Beijing, Grant also trained a group of Chinese experts, including the first Chinese health statistician, Yuan Yijin (Yüan I-Chin), whose work made statistical practices part of public health research in China.

The way statistics were used at the JHSPH can thus be considered the basis for a formal language of statistics, whereas the method employed at the PUMC amounted to developing a local dialect of that language. Experts at the JHSPH did not design a method specific to the Baltimore setting: they conceived of statistics as a universal medium for expressing public health phenomena. In Beijing, on the other hand, the goal was to adapt the "language" of statistical collection to fit the needs and capacities of China.

Through the lens of statistical practices, this chapter touches upon the more general question of how conceptions of the role of statistics in public health science differed between the JHSPH and the PUMC. Though both received Rockefeller money aimed at setting the standard for health research, faculty at the two schools organized their statistical research and training differently. At the JHSPH, Pearl prioritized using biological research to advance statistical theory, and his colleagues Lowell J. Reed and Wade Frost used stochastic simulation to reveal the shared features of epidemics. Grant's conception of health research at the PUMC, however, differed from that of his teachers at the JHSPH. Grant's ambition was to adapt scientific knowledge to the Chinese context by using statistical collection in experiments to develop public health programs that

---

[9] Elizabeth Fee, *Disease and Discovery: A History of the Johns Hopkins School of Hygiene and Public Health, 1916–1939* (Baltimore, MD: Johns Hopkins University Press, 1987), 51–6.

were suitable for China. Upon taking the helm of the department, Grant designed a public health demonstration area where his students could conduct research and be trained in public health administrative procedures, including statistics collection. In that sense, the PUMC was more advanced than the JHSPH, as the PUMC's demonstration area – the Peking First Health Station (PFHS), also known as the Peiping Health Demonstration Station[10] – began its activities in 1925, seven years before the JHSPH set up its Baltimore health demonstration.

## Statistics: Bookkeeping or Scientific Research?

When the Rockefeller Foundation decided to fund an American public health school in 1914, none of its officers had the faintest idea how it should be organized. There were very few such schools in existence, and each had a very different curriculum: some (such as the University of Columbia) were focused on the social and political aspects of public health work, whereas others (including Johns Hopkins) included public health courses within their medical school's curriculum. Meanwhile, the need for trained public health workers had increased as the number of county health units in the US grew from just one, in 1908, to 33 in 1918 (Figure 2.1).

There was also a lack of consensus on statistical practices for public health. Until the 1910s, statistical work in local health offices was considered clerical work that did not require medical or public health knowledge. In county health units across the US, officers who oversaw the compilation of birth and death numbers were variously referred to as "vital statisticians," "health statisticians," "medical statisticians," or even "statistical clerks," with no standardized title or responsibilities apart from amassing numbers concerning births and deaths.[11] Statistical practices were beginning to emerge within public health organizations, but only sporadically.

Despite the lack of a unified title and job description, there was a recognized need for someone to be responsible for calculating numbers in health services. In 1914, during a conference organized by the Rockefeller Foundation's General Education Board to study the need for a new public health school, the New York State Commissioner of

---

[10] In Chinese: 北平市衛生局第一衛生區事務所, *Beipingshi weishengju diyi weisheng qu shiwusuo*.

[11] Thomas Parran and Livingston Ferrand, "Report to the Rockefeller Foundation on the Education of Public Health Personnel," October 28, 1939, 9, RF/1.1/200/185/2222, Rockefeller Archive Center.

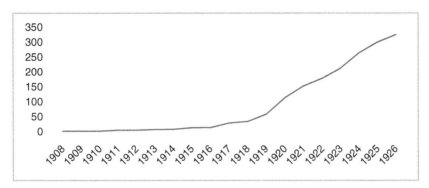

Figure 2.1 Growth in the number of full-time county health organizations (1908–1926).
Note: This figure shows the number of organizations at the close of each year that had been in continuous operation from the date of their opening. Adapted from International Health Board, "Growth in the Number of Full-Time County Health Organisations," n.d., Field Staff/IHB Documents of Record Vol.XI/IHB DR 957, Rockefeller Archive Center. Courtesy of Rockefeller Archive Center.

Health, Hermann Biggs, stated that medical statisticians were "one of the great needs ... of public health service in this country."[12] Biggs gave the conference participants a vivid account of his own experience recruiting a health statistician for his department, concluding that "[t]here are no men, or practically no men, who have had experiences and demonstrated ability in this line, and it is a very, very urgent need."[13] Biggs' words carried considerable weight, as he was a renowned expert who had been involved in public health work in New York since the 1890s.[14] His remarks during the conference were clearly taken seriously: in subsequent plans for the new school – though the priority shifted back and forth several times between science and practical training – a statistical department was always included.

The 1914 conference reached the conclusion that the Rockefeller Foundation should fund a new public health school that would undertake both scientific research and practical training. Wickliffe Rose, then the director of the Rockefeller Foundation's International Health Commission, called for the school to be "an institution of [the] highest

[12] Rockefeller Foundation, "Conference on Training for Public Health Service by Rockefeller Foundation – Committee on Institute of Hygiene," October 16, 1914, 5, RF/1.1/200/184/2214, Rockefeller Archive Center.
[13] Ibid.
[14] Duffy, *The Sanitarians*, 195.

standard, scientific in character, and not neglecting the training for practical service, and further, for it to be scientific in character."[15] Rose thus stressed that among the school's dual missions, science and practical training, science should be the prime standard, and the practical training should itself be scientific.

Discussions on how to set up the statistics department within the new school reveal the tension between science and practical training. The school's two designers, Rose and Welch, did not have the same ideas when it came to statistical practices in public health. Rose, who had led the Rockefeller Foundation's hookworm control campaign in the American South, thought the JHSPH should have a medical statistics department devoted to training public health officers in the methods of organizing statistical collection and analysis within local health units.[16] Rose's administrative experience made him see statistical work in public health as based solely on collecting the number of births, disease cases, and deaths, which was the most common responsibility of statisticians at the time. But Welch, a pathologist by training, paid greater attention to the use of statistical methods in scientific research. He wanted to extend statistical practices in public health to applications in research, probably owing to his training in bacteriological laboratory methods. In his draft design for the school, Welch proposed that "while the various questions connected with the collection and study of vital statistics constitute the most important subject in this field, there are other important applications of statistical science to hygiene."[17] Welch thus advocated that the statistical division should not limit itself to collecting and analyzing vital statistics.

The success of Welch's proposal over Rose's was probably owing to chance. As Elizabeth Fee has documented, Rose only wanted Welch to add comments to Rose's draft for the school, but instead, Welch presented his own draft. Because Welch submitted his draft at the last minute, Rose did not have time to review it before it was presented to, and accepted by, the General Education Board with the title "The Rose–Welch Report."[18] Even though Rose's emphasis on basic statistical training was left out, the JHSPH statistics department did end up providing such training from the beginning.

---

[15] Rockefeller Foundation, "Conference on Training for Public Health Service by Rockefeller Foundation – Committee on Institute of Hygiene," 71–2.

[16] Wickliffe Rose, "School of Public Health," 1916, 4–5, RF/1.1/200/184/2216, Rockefeller Archive Center.

[17] William H. Welch, "Institute of Hygiene," 1915, 12, RF/1.1/200/184/2216, Rockefeller Archive Center.

[18] Fee, *Disease and Discovery*, 40.

Following the acceptance of his proposal, Welch recruited Raymond Pearl as the first director of the statistics department in 1917. Welch's choice was in line with his idea that the department should not focus solely on collecting and analyzing vital statistics. An intellectual descendant of Galton and Pearson, Pearl – who had also been the first chief of the statistical division of the newly established United States Food Administration – was first and foremost a biologist, and had calculated statistical data using logistic curves to demonstrate regularities in heredity.[19] Pearl's research reputation was already established prior to his contact with Welch: after an apprenticeship in Pearson's biometric laboratory in London, he had conducted research into the genetics of domestic animals at the Maine Agricultural Experiment Station and, later, during his service in the Food Administration, had published on food supply and economics in the United States.[20] Pearl's profile as a researcher rather than an administrator made him the ideal candidate for Welch, who gave Pearl full responsibility for organizing the statistics department.

### Of Mice and Fieldwork: A Changing Plan for the JHSPH Statistics Department

The invitation to head a statistics department gave Pearl a great opportunity to conduct biological research, his main interest. Following Pearson's tradition, Pearl added "biometry" to the name of the department, and set his own title as "Professor of Biometry and Vital Statistics."[21] By including both the terms "biometry" and "vital statistics" in his title, Pearl revealed the dual aim of his new department: to conduct biological research based on numerical analysis, and to offer training to administrative statisticians, who mostly dealt with vital statistics collection.

Pearl's design for the department was very much oriented toward biological research. The four research projects he chose for the department were all on topics related to biology: alcoholism and heredity; natural selection in humans (including selective death rates and racial effects); heredity as a factor in lifespan and morbidity; and inbreeding in humans.[22] Pearl took an experimentalist approach and set up a mouse

---

[19] Herbert S. Jennings, *"Biographical Memoir of Raymond Pearl (1879–1940)," National Academy of Sciences of the United States of America Biographical Memoirs Vol. XXII* (Washington, DC: National Academy of Sciences, 1942), 298.

[20] Ibid., 298.

[21] Raymond Pearl, "To William Howell," December 31, 1917, JHUSH O.D.Ja National Research Council School of Hygiene 1917–1921/3/a/5/Pearl, R./Dec 1917–July 1920, Johns Hopkins Medical Archives.

[22] Raymond Pearl, "To Major Greenwood," October 17, 1923, Greenwood, Major (2) 1923/i, Raymond Pearl Papers, American Philosophical Society.

colony to conduct biological research on lifespans. He attached great value to laboratory experiments, believing that a well-designed experiment could reveal the statistical regularities governing all human life.[23] Considering the experimental statistical investigation on the life duration of the mouse "an important feature" of the department, Pearl budgeted for a mouse colony.[24] Although the mouse colony was destroyed in a fire, Pearl still managed to publish *The Biology of Death* (1922), in which he presented a comprehensive discussion on longevity and causes of death based on his work on the colony.

The JHSPH statistics department also conducted mathematical research. Pearl hired Lowell J. Reed, a former assistant professor of mathematics at the University of Maine and director of the Bureau of Tabulation and Statistics at the War Trade Board, to be the department's mathematician.[25] With Reed, Pearl tackled biological questions and mathematical theories by analyzing quantified data in the biological and medical fields. For example, the pair studied patterns of population growth using US census records and conducted an experiment using fruit flies that involved putting the flies in an isolated container and observing changes in their numbers over time; they also used hospital records to study genetic factors behind the morbidity and mortality of tuberculosis patients.[26]

Pearl focused most of his efforts on devising logistic curves to represent regularities in population growth and decline.[27] His methodological presupposition of longevity as a natural law was in total opposition to that of public health workers, who believed that lifespans could be extended through public health interventions. George Whipple's review of *The Biology of Death* sheds light on the disagreement between Pearl and public health experts. As Whipple, a distinguished medical doctor and future Nobel Prize winner, wrote: "health officers will find in it

---

23 Ibid.
24 Raymond Pearl, "Immediate Requirements of the Department of Biometry and Vital Statistics," 1919, 2, JHUSH O.D.Ja National Research Council School of Hygiene 1917–1921/3/a/5/Pearl, R./Dec 1917–July 1920, Johns Hopkins Medical Archives.
25 Johns Hopkins School of Hygiene and Public Health, "Catalogue and Announcement of the School of Public Health, 1919–1920," 1919, 9, The Johns Hopkins University/ School of Hygiene and Public Health/Catalogue and Announcement for 1919–1920 (published in 1919), Johns Hopkins Medical Archives.
26 The American Journal of Hygiene, *The School of Hygiene and Public Health of the Johns Hopkins University*, The American Journal of Hygiene Monographic Series 6 (Baltimore, MD: The American Journal of Hygiene, 1926), 24–5.
27 On Pearl's contributions to the field of eugenics and population control, see, e.g.: Edmund Ramsden, "Carving up Population Science Eugenics, Demography and the Controversy over the 'Biological Law' of Population Growth," *Social Studies of Science* 32, no. 5–6 (2002): 857–99.

much to criticize, little to commend, and nothing to inspire."[28] Indeed, in contrast to most of his colleagues at the JHSPH, Pearl's priority was to discover statistical regularities within the vital conditions of populations (such as longevity, the duration of diseases, and reproductive behavior); he considered improving health and extending longevity to be secondary concerns. Tellingly, Pearl and Reed's most famous co-authored article is on population growth. In it, the two authors contend that their only purpose was "to demonstrate ... the hypothesis here advanced as to the law of population growth, [so] as to make it potentially profitable to continue the mathematical development and refinement of this hypothesis further."[29] The article exemplifies Pearl's priorities when it came to statistical modeling: Pearl and Reed used census records beginning in 1790 to construct a model of US population growth, and concluded that, according to the curve, the population would stop growing once it reached 197 million. (That prediction was proved false when the US population surpassed 197 million in the 1970s.)

Despite his focus on biological research, Pearl did not neglect the mission that Welch and Howell had entrusted to him: training public health workers in statistical skills. Indeed, Pearl set the standard higher than his contemporaries in health administrations. He regarded the ability to compile vital statistics as a basic skill and an insufficient measure of a statistician's competence. Pearl and Greenwood leveled biting criticisms at some well-known statisticians working in public health administration at the time. One striking example is that of Haven Emerson, then representing the American Public Health Association (APHA) in the revision process for the ICD organized by the LNHO. Pearl wrote: "How comes it that Haven Emerson is a member of the International Statistical show? He is no statistician."[30] In a similar vein, Pearl and Greenwood also privately criticized Edgar Sydenstricker, the first statistician at the USPHS and the LNHO, and Otto R. Eichel, of the New York State health department, on the grounds that they were statistically incompetent.[31]

---

[28] George C. Whipple, Review of *The Biology of Death* by Raymond Pearl, *Journal of the American Statistical Association* 18, no. 143 (1923): 926.
[29] Raymond Pearl and Lowell J. Reed, "On the Rate of Growth of the Population of the United States since 1790 and its Mathematical Representation," *Proceedings of the National Academy of Sciences of the United States of America* 6, no. 6 (1920): 287.
[30] Raymond Pearl, "To Major Greenwood," May 2, 1929, I/Greenwood, Major (8) 1929, Raymond Pearl Papers, American Philosophical Society.
[31] For example, Pearl once wrote to Greenwood that "Sydenstricker is a good fellow, ... and he is, at the best, at least second or thrid rate so far as statistics is concerned." (Raymond Pearl, "To Major Greenwood," September 17, 1923, Greenwood, Major (2) 1923/i, Raymond Pearl Papers, American Philosophical Society.)

According to Pearl, students specializing in statistics should acquire knowledge in various domains related to public health work. Citing the way health statisticians were trained in Britain (where he himself had been trained), he devised a curriculum that included biology, statistics, medical geography, the natural history of disease, hygiene, and anthropometry.[32] In his plan for the department, Pearl set forth what he thought it meant to be a good biostatistician, which involved mastering

much more than the customary and traditional official statistics of morbidity and mortality. … [T]he successful leader and practitioner of hygiene and public health in the not distant future must be a man who has been taught to think and reason about every phase of his work quantitatively. The truth that no figure means anything whatever till we know its probably [sic] error must be so ingrained in the mind of every public health worker that it colors every thought or plan that he makes about his work, and lies behind every administrative action he takes.[33]

The quotation captures Pearl's emphasis on integrating mathematical statistics into public health work. Put simply, Pearl considered the theory of errors – a branch of mathematical statistics devoted to forming inferences about a population based on selected samples by estimating the sampling error – to be essential to gauging the real situation. In this sense, Pearl believed statisticians should play a leading role in public health campaigns, as they would design the campaigns in such a way that their effectiveness could be estimated through mathematical statistics. When the Rockefeller Foundation's International Health Board (IHB) asked Pearl to assess its malaria control campaigns in Mississippi, Pearl wrote that, due to the lack of training in quantitative methods, a "vast sums of money are now being virtually wasted in public health work."[34] He further added that because the IHB did not have an overall plan for its malaria control activities, the report based on its fieldwork could not be considered scientific.[35]

Over the following years, Pearl lectured on the general principles of statistics and prepared an outline for laboratory work in which he enumerated the principles of computation and geographical representation.[36] He also offered a workshop entitled "Statistical Clinics" in which

[32] Raymond Pearl, "Plans for the Development of the Department of Biometry and Vital Statistics," 1918, 1, Welch Papers/Papers and Documents of School of Hygiene/Plan for the Development of the Department of Biometry and Vital statistics/100/15, Johns Hopkins Medical Archives.
[33] Ibid.
[34] Ibid.
[35] Ibid.
[36] Raymond Pearl, "Laboratory Outline for Department of Biometry and Vital Statistics," 1920, Welch Papers/Papers and Documents of School of Hygiene/Laboratory Outline for Department of Biometry and Vital Statistics/100/14/1920, Johns Hopkins Medical Archives.

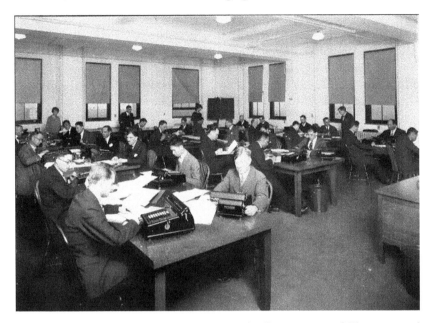

Figure 2.2 Student laboratory at the Department of Biometry and Vital Statistics.
The American Journal of Hygiene, *The School of Hygiene and Public Health of the Johns Hopkins University*, The American Journal of Hygiene Monographic Series 6 (Baltimore, MD: The American Journal of Hygiene, 1926), 23. Courtesy of Rockefeller Archive Center.

he shared his experiences as a biostatistician with students and prepared them for possible difficulties in recording statistics, especially in hospitals and civil administrations.[37] In 1919, Pearl hired Sylvia Louise Parker, who had worked with him at the Maine Agricultural Experiment Station, to take on teaching responsibilities alongside Reed and himself.[38] Reed and Parker led laboratory sessions during which students were taught to use tabulating machines. The biostatistics department provided first-class teaching equipment; in 1926, every student had his or her own adding machine in the laboratory (Figure 2.2).[39] The statistics courses were quite successful. In a report to the Rockefeller Foundation,

[37] Raymond Pearl, "Statistical Clinics," 1922, Welch Papers Corres/ Pearl, R./41/27/Jan 1922–June 1922, Johns Hopkins Medical Archives.
[38] Johns Hopkins School of Hygiene and Public Health, "Catalogue and Announcement of the School of Public Health, 1919–1920," 9, Welch Medical Library, Johns Hopkins University & Medicine.
[39] The American Journal of Hygiene, *The School of Hygiene and Public Health of the Johns Hopkins University*.

John Schapiro called the course of Statistics I "excellent" and "of prime importance for successful health officers."[40]

The department's policy changed in 1925, when Pearl left to establish the Institute of Biological Research, also at Johns Hopkins, with Rockefeller funding. The biological research elements of the department moved with Pearl, as his new institute provided lectures on biology and biological research. At the new institute, Pearl continued to use the curve-fitting method to study population growth and became a key figure in international population-control circles. In his opening speech to the 1927 World Population Conference in Geneva, Switzerland, Pearl presented an experiment he had conducted based on observations of flies in which he had concluded that the flies' rate of reproduction adjusted according to the space and resources available. Pearl then drew a parallel with human reproduction, framing the population growth issue as a question of economy and concluding that it was important to balance population growth with national production.[41]

Reed took over Pearl's professorship in the biostatistics department. Over the following decades, Reed focused on developing statistical methods for epidemiological studies. He changed the department's name to "Statistics Department," dropping "Biometry" and "Vital Statistics." The statistical practices taught in the department also shifted: Pearl's experiments had been aimed at discovering statistical laws through biology, whereas Reed used statistical models to define or explain a phenomenon related to a given population's health conditions. The changes Reed made to the department can be explained in part by his collaboration with Wade Frost, a former USPHS staff member and the director of the JHSPH's epidemiology department since 1919. Welch had originally recruited Frost to teach public health administration and fieldwork methods. Since 1925, Reed and Frost had worked together, using mathematical formulae to explain the life cycle of epidemics and the results of public health fieldwork.

The Great Depression left its mark on Reed and Frost's statistical work, as it substantially decreased the endowment revenue upon which the JHSPH had relied since its founding and forced the school to compete with other public health schools for public funding.[42] The JHSPH also had to meet the government's pressing need for community health workers to work with the ever-growing number of people driven into poverty.

[40] John Schapiro, "Memorandum: School of Hygiene and Public Health, Baltimore," June 14, 1922, RF/1.1/200/186/2231, Rockefeller Archive Center.

[41] Murphy, *The Economization of Life*, 3.

[42] Karen Kruse Thomas, *Health and Humanity: A History of the Johns Hopkins Bloomberg School of Public Health, 1935–1985* (Baltimore, MD: Johns Hopkins University Press, 2016), 15–16.

In 1932, in collaboration with the Baltimore City Health Department, the JHSPH launched the Eastern Health District, a public health system serving 60,000 inhabitants.[43] Reed and Frost's departments were put in charge of conducting census surveys and field investigations in the District, in partnership with the US Census Bureau and the USPHS, to collect birth, death, and morbidity statistics.[44] The statistical practices of the JHSPH were thus closely connected to public health fieldwork of all sorts. For example, Reed and Frost were also associated with the center for syphilis research at Johns Hopkins. This center combined clinical and laboratory work with fieldwork in the Eastern Health District and later became the leading institute in syphilis studies and education.[45]

Classes in the biostatistics department under Reed's directorship continued to cover both the administration and research aspects of statistics. The courses can be loosely divided into five categories: vital statistics registration; mathematics of rates and probability; trends and forecasting raw materials; hospital statistical registration; and epidemiological research.[46] The core curriculum remained identical under Reed, with some minor additions to the elective courses on offer: Statistical Analysis of Small Samples (1938–1940); Genetics (1942–1943, 1946–1947); Dynamics of Population Growth (1944–1946); and Statistical Methods for Laboratory Research (1951–1952).[47]

---

[43] Johns Hopkins School of Hygiene and Public Health, "The Johns Hopkins University School of Hygiene and Public Health Announcements for 1934–1935," 1934, 12, Welch Medical Library, Johns Hopkins University & Medicine.

[44] Ibid.

[45] Parran and Ferrand, "Report to the Rockefeller Foundation on the Education of Public Health Personnel"; Thomas, *Health and Humanity*, 38–9.

[46] Johns Hopkins School of Hygiene and Public Health, "The Johns Hopkins University School of Hygiene and Public Health Announcements for 1934–1935," 28–9, Welch Medical Library, Johns Hopkins University & Medicine.

[47] Johns Hopkins School of Hygiene and Public Health, "The Johns Hopkins University Circular: School of Hygiene and Public Health Catalogue Number 1938–1939," 1938, 32, Welch Medical Library, Johns Hopkins University & Medicine; "The Johns Hopkins University Circular: School of Hygiene and Public Health Catalogue Number 1939–1940," 1939, 33, Welch Medical Library, Johns Hopkins University & Medicine; "The Johns Hopkins University Circular: School of Hygiene and Public Health Catalogue Number 1942–43," 1942, 36, Welch Medical Library, Johns Hopkins University & Medicine; "The Johns Hopkins University Circular: School of Hygiene and Public Health Catalogue Number 1946–1947," 1946, 31, Welch Medical Library, Johns Hopkins University & Medicine; "The Johns Hopkins University Circular: School of Hygiene and Public Health Catalogue Number 1944–1945," 1944, 32, Welch Medical Library, Johns Hopkins University & Medicine; "The Johns Hopkins University Circular: School of Hygiene and Public Health Catalogue Number 1945–1946," 1945, 31, Welch Medical Library, Johns Hopkins University & Medicine; "The Johns Hopkins University: School of Hygiene and Public Health Catalogue Number 1951–1952," 1951, 47, Welch Medical Library, Johns Hopkins University & Medicine.

TOP VIEW

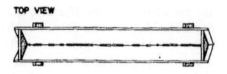

SIDE VIEW

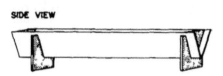

Figure 2.3 Wooden trough representing an isolated community in the Reed–Frost model.
Paul E. M. Fine, "A Commentary on the Mechanical Analogue to the Reed-Frost Epidemic Model," *American Journal of Epidemiology*, 1977, vol. 106, no. 2, 91, by permission of Oxford University Press/ Society for Epidemiologic Research.

The biostatistics department also provided courses co-taught by the epidemiology department. In fact, one of the most important models for explaining the cycle of an epidemic began as one of Reed and Frost's teaching aids. In 1930, the two men designed an analogue mechanical device to serve as "a stochastic simulation of epidemiologic phenomena with non-biological material."[48] The device, later known as the Reed– Frost model, simulates the life cycle of an epidemic within an isolated community. The model (see Figure 2.3) consists of a wooden trough representing an isolated community and balls of different colors representing inhabitants of different immunity status (case, susceptible, immune, and contact neutralizer). By pouring balls randomly into the trough and recording their changes in status (e.g. a susceptible placed next to a case would become a case, whereas a case would become immune no matter what it was placed next to), the model showed students how the number of cases might change over the course of an epidemic.[49] The Reed–Frost model combines the probabilistic tradition of using a container full of different colored balls with epidemiological knowledge about disease transmission and immunity after epidemics. It is also representative of Reed and Frost's statistical practices: instead of conducting biological experiments using mice or flies to construct statistical regularities, as

[48] Paul E. M. Fine, "A Commentary on the Mechanical Analogue to the Reed-Frost Epidemic Model," *American Journal of Epidemiology* 106, no. 2 (1977): 88.
[49] Ibid., 91.

Pearl had done, their work used statistical theory to simulate epidemiological events.

Because the JHSPH's diverse student body included public health officers and researchers from foreign countries, Reed and Frost's teaching aid and their statistical practices became well known in public health schools both in the United States and abroad, despite the fact that the two men never published on their trough-based model.[50] In their 1939 report to the Rockefeller Foundation, public health experts Thomas Parran and Livingston Ferrand praised Reed and Frost's work as "the greatest contribution of Johns Hopkins," because it had made epidemiology the "integrating factor" that united several public health disciplines.[51] As Karen Kruse Thomas has illustrated, the duo's statistical method remained influential during World War II and the postwar years. During the war, the biostatistics department became the JHSPH's major source of financing. Reed, along with Margaret Merrell (who earned her ScD degree from the department in 1930 and was immediately hired as a faculty member), had supervised the research design for penicillin trials and provided statistical expertise to the USPHS and the United States Army Surgeon General during the war.[52] When the war came to an end, the department's influence was visible through its network of alumni, many of whom occupied important positions within the WHO, thus pioneering public health statistical practices across the world.

### Biostatistics Graduates Bring Mathematical Statistics to Public Health Organizations

The JHSPH became an internationally recognized institution not only thanks to the Rockefeller Foundation's generous financial contribution, but also because of the Foundation's policy of sending public health officers to Baltimore for short- and long-term training. From the outset, the school was in charge of organizing four-week courses for health officers in the United States.[53] Officers from American health administrations with different job titles – including "statistician-accountant," and "registrar" – traveled to Johns Hopkins to receive

---

[50] Fine, "A Commentary on the Mechanical Analogue to the Reed-Frost Epidemic Model," 97.
[51] Parran and Ferrand, "Report to the Rockefeller Foundation on the Education of Public Health Personnel," 64.
[52] Thomas, *Health and Humanity*, 44.
[53] Raymond Pearl, "Laboratory Work in Vital Statistics for Intensive Course for Health Officers," 1920, JHUSH O.D. Corres Gaertner-Int 1917-1921/3/a/3/Int./nov. 8-dec. 8 1920, Johns Hopkins Medical Archives.

statistical training.[54] In 1935, the introduction of the Social Security Act set minimum hiring criteria for American public health officers, which led to even more of them being trained at the JHSPH.[55]

From the beginning, the school organized special courses for foreign fellows selected by the Rockefeller Foundation. This mechanism proved to be quite influential. Most statistical fellows would go on to hold important positions in international organizations or research institutes in their home countries. For instance, Spanish statistician Marcelino Pascua went to work for the LNHO after the Spanish health administration failed to offer him a position in 1927. He later worked for the WHO during its early years.[56] Chidambara Chandrasekaran, from India, was recruited by the Population Division within the Social Affairs Section of the United Nations in 1950 directly after his training.[57] The JHSPH also admitted Rockefeller Foundation officers who were pursuing studies in public health, including Fred Soper, an authority on malaria control programs, who led the Pan American Health Organization from 1947 to 1959, and Frederick Russell, the director of the Rockefeller Foundation's International Health Division (formerly the IHB, the name having changed in 1927) during the interwar years.[58] This diverse and impressive student body developed into an international network of public health and statistical experts. Occupying high-level positions in international organizations and national health authorities, these Johns Hopkins alumni formed a chain that linked different health organizations together, enabling them to communicate with one another in a standardized statistical language.

If, to use Theodore Porter's term, quantification is a technology of distance,[59] the making of that distance – abstracting reality into numbers – was never straightforward. The actors who oversaw the fitting of realities into numbers encountered resistance from other experts who had experienced the true situation on the ground. The latter competed with statistical experts for authority when it came to interpreting the numbers, and, as we will see, the statistical experts did not always win. The stories of Persis Putnam and Yves Biraud (also known as Yves-Marie Biraud) are a case in point. These two statisticians, both trained

[54] Parran and Ferrand, "Report to the Rockefeller Foundation on the Education of Public Health Personnel," 9.
[55] Thomas, *Health and Humanity*, 16.
[56] "Fellowship Card: Marcelino Pascua," n.d., RG10.2, Rockefeller Archive Center.
[57] "Fellowship Card: Chidambara Chandrasekaran," n.d., RG10.2, Rockefeller Archive Center.
[58] Fee, *Disease and Discovery*, 79.
[59] Porter, *Trust in Numbers*, ix.

in the JHSPH statistics department in the early 1920s, had to compete with other experts for the authority to interpret data. By the mid-1920s, Putnam was the statistician at the IHB/IHD and Biraud at the LNHO. Their interactions with their non-statistician colleagues are illustrative of the distance separating mathematical statistics from policy-making within the international health organizations in the 1920s.

Putnam joined the IHB in New York following her graduation from the JHSPH biostatistics department with a dissertation entitled "Sexual differences in pulmonary tuberculosis," completed under Reed's direction.[60] She then served as the first and only statistician at the IHB/IHD from 1927 until her retirement in 1948. She was responsible for analyzing reports using statistical methods and invalidated several officers' field reports on malaria control campaigns using Pearson's chi-squared test of significance, a method for gauging possible sampling errors. For example, when reviewing Lewis Hackett's report on a malaria control campaign that involved spraying Paris Green in Italy, Putnam showed that the difference in malaria prevalence rates between the campaign area and other areas was probably due to sampling errors. She further remarked that, owing to the lack of historical records on malaria prevalence rates in the unsprayed areas, the usefulness of the campaign had yet to be demonstrated.[61] She concluded her report by suggesting the establishment of a control group by collecting data from areas in Italy where no malaria program had been implemented. In making this suggestion, Putnam applied mathematical statistical reasoning to an IHB/IHD public health campaign.

As John Farley has chronicled, Putnam's doubts were eventually assuaged as Hackett continued to accumulate data and incorporated control areas into his malaria fieldwork in Sardinia.[62] Hackett and Putnam subsequently co-authored articles on malaria control programs in Italy. However, they continued to face the problem of lack of control data, as inhabitants of the control areas complained, leading the IHD to eventually implement measures in those areas as well.[63]

Putnam's analysis translated fieldwork data into organized scientific language and presented a vision of reality that was independent of the perceptions of officers in the field. This sometimes led to conflict.[64]

[60] "Biofile of Persis Putnam," n.d., Room102/Unit 117/Shelf 4/Box5, Rockefeller Archive Center.
[61] Persis Putnam, "Malaria in Italy: A Statistical Review of Dr. Hackett's Reports," 1927, RG1.1/751/7/81, Rockefeller Archive Center.
[62] Farley, *To Cast Out Disease*, 120.
[63] Ibid., 121–2.
[64] Ibid., 112.

Though Putnam influenced fieldwork methods by encouraging the use of control areas, it remains questionable how much weight her analysis really carried in determining overall disease control measures at the IHB/IHD. Nothing in the archives indicates any changes being made after Putnam invalidated the results of field reports. For example, the IHD carried on with its Paris Green spraying campaign in Italy even after Putnam had pointed out that there was no direct correlation between the drop in the malaria prevalence rate and the spraying.[65] Putnam's work with the IHB/IHD suggests that, although she was given the position of statistician and put in charge of conducting statistical analysis, the power of statistical analysis did not prevail over other considerations.

Yves Biraud, another alumnus of the JHSPH biostatistics department, was a statistical consultant who used mathematical statistics to evaluate a Bacillus Calmette–Guérin (BCG) vaccination experiment in Algeria at the request of the LNHO. As Clifford Rosenberg has documented, Biraud's role was to examine the data collection procedure and carry out a statistical analysis to determine the efficacy of the BCG vaccine.[66] Just as Putnam had observed of Hackett's work, Biraud found that the rule of mathematical statistics invalidated the observations of the experts who had undertaken the campaign. The vaccine's inventor, Camille Guérin, was displeased, as Biraud disqualified the experiment for not being randomly sampled and for lacking a control group. Just as Hackett had done in Italy, Guérin was forced to adjust his fieldwork into a randomized experiment, following which the LNHO's committee of statisticians – led by Biraud – approved the vaccine.[67] The BCG review launched Biraud's career within the international health organizations. He was later enlisted by the LNHO to compile epidemiological information, and he continued to work there until the end of World War II. When the war ended, Biraud was transferred to the WHO as part of the LNHO's epidemiological intelligence service and acted as the main designer of the WHO's statistical work, for which other alumni of the JHSPH biostatistics department were recruited.[68]

While Biraud and his group were at the helm of the WHO's statistical practices, the JHSPH was continuing to train the next generation of public health officers. When the IHD fellowship program dwindled in

---

[65] Ibid., 120–1.
[66] Clifford Rosenberg, "The International Politics of Vaccine Testing in Interwar Algiers," *The American Historical Review* 117, no. 3 (2012): 671–97.
[67] Ibid.
[68] See: "Fellowship Card: Yves Biraud," "Fellowship Card: Marie Cakrtova," "Fellowship Card: Marcelino Pascua," "Fellowship Card: Satya Swaroop," n.d., RG10.2, Rockefeller Archive Center.

1951, the WHO and the US State Department became the major sponsors of fellowships that sent foreign students to study at the JHSPH.[69] This contributed to an increase in the proportion of foreign students at the school, which grew from 20% during the interwar period to 33% after World War II.[70]

The JHSPH biostatistics department transformed Pearson's biometry tradition into applied epidemiological research and lent credence to the use of mathematical statistics for public health research and administration. Most crucially, the department educated a cohort of health statisticians from both inside and outside of the United States, providing a statistical workforce for international health organizations and health authorities across the world. These health statisticians, who had all received the same training, were involved in vital statistics collection, data tabulation, and analysis of fieldwork statistics. Their manner of conducting statistical collection and analysis laid the foundation for statistics to become the lingua franca of public health organizations at different levels throughout the world. Although statistics had gained legitimacy in public health research, the implementation of this shared language was forced to reckon with diverse contexts. The case of interwar China, a major destination of Rockefeller funding, epitomizes how JHSPH-trained experts adapted and innovated statistical practices to fit one such context.

## Advance Science or Save the Country?

In 1922, John B. Grant, having worked for a year at the Rockefeller-funded PUMC as an associate professor of pathology, drew up a plan to establish a public health department at the college. At the time, the Chinese mainland was divided into nine military cliques and lacked a strong central government, let alone a national health system. Only a few sporadic public health initiatives had been implemented, either with the help of foreign powers (usually in treaty ports), military strongmen (such as Yuan Shikai, who established the Beiyang Military Medical Academy in Tianjin in 1902, based on a Japanese model), or missionary associations (such as the Young Women's Christian Association and the Chinese Christian Association, which organized the Joint Council for Public Health Education starting in 1920). Most regulations were nothing more than pieces of paper and had little lasting impact on the local population. Grant, a JHSPH-trained specialist who had worked on hookworm

---

[69] Thomas, *Health and Humanity*, 162–3.
[70] Ibid., 173.

control campaigns in the coal mines of Hunan from 1917 to 1919, called on the Rockefeller IHB to provide funding to establish a public health department at the PUMC.[71]

Grant's design for the department – which emphasized statistics – was undoubtedly inspired by his training at the JHSPH from 1919 to 1920. He had been in Pearl and Reed's biostatistics class, and he kept vivid memories of studying epidemiology with Wade Frost.[72] In Grant's training, biostatistics had been used in conducting biological research, whereas epidemiology had mainly been concerned with developing practical knowledge about epidemic control measures.[73] Generally speaking, Grant valued epidemiology more than biostatistics, since, in his view, epidemiology took community health into account. He complained of being unable to grasp Pearl's lectures and recalled that, as a physician, he had often been shocked by Pearl's doctoral students, who applied the statistical regularity underlying the behavior of flies and mice to human beings.[74]

It is therefore unsurprising that, when devising his public health department at the PUMC, Grant did not seek to implement Pearl's research methods. Instead, he devoted considerable energy to constructing a system for collecting vital and health statistics using methods proposed by Arthur Newsholme, the former principal officer of the United Kingdom Local Government Board and a visiting professor at the JHSPH. It was during his years at the JHSPH that Grant became familiar with Newsholme's statistical methods, which focus mainly on administrative work. In his book *The Elements of Vital Statistics* (1923), Newsholme laid out a comprehensive review of the statistical practices that should be used by health administrations.[75] In contrast to Pearl's mathematical statistics and curve-fitting methods, Newsholme focused on descriptive statistics collected by health administrations, and dedicated only four out of fifty-one chapters to the statistical study of causation.[76]

Grant followed Newsholme's teachings and placed the collection of statistics at the center of his work at the PFHS. Also in line with

[71] Du Lihong, "Zhidu kuosan yu zaidihua: Lan Ansheng zai Beijing de gonggong wei-sheng shiyan, 1921–1925 [Institutional Diffusion and Localization: John B. Grant's Public Health Experiments in Beijing, 1921–1925]," *Zhongyang Yanjiuyuan jindaishi yanjiusuo jikan [Bulletin of the Institute of Modern History Academia Sinica]*, no.86 (2014): 1–47.

[72] Oral History Research Department, Columbia University, "Reminiscences of Dr. John B. Grant (Vol. 1)," 1961, 108, RF/13/1/1, Rockefeller Archive Center.

[73] Ibid.; Fee, *Disease and Discovery*, 133.

[74] Oral History Research Department, Columbia University, "Reminiscences of Dr. John B. Grant (Vol. 1)," 104.

[75] Arthur Newsholme, *The Elements of Vital Statistics in Their Bearing on Social and Public Health Problems* (London: George Allen & Unwin, 1923).

[76] Newsholme, *The Elements of Vital Statistics*, 503–51.

Newsholme's views, Grant did not consider the aim of statistical collection to be the construction of a model for wider application, but rather a means of evaluating the economic feasibility of public health actions.[77] Tellingly, Grant often used business metaphors when describing public health actions. As cited by Du Lihong, a PFHS report noted that public health administration needs statistics to assess its efficiency just as business needs accounting to assess its profit.[78] Grant stressed the importance of public health administration in his designs for both the PUMC public health department and the PFHS. In close collaboration with the department, PFHS would implement public health administration and vital statistics collection in a selected area.

Grant's designs for the PUMC public health department and the PFHS illustrate his vision for how public health research should be conducted in China: by applying scientifically proven theories on Chinese soil. Grant's conception of a Chinese public health school was distinctly different from that of the JHSPH designers. He had no ambition of making universal scientific advances and instead focused on applying existing discoveries to the Chinese context. According to Grant, what was needed in China was not "adding the missing sentences" to explanations of diseases but rather accumulating data to adapt fundamental facts to Chinese fieldwork.[79] He had observed first-hand the absolute lack of epidemiological data regarding disease occurrence in China. To advance scientific research, it was of crucial importance for a medical school to obtain data from local communities.[80] Therefore, Grant's blueprint for the PFHS involved gathering field data in Beijing, based on which the PUMC department of public health could tailor its research and training to Chinese conditions.[81]

Although Grant placed great importance on public health administration, he had good reason to hide this preference from his sponsor, the IHB of the Rockefeller Foundation. The IHB had been increasingly focused on scientific research ever since Frederick Russell had replaced Wickliffe Rose as director in 1923.[82] Also, the Rockefeller Foundation did not place

[77] Oral History Research Department, Columbia University, "Reminiscences of Dr. John B. Grant (Vol. 2)," 1961, 159, RF/13/2/2, Rockefeller Archive Center.

[78] Translated from: Du Lihong, "Zhidu kuosan yu zaidihua," 36.

[79] John B. Grant, "Utilization of a Health Center," December 3, 1923, 3, CMB. Inc/75/528, Rockefeller Archive Center.

[80] John B. Grant, "A Proposal for a Department of Hygiene for Peking Union Medical College," 1923, 42, CMB.Inc/75/531, Rockefeller Archive Center.

[81] Grant, "Utilization of a Health Center," 3; "A Proposal for a Department of Hygiene for Peking Union Medical College," 42.

[82] Farley, To Cast Out Disease, 6.

much importance on public health actions in China, as the Foundation's officers believed that political instability there made it impossible for the government to take over public health work.[83] In order to gain the IHB's financial support, Grant framed the PUMC public health department and the PFHS as serving to advance public health science, and provided few details on the administrative aspect. In his first proposal, submitted in 1923, Grant began by mentioning the need for a department of public health, given the rapid advancement of preventive medicine in recent years.[84] Grant was brief in discussing public health actions but stressed their scientific value. Nonetheless, Grant's first attempt failed. At the time, the IHB was concerned about the rapid growth of the PUMC's budget.[85] Grant repeatedly assured IHB officers that the university's total budget would not exceed $10,000,[86] and in 1924, his second proposal, submitted during a visit to the United States, was finally accepted.[87]

There is, however, a telling discrepancy between Grant's appeals to the IHB and articles published by his Chinese collaborators. Whereas Grant presented scientific research as a key function when discussing his proposals with the IHB, in articles published in Chinese medical and public health journals, his collaborators discussed the department and the PFHS in terms of "saving the country." For example, Jin Baoshan (also known as P. Z. King, Chin Pao-Shan), once an employee of the PFHS and later the director of the National Health Administration (1940–7), underscored the point that calculating birth and death rates could save China and that public health activities could prevent the waste of life, thus helping build a stronger nation.[88] Reflecting the nationalist sentiment of the time, Jin wrote in one of his articles:

There are several ways to save the country, because China has many problems. ... And then there is the problem of public health – the most central of China's weaknesses. ... Civilized countries in Europe and America, thanks to their developed medical sciences and well-equipped public health systems, have a higher average life expectancy. Their populations will serve [society] longer.[89]

[83] Lei, *Neither Donkey nor Horse*, 55–8.
[84] Grant, "A Proposal for a Department of Hygiene for Peking Union Medical College," 2.
[85] Victor Heiser, "Memorandum on Grant's Plan for a Hygiene Program for the P.U.M.C. Submitted by Him October 8th," March 5, 1924, 1, CMB.Inc/75/531, Rockefeller Archive Center.
[86] Oral History Research Department, Columbia University, "Reminiscences of Dr. John B. Grant (Vol. 1)," 128.
[87] Du Lihong, "Zhidu kuosan yu zaidihua," 22–4.
[88] Jin Baoshan, "Beijing zhi gonggong weisheng [Beijing's Public Health]," *Zhonghua yixue zazhi [National Medical Journal of China (Shanghai)]* 12, no.3 (1926): 253–61.
[89] Translated from: Jin Baoshan, "Weisheng yu jiuguo [Public Health and Saving Country]," *Weisheng yuekan [Health Monthly]* 4, no.1 (1934): 2.

According to Jin, lowering the mortality rate through public health administration was key to the country's future. He had indicated in an earlier article that "the only aim of public health administration is to protect the health of the population and reduce the mortality rate."[90] In considering a lower mortality rate as the fundamental aim of public health administration, Jin paved the way for statistical practices becoming essential to Chinese public health administration.[91]

Statistical practices related to birth and death numbers were always presented as being at the center of the new department's responsibilities, no matter the target audience. Specifically, Grant and Jin both stressed the importance of statistics, either for advancing science by gathering data in China or for increasing life expectancy through public health administration. Since its founding in 1925, the PFHS carried out activities that were closely intertwined with the collection and publication of statistics.

### Designing a Dialect: The Chinese List of Causes of Death

The PFHS employed physicians, nurses, sanitary inspectors, and clerks and provided basic medical care to inhabitants living in a specific district (home to 58,605 people) with the aim of decreasing the mortality rate there.[92] The Station's first major undertaking was to establish a birth- and death-reporting system. That system did not arise in a vacuum: as Yang Nianqun has shown, prior to the founding of the PFHS, the management

---

[90] Translated from: Jin Baoshan, "Xiwang yu Beijing weisheng dangju zhe [Plea to the Peking Public Health Authority]," *Zhonghua yixue zazhi [National Medical Journal of China (Shanghai)]* 14, no. 5 (1928): 4.

[91] Grant and his associates were not the only public health experts to adopt different rhetorical strategies for different audiences. Wu Liande, who contributed to controlling the 1910 plague epidemics in northern Manchuria and who served as a Chinese representative to the LNHO, also adopted mixed rhetorical strategies when advocating that foreign powers should transfer maritime quarantine authority to the Republic of China's government. When communicating with foreign powers, Wu presented a Chinese takeover of maritime quarantine authority in terms of the Chinese government's efforts to implement up-to-date public health administration. Vis-à-vis the Chinese public, however, Wu presented the takeover as a matter of Chinese sovereignty. (Yang Xiangyin and Wang Pong, "Minzu zhuyi yu xiandaihua: Wu Liande dui shouhui haigang jianyiquan de hunhe lunshu [Nationalism and Modernization: The Mixed Discourse of Wu Liande Regarding the Takeover of Maritime Quarantine]," *Huaren huaqiao lishi yanjiu [Journal of Overseas Chinese History Studies]*, no. 1 (2014): 51–60.)

[92] John B. Grant, "Second Annual Report, Peking Health Station,1926–1927," 1927, 16, RF/5/3.601J/219/2735, Rockefeller Archive Center; Bullock, *An American Transplant*, 145.

of births and deaths in the district had been the responsibility of traditional midwives and feng shui masters (*yin yang shen*), whom the inhabitants called upon to organize rituals signifying the arrival of a newborn or
the death of a family member.[93] This meant that only midwives and feng
shui masters were kept abreast of the total number of births and deaths.
Despite the legal requirement for every household to report births and
deaths to the municipal police, this was seldom followed.

The establishment of the PFHS, which was subordinated to the
police, changed the situation. With police support, the PFHS obtained
the backing of the local authorities to roll out a new vital statistics collection system in the district selected. By introducing a stricter law, under
which required deaths had to be reported at the police station in order
to obtain permission for burial, and by working to discredit traditional
midwives and feng shui masters, the PFHS gradually integrated itself
into the local social net and eventually became the main organization
handling the inhabitants' birth and death information.[94] Through its
partnership with the municipal police, the PFHS was informed as soon
as a birth or death was reported by inhabitants. The PFHS then sent its
medical staff to carry out a home visit to establish the cause of death or
verify the condition of the newborn.[95]

This statistical collection system depended on an interpersonal network that Grant and his collaborators fostered with the municipal police.
Grant and one of his students at the PUMC, Fang Yiji (Fang I-Chi, I. C.
Fang), used informal channels to obtain political backing for their public
health measures.[96] Grant also offered internships with the title of "political appointee" to candidates recommended by Chinese officials in order
to consolidate his relationship with the local authorities.[97]

The PFHS's statistical work also involved an effort to align Chinese
vital statistics with international standards. Grant and his colleagues
Huang Zifang (Huang Tse-Fang), of the Central Epidemic Prevention

[93] Yang Nianqun, "'Lan Ansheng moshi 'yu minguo chunian Beijing shengsi kongzhi
kongjian de zhuanhuan."
[94] Here I rely mostly on two scholarly accounts: ibid.; Yang Nianqun, "Minguo chunian Beijing de shengsi kongzhi yu kongjian zhuanhuan [Birth and Death Control
and the Transformation of Space at the Beginning Years of the Republic of China],"
in *kongjian jiyi shehui zhuanxing*: "xin shehui shi" yanjiu lunwen jingxuan ji *[Space,
Memory, Transformation of Society]: Compilation of New Social History Papers* (Shanghai:
Shanghai People's Publishing House, 2001).
[95] Jin Baoshan, "Beijing zhi gonggong weisheng."
[96] Fang later became one of the directors of the PFHS and was personally acquainted
with the chief of the municipal police. Oral History Research Department, Columbia
University, "Reminiscences of Dr. John B. Grant (Vol. 2)," 191.
[97] Ibid., 205.

Bureau, and Xu Shijin (Hsu Shih-Chin), of the PUMC, worked to adapt the ICD into the Chinese language. Their efforts went beyond translation, as they also endeavored to cross-reference Chinese lay terms with the ICD's medical vocabulary. The trio estimated that it would take two generations to fully implement the ICD, which comprised over 200 rubrics.[98] They therefore focused on creating a list of causes of death for use in China that had only twenty rubrics; this made it longer than the Indian list (eight rubrics) and shorter than that used in Japan (sixty-one rubrics).[99]

Previously, causes of death had been reported using either a vague descriptor such as "stomach ache," "skin trouble," or "eye trouble," or with etiological terms drawn from Chinese medicine such as "witchy wind," "seasonal wind," or "lung weakness": neither type was very useful to foreigners seeking to understand the health situation in China.[100] To decrypt commonly used lay terms and make them fit the ICD rubrics, the PFHS carried out a year-long field survey. Over the course of 1925, PFHS physicians registered every reported death using both ICD terms and the terms used by the deceased's relatives to describe the cause of death.[101] A total of 104 lay terms were recorded for the 116 deaths that occurred that year, with some terms recurring more than once. Based on these results, Grant, Huang, and Xu drew up a list of twenty-five rubrics (hereafter, "the Chinese list").[102] They further double-checked the reliability of the Chinese list by keeping notes on which terms inhabitants used to describe their relatives' causes of death and by asking physicians to check those terms against the ICD using the Chinese list. It turned out that 90% of causes of death were correctly reported using the Chinese list.[103]

The reporting system put in place by the PFHS faced resistance from local inhabitants despite the legal requirements.[104] At first, police officers were responsible for reporting the causes of death provided by feng shui masters or relatives of the deceased, following a check by a PFHS

---

[98] John B. Grant, T. F. Huang, and S. C. Hsu, "A Preliminary Note on Classification of Causes of Death in China," *National Medical Journal of China (Shanghai)* 13, no. 1 (1927): 2.

[99] Ibid., 2.

[100] Ibid., 5–6.

[101] Oral History Research Department, Columbia University, "Reminiscences of Dr. John B. Grant (Vol. 1)," 67.

[102] Oral History Research Department, Columbia University, "Reminiscences of Dr. John B. Grant (Vol. 2)," 199; Grant, Huang, and Hsu, "A Preliminary Note on Classification of Causes of Death in China," 16–19.

[103] Grant, Huang, and Hsu, "A Preliminary Note on Classification of Causes of Death in China," 2–3.

[104] Yang Nianqun, "'Lan Ansheng moshi 'yu minguo chunian Beijing shengsi kongzhi kongjian de zhuanhuan," 106–9.

physician.[105] It took less than a year for the PFHS staff to realize that most people did not report births and deaths to the police. The PFHS was forced to opt for a more direct approach: its staff carried out home visits in every household in the district and communicated with coffin dealers to collect death numbers. From 1927 onwards, sanitary inspectors were also put in charge of reporting births and deaths to the PFHS,[106] thus reducing the role played by the police. Statistical practices became more and more standard and health inspectors/statisticians gained broader responsibilities within the PFHS. In 1931, six years after the PFHS was founded, its staff concluded – by comparing their numbers with those of feng shui masters and coffin dealers – that "the reporting of adult deaths was not far from complete."[107]

## Overarching Quantification at the PFHS

Despite local resistance to statistical collection, quantification work quickly expanded within the administration of the PFHS. This trend can be observed in the Station's annual reports: the first included only mortality rates, the socioeconomic situation of the dead, and the types of medical services they had received; the fifth annual report, however, quantified every aspect of the PFHS's work in numerous tables setting forth the quantity of every public health service provided.[108] For example, in the fourth annual report, published in 1929, visits by public health nurses were categorized in detail with pie charts (see Figure 2.4) that broke down visits by the type of service provided.[109]

The PFHS's annual reports were published in both Chinese and English, and were not only sent to the Rockefeller Foundation headquarters in New York but also made available to Chinese public health officials. As Theodore Porter has rightfully observed, when community ties are weak, numbers can inspire trust through their mechanical objectivity, i.e. when it can be shown that numbers have been collected according to certain rules.[110] In the case of the PFHS, the community

---

[105] Grant, "Second Annual Report, Peking Health Station, 1926–1927," 13.
[106] I. C. Fang, "Annual Report on Vital Statistics and Communicable Diseases Control for the Year 1928–1929," 1929, 4, CMB.Inc/67/470, Rockefeller Archive Center.
[107] Li Tingan, "The Sixth Annual Report of the Peking First Health Station, 1930–1931 – Annual Report of Vital Statistics and Communicable Diseases Control," 1931, 17, CMB.Inc/67/472, Rockefeller Archive Center.
[108] Peking First Health Station, "The Fifth Annual Report of the Peking First Health Station, 1929–1930," 1930, CMB.Inc/67/471, Rockefeller Archive Center.
[109] Peking First Health Station, "The Fourth Annual Report of the Peking First Health Station, 1928–1929," 1929, 89, CMB.Inc/67/470, Rockefeller Archive Center.
[110] Porter, *Trust in Numbers*. See page 4 for Porter's discussion of mechanical objectivity.

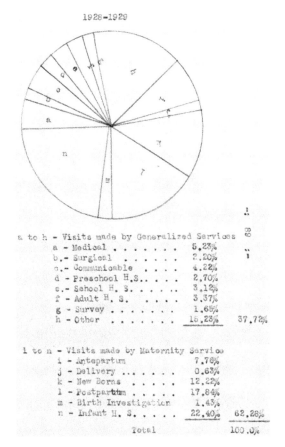

Figure 2.4 Pie chart of visits by Peking First Health Station public health nurses (1928–1929).
Peking First Health Station, "The Fourth Annual Report of the Peking First Health Station, 1928–1929," 1929, 89, CMB.Inc/67/470, Rockefeller Archive Center, 89. Courtesy of Rockefeller Archive Center.

in question was the Rockefeller Foundation, the municipal police in Beijing, and the PUMC staffers. This was indeed a group of actors who did not have much in common in terms of methods and training. The authors of the PFHS reports therefore had to rely on numbers to inspire trust in their readers, some as far off as New York, some 11,000 kilometers away.

The report writers tailored the way they presented numbers to their intended audience. For instance, in the English version of the fifth annual report, Grant used the appraisal form promoted by the APHA

| | 1929-1930 | 1928-1929 | 1927-1928 |
|---|---|---|---|
| Administration (100)ˣ | 95 | 46 | 78 |
| Statistics (40) | 32 | 29 | 33 |
| Laboratory (25) | 22.3 | 20 | 20 |
| Communicable Disease Control (135) | 21.6 | 20 | 0 |
| Sanitation (230) | | | |
| Water (70) | 20.3 | 16 | 20 |
| Sewage (60) | 10 | 5 | 6 |
| Foods & Beverages (40) | 0 | 0 | 0 |
| Sanitary Inspection (40) | 36 | 40 | 10 |
| Refuse (20) | 9.3 | 17 | 15 |
| Control of Medical Practice (60) | 22.8 | 12 | 0 |
| Health Education (10) | 7.3 | 5 | 5 |
| Medical Relief (170) | ˣˣ 163 | ˣˣ170 | 110 |
| Practice of Medicine (130) | 108 | 115 | 38 |
| Personal Hygiene (55) | 26.6 | 30 | 30 |
| Preventive Medicine (40) | 18.8 | 17 | 23 |
| Recreation (5) | 3.8 | 0 | 3 |
| Special Activities | 61.8 | 17 | 15 |
| | 658/1000 | 559/1000 | 403/1000 |

x - Figures in brackets are standard values in the City Public Health Appraisal form by John B. Grant and P. Z. King.

xx - This increase is solely due to redistricting of the city Wards whereby the Peiping Union Medical College Hospital was included in the Demonstration District.

Figure 2.5 Health appraisal of the Peking First Health Station (1927–1930).
Peiping Health Demonstration Station, "The Fifth Annual Report of the Peiping Health Demonstration Station for the Year Ending June 30, 1930," 7. Courtesy of Rockefeller Archive Center.

to summarize the PFHS's activities (see Figure 2.5). Specifically, the APHA form attributed 1,000 points to all functions considered necessary for a public health service (such as home visits and school health education).[111] In the United States, experts were asked to evaluate the public health administration in each community by giving scores to

[111] For the history of APHA appraisal forms and their transfer to Europe, see, e.g.: Lion Murard, "Atlantic Crossings in the Measurement of Health: From US Appraisal Forms to the League of Nations' Health Indices," in *Medicine, the Market and the Mass Media: Producing Health in the Twentieth Century*, edited by Virginia Berridge and Kelly Loughlin (London: Routledge, 2004), 19–54; Lion Murard, "La santé publique et ses instruments de mesure: des barèmes évaluatifs américains aux indices numériques," in *Body Counts: Medical Quantification In Historical And Sociological Perspectives/La Quantification Médicale, Perspectives Historiques et Sociologiques*, eds. Gerard Jorland, Annick Opinel, and George Weisz (Montreal: McGill-Queen's University Press, 2005), 266–93.

every item on the form. The APHA also organized competitions, in which communities were invited to compete for the best score, with funding awarded to the winning community. Just as the PFHS had worked to adapt the ICD, Grant and Jin adapted the APHA appraisal form for "large Chinese cities."[112] The form became a central piece of reporting, as Grant opened the fifth annual report by stating that the PFHS had made major progress, citing an improvement in the appraisal score (see Figure 2.5).[113] By using an adapted APHA appraisal form, Grant and Jin were clearly addressing an English-speaking readership acquainted with American public health work. However, the way the form was presented raised more questions than it resolved, as there was no mention of the scoring criteria, except for a simple note that the scores had been decided by three clerkship students from the PUMC.[114] Tellingly, Grant and Jin did not include the form in the Chinese version of the report.[115]

Grant's management style was another factor behind the overarching quantification employed at the PFHS. As Du Lihong has documented, Grant ran the PFHS like a business: facilities and human resources were allocated with the aim of achieving optimal health returns.[116] Another telling example of Grant's strategy was his decision not to focus on tuberculosis control. He argued that tuberculosis was closely related to overall economic conditions, whereas gastrointestinal diseases responded more "readily to the influence of public health measures."[117] Seeking to maximize the PFHS's impact as quickly as possible, Grant left tuberculosis on the sidelines of the Station's agenda.

Though quantitative rationale was quickly taken up in the PFHS's annual reports, such numbers-based arguments were generally simple and brief, as in the appraisal form described above. Because no extended social surveys had actually been conducted, the report writers could only speculate as to the reasons behind changes in mortality rates. All of the Station's statistics were purely descriptive, with no way to tell if changes were mathematically significant (the standard set by Grant's teachers at

---

[112] John B. Grant, "Third Annual Report of the Peking Health Demonstration Station, for the Year Ending June 30, 1928," 1928, 3, RF/5/3.601J/219/2736, Rockefeller Archive Center.

[113] Peiping Health Demonstration Station, "The Fifth Annual Report of the Peiping Health Demonstration Station for the Year Ending June 30, 1930," 1.

[114] Peiping Health Demonstration Station, 7.

[115] Peking First Health Station, "Beiping shi gonganju diyi weisheng qu shiwusuo diwunian nianbao [The Fifth Annual Report of the Metropolitan Police Department's First Health Station]," 1930.

[116] Du Lihong, "Zhidu kuosan yu zaidihua," 36.

[117] Lei, "Habituating Individuality," 253.

Johns Hopkins).[118] Despite the intentions behind Grant's design, statistical practices slowly became disassociated from policy at the PFHS. As Li Tingan (Lee Ting-An) – another graduate of the PUMC public health department who later earned his medical degree at Harvard – showed in the 1932 PFHS annual report, statistical practices were a routine task with no strategic implications. Inspectors were aware of missing reporting of births and deaths and more initiatives were needed to improve the situation.[119]

### Mathematical Statistics and the PUMC Statistical Laboratory

Grant was aware of the limitations of his statistical knowledge. He therefore convinced the China Medical Board, the Rockefeller agency that sponsored the PUMC, to fund a fellowship for one of his staff to learn statistical techniques in the United States. Grant had another reason for wanting to improve statistical practices: unlike at the JHSPH, there was no consensus at the PUMC as to the need for a public health department, and Grant had to defend the department's existence. The PUMC placed great emphasis on medical science, and Grant decided that statistical skills would be the public health department's *raison d'être*. He proposed that the department should have a statistician who oversaw statistical analysis for all research conducted at the PUMC.[120] Grant believed that the possibility of conducting statistical research would attract students to choose public health as their specialization.[121]

In 1927, Grant wrote to Gist Gee, the Rockefeller Foundation's adviser in China,[122] to request that a fellowship in biostatistics be established. In his letter, Grant stressed the growing demand for statistical analysis, both from PUMC medical researchers and from the Chinese public health administration. Citing the partnership between the JHSPH

[118] Sun Yun Chen, "Sixth Annual Report of the Peiping Health Demonstration Station, for the Year Ending June 30, 1931 – Annual Report of Vital Statistics and Communicable Diseases," 6; I. C. Yuan, "The Seventh Annual Report of the Department of Hygiene and Public Health in Cooperation with the Peiping Health Demonstration Station for the Year Ending June 30, 1932 – Annual Report of Vital Statistics and Communicable Disease Control," 1930, 3, CMB.Inc/67/471, Rockefeller Archive Center.
[119] Li Tingan, "A Critical Study of the Work of the Health Station First Health Area, Department of Public Health, Peiping for the Years 1925–1931 with Suggestions for Improvement," January 1932, 37–9, Peking Union Medical College Archives.
[120] John B. Grant, "Subject: Statistician," December 6, 1927, 1, CMB.Inc/77/541, Rockefeller Archive Center.
[121] Ibid., 1.
[122] On Gee's work in China, see: William Joseph Haas, *China Voyager: Gist Gee's Life in Science* (Armonk, NY: M.E. Sharpe, 1996).

biostatistics department and the Johns Hopkins University hospital, Grant claimed that "much of medical knowledge is the result of accumulation of day-by-day data subjected to careful analysis": having a statistician in the public health department, Grant argued, would likewise be essential for interpreting the medical records accumulating at the PUMC hospital. Like his teachers Pearl and Reed, Grant asserted that a true statistician should not merely collect statistics – which could be done by a clerk – but should also be able to interpret the numbers.[123] Grant hoped that the future Rockefeller fellow, having acquired statistical knowledge under Pearl and Reed at the JHSPH, would become an authority on medical statistics and develop statistical practices for both research and administration.[124]

The Rockefeller Foundation accepted Grant's quest for a fellowship as well as his choice of candidate: Yuan Yijin (I. C. Yuan), a PUMC graduate employed at the PFHS. Grant mentioned that Yuan had "a mathematical trend in a somewhat judicial and philosophical mind, a liking for the abstract combined at the same time with a practical outlook," which would make him a good public health statistician.[125] In 1929, Yuan was awarded a two-year fellowship to study statistics at the JHSPH.

Yuan's training in the United States was no different from that of his contemporaries. His curriculum was co-designed by Grant and Reed and comprised two parts: coursework in biostatistics research, and an internship in public health administration. He spent most of his stay working with Reed in the statistical laboratory of the JHSPH. Following Reed's lead, Yuan familiarized himself with mathematical theories, such as calculus and the law of probability, and learned how to operate IBM counting and sorting machines. For his administrative training, Yuan spent a summer interning in Albany, New York, where he gained knowledge about the routine work of collecting vital statistics and the importance of enforcing legislation on birth and death registration.[126] Yuan obtained a Certificate of Public Health after one year and a Diploma of Public Health at the end of the second year of the fellowship.[127]

Reed had designed a third-year curriculum to train Yuan's capacity for "tak[ing] an applied problem and translat[ing] it into its mathematical

[123] Grant, "Subject: Statistician," 2.
[124] Ibid., 2.
[125] Ibid., 2.
[126] I. C. Yuan, "To Miss Eggleston," November 17, 1929, CMB.Inc/77/541, Rockefeller Archive Center.
[127] W.S.C., "Interviews," February 26, 1929, CMB.Inc/77/541, Rockefeller Archive Center.

statement," an ability needed for pursuing a PhD.[128] Reed explained that once Yuan was fully trained, he could finish his dissertation by focusing on a specifically Chinese problem upon returning home.[129] Yuan was equally ambitious in terms of advancing his mathematical knowledge. He wrote to Grant insisting that he was not satisfied with being the mathematical consultant that Grant had first envisioned; instead, he wished to become a researcher specializing in human biology and the mass phenomena of diseases.[130]

Despite Reed and Yuan's pleas, however, Grant and Roger Greene, the acting director of the PUMC, refused to extend the fellowship for a third year, stating that China was in urgent need of a public health statistician.[131] The IHD's director, Frederick Russell, sided with Grant and Greene. This rejection reflects the kind of science accorded priority by Rockefeller officers in China. When consulted by Grant, Russell agreed that Yuan should return to China and be oriented toward specifically Chinese problems.[132] Unlike Reed, who was focused on epidemiological theory, Grant and Greene preferred applied science: the kind of science in which research results could be directly applied to Chinese policymaking in order to improve health conditions in the country. As Grant had explained in his memorandum when seeking to establish a department of public health, it was not about "adding the missing sentences" to proven facts but testing proven facts to determine public health strategies that were adapted to China.[133]

Yuan's return home in 1931 marked the beginning of a new era of health statistical practices in China. He established the first statistical laboratory with an IBM computing system, with funding from the China Medical Board. Yuan prepared a memo to Grant setting forth the extensive scope of a statistician's work, from introducing statistical methods to medical research, to organizing hospital records, to teaching clerks and staff about the chi-squared test, probability, and correlation.[134] Yuan's

---

[128] Lowell J. Reed, "To Grant," January 29, 1930, CMB.Inc/77/542, Rockefeller Archive Center.

[129] Lowell J. Reed, "To Miss Eggleston," January 28, 1930, CMB.Inc/77/542, Rockefeller Archive Center.

[130] I. C. Yuan, "To Grant," July 1, 1930, CMB.Inc/77/542, Rockefeller Archive Center.

[131] John B. Grant, "To Reed," July 3, 1930, CMB.Inc/77/542; "To Heiser," June 27, 1930, CMB.Inc/77/542, Rockefeller Archive Center.

[132] Grant. "To Heiser," June 27, 1930.

[133] Grant, "Utilization of a Health Center," 3.

[134] I. C. Yuan, "To Grant: Memorandum of the Scope of Work of a Medical Statistician," March 18, 1930, 3, CMB.Inc/77/542, Rockefeller Archive Center. On the IBM purchase: Rollin C. Dean, "To Greene: Tabulating Equipment," April 22, 1931, CMB. Inc/77/542, Rockefeller Archive Center.

view of the statistician's role was very much in line with Reed's. Accordingly, Yuan was involved in teaching, research, and public health administration at the PFHS.

Yuan's contribution to research was also similar to Reed's. He collaborated with other departments at the PUMC, such as physiology and biochemistry, to conduct statistical analysis on the numbers collected during their experiments. One of Yuan's most famous publications was his statistical analysis – conducted for Robert Lim of the physiology department – of research on acidity variation in the gastric juice of pouch dogs. Yuan also planned to perform statistical analysis on mouse colony research conducted by the biochemistry department. Coincidentally – or perhaps ironically – just as with Pearl's project at the JHSPH, the study in question was cut short by a fire that killed a quarter of the mice in the colony.[135]

In terms of administration, Yuan served first as a consultant then as a core staff member at the PFHS, where he made efforts to implement mathematical statistics. Yuan was disappointed that the vital statistics collected at the Station were merely descriptive and did not pass statistical tests based on the laws of probability. Arguing that investigations should be more "mathematical" as medical science advanced,[136] Yuan unified various statistical surveys and hired four extra statistical investigators,[137] two of whom were responsible for compiling statistical tables.[138] Yuan's responsibility also extended to administrating the entire Station's statistical work: he was responsible for reviewing the statistics in annual reports and deciding upon scores on the APHA appraisal form with Grant.[139]

Yuan's teaching responsibilities were overarching. He organized statistical training for medical students at the PUMC and statistical investigators at the PFHS. He also taught mathematical statistics to students specializing in sociology at Yenching University,[140] which not only was at

---

[135] I. C. Yuan, "The Eighth Annual Report of the Peking First Health Station, 1932–1933 – Annual Report of Medical Statistics," 1933, 15, RF/5/3.601J/220/2741, Rockefeller Archive Center.

[136] Ibid., 1.

[137] The names and the educational level of these statistical investigators remain unknown. However, they were personally trained by Yuan at the PFHS before undertaking their duties.

[138] I. C. Fang, "The Eighth Annual Report of the Peking First Health Station, 1932–1933 – Annual Report of Vital Statistics and Communicable Diseases Control," 1933, 25, RF/5/3.601J/220/2741, Rockefeller Archive Center.

[139] Li Tingan, "The Sixth Annual Report of the Peking First Health Station, 1930–1931 – Annual Report of Vital Statistics and Communicable Diseases Control," 6.

[140] Peking First Health Station, "The Ninth Annual Report of the Peking First Health Station, 1933–1934," 1934, 22–3, CMB.Inc/67/473, Rockefeller Archive Center.

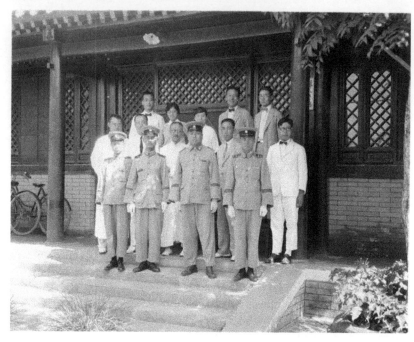

Figure 2.6 The first cohort of Peking First Health Station sanitary inspectors, photographed in front of the Peking Union Medical College. Peking First Health Station, "The Third Annual Report of the Peking First Health Station, 1927–1928," 1928, 26–7, RF/5/3.601J/219/2736, Rockefeller Archive Center. Courtesy of Rockefeller Archive Center.

the center of the Chinese Social Survey Movement in the 1920s but also collaborated with the Rockefeller Foundation's China Program in the 1930s with the aim of rebuilding Chinese society through agriculture, economic measures, public health, and social work.[141]

Yuan's statistical practices at the PFHS came up against similar hurdles to those faced by his predecessors. Local inhabitants were reluctant to collaborate with sanitary investigators from the PFHS, who often presented themselves as authorities in the streets of Beijing, wearing uniforms very similar to those worn by the military (see Figure 2.6).

---

[141] For more on the Chinese Social Survey Movement, see, e.g.: Lam, *A Passion for Facts*. For historiographies regarding the Rockefeller Foundation's China Program, see, e.g.: Frank Ninkovich, "The Rockefeller Foundation, China, and Cultural Change," *The Journal of American History* 70, no. 4 (1984): 799–820; Socrates Litsios, "Selskar Gunn and China: The Rockefeller Foundation's 'Other' Approach to Public Health," *Bulletin of the History of Medicine* 79, no. 2 (2005): 295–318.

Locals remained skeptical. This conflict between the investigators and the local population came to a head when a street fight broke out in 1934:[142] two newspaper vendors were yelling in the street when a statistical investigator named Yin intervened. Yin wanted to remove one of the two vendors from the street, but the latter did not obey, which turned into a fight involving Yin. The episode made it clear that Yin, though merely a statistical investigator, considered himself as something like a policeman. The street vendors certainly did not recognize his authority to intervene. The episode is emblematic of the disconnect between statistical workers and the populations they were investigating. Humorous popular sayings were also circulating in Beijing that recounted locals' reactions to the inspectors. Nearly all started with inspectors asking routine questions, such as if someone was ill in the family. Such questions were considered inappropriate, disturbing locals and leading them to poke fun at the inspectors or even threaten them, causing them to flee the premises.[143]

Although Yuan's service at the PFHS ended with the Japanese invasion in 1937, he continued to work as a statistical specialist for the rest of his career: he was the head of the epidemiology division of the Central Field Health Station during the war, then worked as a researcher at Academia Sinica, eventually going on to become the WHO's statistical expert on tuberculosis.[144] His career path is illustrative of the increasingly central role of statistics in public health research and administration in China.

*

When one juxtaposes the work of the JHSPH and that of the PUMC, a complete picture of the circuit through which statistical practices in research were transferred between the United States and China emerges. This circuit had a number of significant features. First, there

---

[142] Beijing Bureau of Health, "Beiping shi weishengju guanyu Bai Liude Wang Wei erming ouda benju tongji yuan Yin Zhijie qing yifa chengjie [Peiping Bureau of Health's Appeal Concerning Disciplining Bai Liude and Wang Wei for Their Assault on its Statistician Yin Zhijie]," December 27, 1934, J181-021-29355, Beijing Municipal Archives.

[143] Yu Xinzhong, "Fuza xing yu xiandaixing: wan Qing jianyi jizhi yinjianzhong de shehui fanying [Complexity and Modernity: Social Reactions Toward the Establishment of Quarantine Measures in the Late Qing Dynasty]," *Jindaishi Yanjiu [Modern Chinese History Studies]* 188, no. 2 (2012): 56–7.

[144] Over the course of his career, Yuan worked in: Czechoslovakia, Poland, Syria, Israel, Malta, Tunisia, Ecuador, Austria, Morocco (and Tangier, an autonomous city at the time), Greece, and Yugoslavia (WHO, "Bureau de Recherches sur la Tuberculose (Copenhague)," November 10, 1952, 36, EB11/12, WHO Library).

were clear differences of opinion regarding the definition of public health science. The JHSPH biostatistics department prioritized using mathematical statistics for biological research (1917–1925) and later epidemiological research. At the PUMC, however, statistical practices were used to collect quantified data in China and then apply and adapt proven scientific facts to the Chinese context. Public health science at the PUMC was pursued purely in the interest of improving the health of the Chinese population. Grant thus launched statistical collection at the PFHS – a public health administration station – instead of establishing a mouse colony or using census data, as Pearl and Reed had done. The PFHS rolled out a vital statistics reporting system within its jurisdiction, and its experts worked to adapt established standards, such as the ICD and the APHA appraisal form, to the Chinese context.

The second important feature of the circuit of transferal was the time interval involved. The transfer took place in two stages, led first by Grant and then by Yuan. The two men studied at the same institution but almost ten years apart, and so had distinctly different visions of biostatistics. Grant rejected Pearl's focus on biological research and instead adhered to Newsholme's statistical practices; his major focus was on setting up a statistical reporting system. In contrast, when Yuan arrived at the JHSPH, Pearl had left the biostatistical department, and Yuan was trained by Reed in his statistical laboratory. Yuan spent two years studying mathematical statistics and their applications to medical and public health research. When Yuan returned to China, his practices came to be implemented at the PFHS. As the following chapter will show, however, Grant's statistical practices had already spread to other provinces – his students had begun to occupy important positions in public health administrations throughout China.

This brings us to the third feature: both schools spread their statistical practices via their alumni. At the JHSPH, Reed's influence survived World War II and was taken up at the WHO, whereas Grant's views on statistics were spread by his students at the PUMC. The students of both schools, having learned to speak the language of statistics, later became public health officials in various public health administrations. As previously discussed, statistical experts in New York, Geneva, and Beijing either competed with other experts for interpretative authority or faced resistance from those being surveyed. Nevertheless, numbers were gaining ground in fieldwork and reporting. As the case of the PFHS shows, collecting and reporting numbers had become routine for field researchers, despite the difficulties they encountered on the ground.

The differences in how statistics were used at the two schools reflect how – despite being a sort of lingua franca used by actors with similar training – statistics were nonetheless used differently depending on experts' conception of scientific research. In the end, the two schools' plans to use statistics to orient public health programs were only partially implemented. In the following chapters, I will describe other circuits through which statistical practices were implemented with different sponsors, as well as the ways in which graduates of the JHSPH and the PUMC deviated from what they had been taught.

# 3 The Language of Health Administrations
## The League of Nations Epidemiological Intelligence Service

The end of World War I offered a new opportunity for the Rockefeller Foundation to bring public health statistics onto the international political stage. The signing of the Treaty of Versailles (1919) and the establishment of the League of Nations (1920) marked the start of a new era of internationalism based on a nation-state system that provided an institutional framework for international collaboration.[1] The countries that emerged victorious from the war responded favorably to calls from various socioeconomic sectors to initiate international collaboration to resolve the problems created by industrialization. In so doing, they hoped to contain the Bolshevik Revolution by offering an alternative to Marxist internationalism.[2] The League of Nations, founded as part of this wave, was conceived as a platform for member countries to coordinate with one another, and public health matters were among the topics for coordination. Specifically, the League's first public health mission was in response to the Polish government's request for assistance in combating the typhus epidemic raging through Eastern Europe and Russia after the war. That mission contributed to the decision, in 1922, to create a permanent health organization within the League of Nations – what would become the League of Nations Health Organization (LNHO).[3]

The Rockefeller Foundation was also active in Europe immediately after World War I, carrying out health philanthropy in several European countries.[4] The LNHO's intergovernmental nature provided the Foundation with the legitimacy it needed to collect and communicate

---

[1] For discussions on nationalism and internationalism, see, e.g.: Benedict Anderson, *Imagined Communities: Reflections on the Origin and Spread of Nationalism* (London: Verso, 2006); Isabella Löhr and Roland Wenzlhuemer, eds., *The Nation State and Beyond: Governing Globalization Processes in the Nineteenth and Early Twentieth Centuries* (Heidelberg: Springer, 2013); Sluga, *Internationalism in the Age of Nationalism*.

[2] Sluga, *Internationalism in the Age of Nationalism*, 45, 50.

[3] The Provisional Health Committee met for the first time in August 1921. The decision to create a permanent organization was formalized in 1922.

[4] Ludovic Tournès, *Les États-Unis et la Société des Nations (1914–1946): le système international face à l'émergence d'une superpuissance* (Bern: Peter Lang, 2016), 154–5.

vital and health statistics in different countries: statistics could be used to grasp the latest epidemiological developments, although most governments considered such information too sensitive to share with other governments. The Foundation, in parallel to its investments in the Johns Hopkins School of Public Health (JHSPH) and the Peking Union Medical College (PUMC) – neither of which provided the opportunity to collect international statistics – earmarked funding for an epidemiological intelligence and public health statistics service (hereafter, "epidemiological intelligence service") within the LNHO.

This chapter will focus on the LNHO and its epidemiological intelligence service, which represented a crucial circuit through which epidemiological reporting practices were transferred from the LNHO's headquarters in Geneva to other parts of the world, which then reported back to Geneva. This service has already attracted some scholarly attention. Historians have written about the LNHO's institution-building, the service's technological infrastructure, and the influence of geopolitics on the service.[5] This chapter complements such work by examining the LNHO's efforts to standardize statistical practices. Officially inaugurated in 1923, the LNHO's epidemiological intelligence service was responsible for promulgating standardized procedures for statistical collection and advocating that member countries integrate statistical collection into their health authorities. The LNHO's first director-general, Ludwik Rajchman, had a clear aim in doing so: instead of focusing on advancing science or forging diplomatic regulations like the service's predecessors (i.e. the International Statistical Institute [ISI] and Office international d'hygiène publique [OIHP]),[6] the LNHO was to concentrate on convincing national health administrations to integrate standardized statistical practices into their operations. The endeavor quickly made an impact. As early as 1926, the epidemiological intelligence service was covering five continents, with 116 countries providing epidemiological information on plague, cholera, yellow fever, typhus, smallpox and more, as well

[5] See, e.g.: Lenore Manderson, "Wireless War in the Eastern Arena: Epidemiological Surveillance, Disease Prevention and the Work of the Eastern Bureau of the League of Nations Health Organisation," in *International Health Organisations and Movements, 1918–1939*, ed. Paul Weindling (Cambridge: Cambridge University Press, 1995), 109–33; Borowy, *Coming to Terms with World Health*, sec. II; Heidi J. S. Tworek, "Communicable Disease: Information, Health, and Globalization in the Interwar Period," *The American Historical Review* 124, no. 3 (2019): 813–42.
[6] On the ISI and OIHP's endeavors in this regard, see, e.g.: Brian, "Statistique administrative et internationalisme statistique pendant la seconde moitié du XIXe siècle"; Huber, "The Unification of the Globe by Disease? The International Sanitary Conferences on Cholera, 1851–1894."

as statistics on birth rates and general and infant mortality in 696 cities.[7] The service was also the longest-living function within the LNHO, surviving World War II to set the example for the WHO's statistical work.

The LNHO's epidemiological reporting system provides insights into the relationship between statistics and authorities at the international level. Reflecting Theodore Porter's argument that quantification is often the resort of authorities vulnerable to outsiders,[8] in this chapter I show how the LNHO's founding members used statistics to establish the organization's authority when it came to international health collaboration. LNHO staff set statistical reporting standards on a purely administrative level, without attempting to enforce compliance or claiming to be scientific.[9] Their goal was to teach national health administrations to speak the language of statistics.

The epidemiological intelligence service eventually brought together various regional authorities within a single platform for sharing epidemic statistics. The system was not established all at once but was a patchwork that grew out of negotiations with myriad stakeholders all over the world. As this chapter will detail, the service had to negotiate both with other organizations and government authorities. In Asia, where most polities were under European colonial rule, the LNHO positioned itself as an alternative to the European-led OIHP. In doing so, the LNHO sought to collaborate with countries such as China that were suspicious of imperial influence. The making of a statistical reporting system added another layer to the LNHO's aim to construct an inter-colonial medical system, as convincingly illustrated by Tomoko Akami.[10] While Akami describes how the LNHO integrated and utilized an existing inter-colonial network, the Far Eastern Association of Tropical Medicine, this chapter, with a focus on the LNHO's statistical reporting system, will demonstrate that the LNHO also sought to bring solutions directly to the local authorities, transcending the colonial system in the region.

---

[7] International Health Board, "Minutes of the International Health Board: Working Program for 1927," April 11, 1926, 26386, RF/1.1/100/20/164, Rockefeller Archive Center.

[8] Porter, *Trust in Numbers*, 8.

[9] The LNHO did use statistics for scientific activities outside its reporting system. The case of Yves Biraud and the approval of the Bacillus Calmette–Guérin (BCG) vaccine is a telling example. See Chapter 2 and Rosenberg, "The International Politics of Vaccine Testing in Interwar Algiers."

[10] Tomoko Akami, "A Quest to be Global: The League of Nations Health Organization and Inter-Colonial Regional Governing Agendas of the Far Eastern Association of Tropical Medicine 1910–25," *The International History Review* 38, no. 1 (2016): 1–23. For other discussions regarding colonial health, its relation with the international health, see, e.g.: Anderson, *Colonial Pathologies*; Packard, *A History of Global Health*.

I will conclude by spotlighting the Chinese context, to show how the LNHO's statistical standards were received and implemented at the country level – in particular, how the Chinese Nationalist government saw the LNHO's statistical work as a means of recovering the sovereignty the country had lost under the unequal treaties imposed on it.[11]

## The Origins of the LNHO Epidemiological Intelligence Service

When the League of Nations established a special commission to contain the typhus epidemic in Eastern Europe, it soon became clear that there was a dire need for vital and health statistics to be standardized across countries.[12] Composed of well-known public health experts – with Ludwik Rajchman, the founder of Poland's first bacteriological laboratory,[13] at the helm – the commission sent a team to visit Russia and Ukraine to collect statistics on typhus and malaria prevalence rates in 1921.[14] This was when the League's experts came to acknowledge the barriers preventing epidemiological information from being useful in different countries. Every country had its own procedure for recording births and deaths. There was no centralized intergovernmental channel for health statistics: the OIHP collected epidemiological information only from its member countries, and the League of Red Cross Societies obtained epidemic reports through unofficial channels.[15] Most national authorities acquired numbers on epidemic cases through diplomatic channels, and some from colonial offices.[16]

The League was quick to include statistics within its purview. In 1921, the League's First Provisional Health Committee agreed to integrate the

---

[11] On the Chinese government's strategies for recovering sovereignty, see, e.g.: Kirby, "The Internationalization of China."

[12] Although the main target was typhus, the League of Nations also gathered information on other epidemics, such as cholera and relapsing fever (see Borowy, *Coming to Terms with World Health*, 88).

[13] Tournès, *Les États-Unis et la Société des Nations (1914–1946)*, 150.

[14] Paul Weindling, "German Overtures to Russia, 1919–1925: Between Racial Expansion and National Coexistence," in *Doing Medicine Together: Germany and Russia between the Wars*, eds. Susan Gross Solomon, German and European Studies 4 (Toronto: University of Toronto Press, 2006), 43–4. The commission included Emil Roesle, of the German Imperial Office of Health, and Norman White, then the assistant director-general of the Indian Medical Service, to name just two of its more prominent members.

[15] League of Nations, "The League of Nations Provisional Health Committee Minutes of the First Session," August 25, 1921, 18–21, C.400. M. 280.1921.III, League of Nations Archives.

[16] Ibid., 18–21.

statistical bureau of the League of Red Cross Societies,[17] and later that year, the League of Red Cross Societies transferred the entire bureau – including its adding machines, reports, and statistician Knud Stouman – to the League.[18] The OIHP and LNHO subsequently reached an agreement to share epidemiological information. The LNHO thus acquired the capacity to issue epidemiological reports and became part of the channels for epidemic case reporting.

The typhus control commission to Eastern Europe and the ensuing Warsaw Conference, in Spring 1922, further consolidated the consensus that international collaboration was needed to contain epidemics, that health information should be shared among countries,[19] and that the LNHO would be in charge of carrying out the decisions made during the conference.[20] This consensus was crystalized into an agreement signed by the People's Health Commissariats of the Russian, Ukrainian, and White Russian Republics, and the League's representative.[21] The decisions cemented statistical surveys on Eastern European epidemics and policy suggestions as the LNHO's two core missions.[22] Notably, the Warsaw Conference was first and foremost European. Its official name was the European Health Conference, and it included representatives from twenty-six European countries, with Turkey and Japan being the only non-European participants.[23]

The LNHO's ambition to become the center of international epidemic statistics reporting went beyond typhus in Eastern Europe. To advance that aim, Rajchman, then the LNHO director-general, sought funding from the Rockefeller Foundation to found the epidemiological intelligence service within the LNHO.[24] Underscoring the need for international cooperation, Rajchman justified the need for the Service to

---

[17] Ibid.
[18] Claude H. Hill, "To Eric Drummond," October 20, 1921, 12B/16902/14212/R823/1921, League of Nations Archives.
[19] League of Nations, "European Health Conference Held at Warsaw from March 20th to 28th, 1922," April 3, 1922, 11. http://archive.org/details/europeanhealthco00euro.
[20] Ibid., 8.
[21] Norman White, "Agreement between the LNHO and People's Health Commisariats of the Russian, Ukrainian and White Russian Republics," May 1, 1922, 12B/20492/20492/R830/1922, League of Nations Archives.
[22] Wickliffe Rose, "To Rajchman," July 31, 1922, 12b/21836/21836/R839/1923, League of Nations Archives.
[23] League of Nations, "European Health Conference Held at Warsaw from March 20th to 28th, 1922," 4.
[24] Rajchman also requested that the IHB fund health worker exchange programs (League of Nations, "C.H.16, Correspondence Between the Health Section of the Secretariat and the Rockefeller Foundation," July 10, 1922, 12b/21836/21836/R839/1922, League of Nations Archives).

Wickliffe Rose, director of the Rockefeller's International Health Board (IHB), in the following manner:

> In order to secure such cooperation [real collaboration in various health adminis-
> trations], it is necessary, on the one hand, to prove the usefulness and efficiency
> of the international public health work and, on the other hand, to lay foundations
> on which a spirit of cooperation may be built up. … Epidemiological Intelligence
> and Public Health Statistics … would demonstrate the practicability and the
> indispensability of international health work.[25]

Rajchman's views on the role of the future statistical service thus went beyond the practicalities of epidemic control and extended to laying a foundation for "a spirit of cooperation." By exchanging statistical information, countries were expected to generate a consensus to serve as the basis for cooperation in public health.

The LNHO's proposal was attractive to the trustees of the IHB, not only because it promised to promote collaboration among countries in line with the IHB's ethos, but also because it was not politically sensitive. The Warsaw Conference resolutions had demonstrated that European countries widely accepted the necessity of exchanging information on epidemics, and there was no risk that the IHB's involvement would be viewed as political interference. Nor would it be difficult to attract financial support from governments to supplement (and eventually replace) the Rockefeller funding. This was a necessity for the Rockefeller Foundation, and the reason why its funding was always contingent on there being a demonstration element.[26] Specifically, the Foundation only provided financial aid to initiate a given program when there was the possibility of demonstrating its effectiveness to local authorities and inducing them to take over the program in question.[27] The aid provided to the LNHO epidemiological intelligence service was no exception. Rose explicitly stressed the importance of the demonstration principle to Selskar Gunn, the director of the Europe Office of the Rockefeller Foundation and the man in charge of coordination between the LNHO and the Foundation:

> The Board is disposed to aid the League in maintaining [the epidemiologi
> cal intelligence service] for a period of five years with a view to demonstrating
> its usefulness. It is to be hoped that within that time it will have become so

---

[25] Ludwik Rajchman, "To Wickliffe Rose," May 2, 1922, 4, 12b/21836/21836/
R839/1922, League of Nations Archives.

[26] League of Nations, "C.H.16, Correspondence Between the Health Section of the
Secretariat and the Rockefeller Foundation," 6.

[27] Darwin H. Stapleton, "Malaria Eradication and the Technological Model: The
Rockefeller Foundation and Public Health in East Asia," in *Disease, Colonialism, and
the State: Malaria in Modern East Asian History*, ed. Ka-Che Yip (Hong Kong: Hong
Kong University Press, 2009), 71–84.

serviceable that the governments which are supporting it will regard it as indispensable and will provide the funds necessary for its continuance and further development.[28]

The IHB trustees agreed, in May 1922, to fund the LNHO's epidemiological intelligence service over a period of five years.[29] And despite Rose's emphasis on the demonstration principle, the IHB continued to provide supplementary funding after the five years were over.[30] In the original agreement, the IHB granted $32,000 to the service for the period from 1923 to 1927.[31] That pledge was later renewed, and the IHB eventually added more grants for "special work in vital and public health statistics" and the "Epidemiological Bureau in the Far East."[32] At the end of 1927, the IHB again renewed its financial endorsement for another seven years. From 1923 to 1929, a total of $350,700 was granted to the service. Despite some changes in the sums accorded, the Rockefeller Foundation's financial support to the service lasted until 1937.[33]

With the Rockefeller Foundation's support, Rajchman devised the epidemiological intelligence service as an independent entity based in Geneva and focused on harmonizing national health administrations' practices regarding the collection and reporting of vital and health statistics. Rajchman's plan can be understood, in part, as a competition for authority with the United Kingdom, by that time the most advanced country when it came to vital and health statistics. This can be seen in the fact that Rajchman and the majority of the League of Nations Health Committee (which acted as the LNHO's executive body) rejected two proposals from Sir George Buchanan, a committee member who was a senior officer at the British Ministry of Health. Buchanan's first proposal was for the British ministry, as well as those of the United States and Italy, to offer expertise to the epidemiological intelligence service, as these countries were pioneers in statistical practices for health administration and research. In response, Rajchman expressed the desire to take preliminary steps to

---

[28] Wickliffe Rose, "To Gunn," November 12, 1922, 12b/26222/21836/R839/1923, League of Nations Archives.

[29] The IHB also agreed on funding the LNHO's health personnel exchange programs (Wickliffe Rose, "To Arthur Sweetser," Private, July 27, 1922, 12b/26117/21836/R839/1923, League of Nations Archives).

[30] International Health Board, "League of Nations Health Section," December 13, 1933, 33340, RF/1.1/100/20/164, Rockefeller Archive Center.

[31] Tournès, Les États-Unis et la Société des Nations (1914–1946), 160.

[32] International Health Board, "Minutes of the International Health Board: Working Program for 1926," June 11, 1924, 24341, RF/1.1/100/20/164, Rockefeller Archive Center.

[33] Tournès, Les États-Unis et la Société des Nations (1914–1946), 170.

appoint a Geneva-based director of the service, without going through time-consuming consultations with three governments, as Buchanan had proposed.[34] Buchanan's second proposal was to devise the epidemiological intelligence service as a research institute for conducting epidemiological investigations in different countries. This proposal was also rejected, and Rose instructed Gunn that the IHB grant was intended to create an independent center for epidemiological intelligence, rather than to sponsor such an institute.[35] By rejecting Buchanan's proposals, the LNHO retained centralized control over its epidemiological intelligence service.

Despite the conspicuous influence of the IHB in formulating the LNHO's plan of action, IHB officers Rose and Gunn endeavored not to reveal the power dynamics at play, so as to avoid the LNHO's member countries accusing them not only of providing the money but also of leading the work.[36] Rose therefore refused to send a Rockefeller representative to attend Health Committee meetings, in order to maintain a purely financial relationship between the IHB and the LNHO.[37] The appointment of Edgar Sydenstricker as director of the epidemiological intelligence service was also a source of concern for Rose and Gunn. Upon reading the minutes of the Health Committee meeting in which Rajchman presented his choice of Sydenstricker and mentioned Rose's support for his candidacy, Gunn wrote to Rajchman assuring him that Rose had suggested Sydenstricker without any outside pressure whatsoever and noted that Rose was afraid of giving the impression that the Rockefeller Foundation was directing the work of the LNHO through its financial support.[38] Rajchman explained in response that he was aware of the IHB's position, which was why he had also cited the support of Hugh Cumming of the United States Public Health Service (USPHS) for Sydenstricker, to disguise the fact that his choice was based entirely on Rose's recommendation.[39]

Despite Rose and Gunn's repeated denials, it was clear that Rockefeller funding affected the LNHO's statistical policies more than the IHB was willing to admit. From the very beginning, most of the statisticians at the epidemiological intelligence service were either American public health

---

[34] League of Nations, "Minutes of the Fourth Session Held at Geneva, August 14th to 21st, 1922," September 1, 1922, 40–1, 12B/26449/126/R811-2/1923, League of Nations Archives.

[35] Wickliffe Rose, "To Gunn," November 12, 1922.

[36] Selskar Gunn, "To Rajchman," December 11, 1922, 12b/26222/21836/R839/1923, League of Nations Archives.

[37] Ibid.

[38] Selskar Gunn, "To Rajchman," December 5, 1922, 12b/26222/21836/R839/1923, League of Nations Archives.

[39] Ludwik Rajchman, "To Gunn," December 7, 1922, 12b/26222/21836/R839/1923, League of Nations Archives.

officials or health statisticians educated in the United States. For more than two decades, because these American or American-educated statisticians endeavored to implement statistical practices in the health administrations of the League's member states, the American public health system had considerable visibility, despite the United States not being a member of the League. In addition, along with the Milbank Memorial Fund, the Rockefeller Foundation financed American officers' travel expenses when they went to Europe to participate in LNHO conferences, and owing to that support, American public health officers were included in discussions about international standards regarding health statistics, including the International List of Causes of Death (ICD).[40]

## Harmonizing Statistical Practices Across National Health Administrations

Once the institutional framework for the epidemiological intelligence service was decided upon, all that remained was to recruit the personnel to put the blueprint into practice. Representatives of the Rockefeller Foundation, Rajchman, and the League of Nations Health Committee all agreed that the director of the new service should be given free rein to organize its missions. They aimed to recruit a highly qualified expert who came recommended by renowned experts in the field.[41] The choice was between Edgar Sydenstricker, the first statistician at the USPHS, and Major Greenwood, a well-known, Pearson-trained statistician and researcher at University College, London. Although Greenwood had an excellent reputation in the field of epidemiological research, Sydenstricker's candidacy prevailed because he had the support of the Rockefeller Foundation, as mentioned above. In a letter, Rose stated that Sydenstricker was the "best man in [the United States] for this post," as he had built up the statistical office of the USPHS.[42] But he also forwarded references from Hugh Cumming (the chief of the USPHS) and Raymond Pearl (another well-known, Pearson-trained biostatistics professor, at the JHSPH) to support Sydenstricker's candidacy.[43] Upon Rose's forceful recommendation, Rajchman borrowed Sydenstricker from the USPHS for one year.[44]

[40] LNHO, "Report to the Council on the Work of the Twenty-First Session of the Health Committee," June 7, 1934, 2, C.283.M.97.1934.III, League of Nations Archives.
[41] League of Nations, "Minutes of the Fourth Session Held at Geneva, August 14th to 21st, 1922."
[42] Wickliffe Rose, "To Rajchman," July 18, 1922, 12b/26117/21836/R839/1923, League of Nations Archives.
[43] Ibid.
[44] Ludwik Rajchman, "To Gunn," December 7, 1922, 12b/26222/21836/R839/1923, League of Nations Archives.

Sydenstricker's work at the epidemiological intelligence service was intensive, as he had only a one-year assignment (with a two-month extension) to complete it. He devised the service to manage epidemiological information sent in by the LNHO's member states. Instead of seeking to advance the general statistical ability of officials, Sydenstricker prioritized the standardization of the statistical collection procedures used by national health authorities. The remarks of an outside observer at the time provide a good illustration of Rajchman and Sydenstricker's strategy in standardizing statistical practices: Major Greenwood complained that the LNHO's statistics programs were superficial. He wrote to his friend and colleague Raymond Pearl:

> Far too much of the Rockefeller money is spent in violently dashing about Europe having buns with the "best people" and drawing up programmes of futile get-learned-quick courses. If you and I would only draw up a nice little course THE Whole THEORY AND PRACTICE OF VITAL STATISTICS MEDICAL STATISTICS AND BIOMETRY, COMPLETE IN SIX REELS WITH INCIDENTAL MUSIC, the film rights would make us rich men.[45]

Despite its sarcastic tone, Greenwood's criticism does shed light on the LNHO's strategy for implementing statistical practices in its member states' health administrations: the organization sought to quickly convince national health authorities to implement statistical practices and harmonize them across countries. The epidemiological intelligence service had no intention of providing complete training to health statisticians. For that reason, the LNHO turned down Greenwood's proposal for an international school in Geneva.[46] Pearl, the founding director of the Rockefeller-funded biostatistical department of the JHSPH, also confessed to Greenwood after a meeting with Sydenstricker that he could not "work up any enthusiasm at all about these international statistical policies."[47]

In concrete terms, Sydenstricker's plan was to create fora and channels for various countries' health statisticians to become familiar with each other's practices. After three months spent traveling to confer with statisticians in London, Paris, and Brussels, he submitted a memorandum to the League of Nations Health Committee in February 1923 in which he listed the major goals for the Service: put succinctly, these were

[45] Original capitalization. Major Greenwood, "To Raymond Pearl," August 5, 1923, Greenwood, Major (2) 1923/i, Raymond Pearl Papers, American Philosophical Society.
[46] Pearl, "To Major Greenwood," September 17, 1923, Greenwood, Major (2) 1923/i, Raymond Pearl Papers, American Philosophical Society.
[47] Raymond Pearl, "To Major Greenwood," April 12, 1924, Greenwood, Major (3) 1924, Raymond Pearl Papers, American Philosophical Society.

to publish epidemiological reports and to standardize statistical practices among health authorities.[48] The key to both missions was to make health officials aware of the importance of using statistics to communicate. Sydenstricker then defined two approaches to achieving these goals: first, publishing handbooks presenting every member state's statistical practices; and second, organizing collective studies and exchange programs for national health statisticians. Although Sydenstricker was the author of both approaches, they were also in line with Rajchman's original proposal, which emphasized the promotion of mutual understanding among countries in order to advance international collaboration. Tellingly, the collective studies and exchange program that Sydenstricker put forward were already part of Rajchman's proposal to the IHB in 1922.

Sydenstricker's first approach was to devise handbooks to serve as guidelines for statisticians wishing to use a given country's statistical data. These handbooks formatted local know-how on vital and health statistics collection. Sydenstricker mandated two statisticians from the United Kingdom, Major Greenwood and Major Edge, to compile statistical handbooks on "significant" countries (i.e. European and North American countries). Work on other countries' handbooks was done directly by statistical officials from the countries in question. Although every handbook had a different author, they all had the same table of contents. Each handbook started by giving basic information about the country, followed by a historical background of the official machinery for collecting vital statistics. Afterwards, a detailed description was offered on the procedure for registering births, marriages, and deaths, including official forms, job titles of responsible officers, and the relevant civil laws on the protection of personal information. Finally, each handbook ended with a chapter dedicated to the country's epidemic reporting system and health statistics, allowing for a basic understanding of vital and health statistics in the country. By providing essential knowledge about statistical practices in different countries, the handbooks served as dictionaries of a sort that helped health officials decipher statistical data from the country in question.

Sydenstricker's second approach was to organize study groups and exchange programs for government health statisticians, through which national statistics officers could share their experiences and agree upon

[48] Edgar Sydenstricker, "Annex 5. The Work of the Service of Epidemiological Intelligence and Public Health Statistics, Minutes of the First Session Held at Geneva, February 11th to 21st, 1924," February 14, 1924, 103, C.10.M.7.1924 III, League of Nations Archives; International Health Board, "IHB Minutes: League of Nations – General Policy and Interchanges," May 20, 1924, 24128, RF/1.1/100/20/164, Rockefeller Archive Center.

a standard procedure for collecting and analyzing statistics. When studied closely, Sydenstricker's network of statistics officials was not homog-
enous but was organized into tiers based on countries' varying levels of
statistical capacity (See Figure 3.1).

The top tier officials were exclusively from Western Europe, Scandi-
navia, and North America.[49] They were invited by the LNHO to take
part in study groups and commissions to draft international standards
regarding vital statistics collection. In 1924, the epidemiological intelligence service established four study groups on joint causes of death,
standard million population, age and sex classification, and stillbirths,
respectively. Each group comprised four to five statistical experts working for either national health authorities or research institutes, while the
epidemiological intelligence service served as the secretariat of these
groups and was in charge of correspondence among participants.[50] The
study groups included some of the best known statisticians at that time,
such as Raymond Pearl of the JHSPH, Emile Roesle of the German
Imperial Office of Health, and Henri Methorst, then director of the Central Statistical Bureau of the Netherlands and the permanent bureau of
the ISI. After a year of correspondence, the four study groups compiled
memoranda that served as discussion materials for statistician exchange
programs: the second tier of Sydenstricker's network.

Sydenstricker devised this second tier to consist of national statisticians from LNHO member states – ranging from Eastern Europe to
Latin America – whose statistical practices were not well recognized by
the organization.[51] The LNHO invited these statisticians to participate
in exchange programs so that they could be included in discussions on
standards prepared by the participants of the study groups (the top tier).
Sydenstricker also proposed making the second-tier statisticians intermediaries between the LNHO and their respective national health authorities. Citing a Provisional Health Committee resolution, Sydenstricker

[49] The nationalities of the seventeen experts involved in the study groups were: Austrian,
Canadian, Danish, French, German, Italian, Dutch, Swedish, Swiss, British, and
American (LNHO, "Health Committee: Minutes of the Fourth Session," April 1925,
89–92, C.224,M.80,1925, III., League of Nations Archives).

[50] Otto R. Eichel, "C.H.241, Work of the Epidemiological Intelligence Service,"
September 29, 1924, C.588.M.202.1924II, League of Nations Archives.

[51] The participating countries in the first session were: Brazil, Bulgaria, Czechoslovakia,
Hungary, the Kingdom of Serbs, Croats and Slovenes, Norway, Poland, and Russia.
Countries participating in the second session largely overlapped with those of the
first: Bulgaria, Cuba, Czechoslovakia, Estonia, Hungary, Romania, Russia, the
Kingdom of Serbs, Croats and Slovenes, and Ukraine (LNHO, "Health Committee:
Minutes of the Fourth Session," 92; Edgar Sydenstricker, "Annex 5. The Work of the
Service of Epidemiological Intelligence and Public Health Statistics, Minutes of the
First Session Held at Geneva, February 11th to 21st, 1924," 111).

wrote that one of the purposes of exchange programs was to strengthen ties between the epidemiological intelligence service and member states' statisticians.[52]

The first two exchange programs took place in 1923 and 1924. Participants were to introduce their local practices to the LNHO statistical forum with the goal of reaching a consensus, and then apply that consensus to their own health administrations. In both sessions, participants presented their own statistical practices; Sydenstricker and statistical experts from Western Europe then offered comments based on the presentations. The LNHO later organized a trip for participants to visit countries with advanced public health administrations, i.e. the Netherlands, Switzerland, France, and the United Kingdom. The exchange program participants then exchanged views once more in Geneva after the trip and submitted final reports to the LNHO. Both sessions succeeded in raising officials' awareness, but no concrete standard for statistical collection was agreed upon. The only consensus reached during these two sessions was that procedures for collecting statistical data were extremely varied across countries and special efforts would be needed to standardize them.[53]

The third exchange program differed from its antecedents on two counts. First, the participants in the third session were all chief statistical officers from countries with more advanced statistical practices.[54] Most had been involved in the study groups or had briefed the participants of the two previous sessions. Second, the destination for the exchange was the Scandinavian countries, rather than the Western European countries visited in the previous programs. Knud Stouman, a member of the LNHO's statistical staff, recruited participants and selected the destination based on the particular nature of Scandinavian vital statistics work.[55] The Scandinavian countries had their own list of the causes of death and were preparing to revise it in 1926. Stouman argued that because the Scandinavian countries had well-trained medical officers but had not implemented the ICD, they were the ideal site for a demonstration.[56]

[52] Sydenstricker, "Annex 5. The Work of the Service of Epidemiological Intelligence and Public Health Statistics, Minutes of the First Session Held at Geneva, February 11th to 21st, 1924," 111.

[53] Ibid., 111–14; LNHO, "Health Committee: Minutes of the Fourth Session," 92.

[54] LNHO, "Health Committee: Minutes of the Fifth Session," October 1925, 67, C.647,M.236,1925, III., League of Nations Archives.

[55] Knud Stouman, "Note on International Nomenclature of Causes of Death," January 16, 1925, 13, 12b/34767/32528/R920/1924, League of Nations Archives.

[56] Knud Stouman, "Memorandum on Expert Groups on Comparability of Mortality Statistics," January 16, 1925, 13, 12b/34767/32528/R920/1924, League of Nations Archives.

Stouman's reasoning is illustrative of the LNHO's ambition to include the Scandinavian countries within the network of its epidemiological intelligence service, making it the real center of all international vital and health statistical reporting.

The third exchange ended with an eight-session conference organized by the LNHO in Geneva, during which a set of resolutions was issued that contained recommended standard procedures for collecting and analyzing vital and health statistics. The conference also set the ground rules governing the division of labor between statisticians and medical doctors in terms of vital statistics collection. This time, the participants succeeded in reaching a consensus on statisticians' role in compiling vital and health statistics. A statement made by S. Rosenfeld, Chief of the Statistical Bureau of the Health Administration of Austria, was illuminating as to the statisticians' stance. He quoted Jacques Bertillon, the author of the original classification of causes of death, who had once said it "was necessary for statisticians to have confidence in their work." Rosenfeld went on to stress that "the work of statisticians [had] already [shown] that it was possible to establish general rules for the tabulation of statistics."[57] As for statistical collection, he made the suggestion (which met with approval) that doctors should be put in charge of recording causes of death among their patients (i.e. serve as witnesses of the facts), whereas statisticians were to be responsible for observing general statistical regularities in deaths.[58] It was also agreed that statisticians should not be considered medical professionals but should nonetheless be included in discussions of medical problems. This division of labor laid the foundation for the LNHO's subsequent statistical endeavors. Over the following decades, the LNHO established a commission of expert statisticians to implement statistical methods into studies on cancer, the BCG vaccine, and morbidity, among others.

No known sources specify the extent to which the participating countries adopted the statistical standards promoted during the three exchange sessions. Nevertheless, the exchanges clearly did inform governments of the importance of communicating their statistics to the epidemiological intelligence service. The League of Nations Health Committee began to receive epidemiological reports in 1924 that covered a larger geographical range

---

[57] LNHO, "The Third Collective Study of Medical Statistics, Final Conference, Provisional Minutes of Fourth Meeting," August 24, 1925, 8, C.S.III/P.V.6, League of Nations Archives.

[58] Ibid., 11.

Table 3.1 *LNHO tiered network for statistical standards*

|  | First tier | Second tier |
|---|---|---|
| Composition | • Officials and researchers from Western Europe, Scandinavia and North America | • Statisticians from LNHO member states where local statistical practices were not well recognized |
| Part played in LNHO statistical work | • Compile statistical handbooks on "significant" countries<br>• Participate in study groups and commissions<br>• Prepare discussion materials for exchange programs<br>• Participate in third exchange program | • Compile statistical handbooks on their respective countries<br>• Participate in first and second exchange programs |

than the OIHP reports.[59] In 1926, the reports published by the service came from five continents, with 116 countries providing epidemiological information on plague, cholera, yellow fever, typhus, smallpox, birth rates, infant mortality, and more, in a total of 696 cities.[60] In 1927, member states were reportedly satisfied with the LNHO's epidemiological reports.[61] Public health schools, including those at Johns Hopkins and Harvard University, included the LNHO's monthly reports in their syllabi.[62]

It is worth noting that George Buchanan remained an unflagging critic of the reports. His criticism of the use of maps to represent epidemic cases is illustrative of ongoing rivalries when it came to epidemiological reporting. Specifically, he complained that using maps – which provided information at a glance – would be unfair to the United Kingdom. As a country that boasted one of the best-organized epidemic reporting systems in the world, he claimed that such maps would give the misleading impression that the United Kingdom had more epidemic cases than other countries just because its reporting system was robust and

[59] LNHO, "Minutes of the Health Committee First Session," February 11, 1924, C. 10. M. 7. 1924. III, League of Nations Archives, cited in: Borowy, *Coming to Terms with World Health*, 107.
[60] International Health Board, "Minutes of the International Health Board: Working Program for 1927," 26386.
[61] LNHO, "Health Committee Ninth Session," March 1927, 22, C. 107. M. 38. 1927. III, League of Nations Archives.; "Health Committee 19th Session," October 10, 1932, 14–15, C. H./19 session/P.V., League of Nations Archives.
[62] LNHO, "Health Committee 19th Session," 14–15.

covered more territory. Once again, Buchanan's views were at odds with the position of other members of the Health Committee.[63] Buchanan's remark nonetheless pointed to a crucial lingering question when it came to statistical reporting: whether increasing numbers could be taken at face value, or whether they were the result of increased attention or capacity when recording cases.

## The LNHO Takes Over the Revision of the ICD

The epidemiological reporting discussed above is illustrative of the tiered system within which statisticians of different countries were given an uneven say in dictating statistical collection procedures. Similarly, the evolution of the LNHO's ICD highlights the ambitions of individual countries and Europe-based international organizations to gain influence. As early as 1923, the LNHO's three statisticians – Edgar Sydenstricker, Otto R. Eichel, and Knud Stouman – took ICD revisions into account as part of their efforts to standardize vital statistics collection, despite the fact that the ISI still officially oversaw revisions. Sydenstricker and his colleagues were all experienced statistical officials; as discussed above, they focused their discussions on administrative procedures, including who should be put in charge of registering causes of death, how death certificates should be sent to the national administration, and how causes of death should be tabulated in histograms.[64]

The LNHO statisticians discussed points that were completely different from those covered in the three previous revision meetings, which had taken place in 1900, 1909, and 1920. Those meetings had been organized by the ISI and convened by the French government at the suggestion of a French statistician, Jacques Bertillon, who had proposed the idea of the ICD during a meeting of the ISI in 1893. Attended by researchers and medical doctors whose core concern was scientific research, the early meetings focused on how to integrate new pathological discoveries into the list and how to categorize various causes of death. At the end of the third meeting, the ICD comprised 205 rubrics with an abridged list of ninety rubrics. Up until the 1920s, the ICD's reception was uneven in different regions of the world. For instance, Ana María Carrillo and Anne-Emanuelle Birn have shown that Bertillon's list enjoyed early success

---

[63] League of Nations, "Minutes of the Fourth Session Held at Geneva, August 14th to 21st, 1922," 10–16, cited in: Borowy, *Coming to Terms with World Health*, 104–5.

[64] Sydenstricker's emphasis on the administrative aspect of the ICD is also documented by Borowy, "Counting Death and Disease: Classification of Death and Disease in the Interwar Years, 1919–1939," 460.

in the Americas thanks to an endorsement from the American Public Health Association (APHA) in 1898. At APHA's recommendation, the United States, Canada and Mexico – the APHA member countries at that time – all applied Bertillon's list when collecting mortality statistics in their censuses of 1900/1901.[65] Outside of the Americas, however, only a few countries (mostly in Europe) adopted the complete list. Others used only the abridged list, if they made use of the ICD at all.[66]

Iris Borowy offers a vivid description of the rivalry between the LNHO and the ISI regarding the leadership of the ICD revisions during the LNHO's early years. She argues that, despite their differences, collaboration between the two organizations was inevitable as they shared many expert members.[67] The League of Nations Health Committee eventually agreed that the LNHO should be responsible for revising the ICD in coordination with the ISI and the French government. Following an intensive correspondence, the LNHO and the ISI decided on a division of labor for the upcoming revision conference.[68] The ISI would serve in a consulting capacity, while the LNHO would take over as the main organizer.[69] In 1927, the LNHO and the ISI co-organized a mixed commission to discuss countries' vital statistics systems and collect materials for the 1929 revision conference.[70]

When the LNHO eventually partnered with the ISI and took over responsibility for preparing the revision conferences, some considered it an opportunity to overhaul the ICD, especially certain American officials who had felt marginalized in the decision-making process during previous revisions. Once the LNHO took over, American experts William H. Davis, the chief statistician for vital statistics at the United States Census Bureau, and Haven Emerson, director of APHA, corresponded with the LNHO on ICD-related matters and took an active part in the study groups and conferences.[71] In addition, the

---

[65] Ana María Carrillo and Anne-Emanuelle Birn, "Neighbours on Notice: National and Imperialist Interests in the American Public Health Association, 1872–1921," *Canadian Bulletin of Medical History* 25, no. 1 (2008), 243–4.

[66] LNHO, "C.H. 357. The International Nomenclature of Causes of Death," September 29, 1925, 12B/43806/22685/R842/1925, League of Nations Archives.

[67] Borowy, "Counting Death and Disease: Classification of Death and Disease in the Interwar Years, 1919–1939," 465.

[68] For the details of the discussions, see: ibid.

[69] LNHO, "Health Committee Eighth Session," November 27, 1926, 70, C. 610. M. 238- 1926. III, League of Nations Archives.

[70] Eric Drummond, "To Aristide Briand," November 4, 1927, 12b/51488/22685/ R842/1926; "To Aristide Briand," November 28, 1927, 12b/51488/22685/R842/1926, League of Nations Archives.

[71] International Health Board, "IHB Minutes: Delegate to Interchange of Vital Statisticians- Appropriation," May 20, 1924, 25196, RF/1.1/100/20/164, Rockefeller Archive Center.

Scandinavian countries, which had their own list of causes of death, were still hesitant about adopting the ICD. For them, the LNHO taking over the ICD was an opportunity for their system to be taken into account in future revisions, which would help them to adapt it. Indeed, it was at the urging of APHA and the Scandinavian countries that the LNHO sought to undertake revisions to the ICD in the first place.[72]

The 1929 revision conference marked a turning point for the ICD in that it became intergovernmental. Because the conference was held within the LNHO framework, countries sent delegates to participate in the revisions for the first time. A total of thirty-eight countries were represented.[73] Participants agreed on a definition of stillbirth and its registration procedure, which remained in place until the 1960s.[74] The success of the fourth revision was fleeting, however, as the fifth revision conference in 1938 was undermined by hostility between countries. Only the United Kingdom sent a representative with diplomatic power to the 1938 conference, and other countries were reluctant to endorse the new version of the ICD. This situation spurred Yves Biraud, an alumnus of the JHSPH and a statistician at the LNHO, to urge the members of the Health Committee to promote the ICD in their respective countries.[75] Given the outbreak of World War II, this appeal met with little success.

### The Epidemiological Intelligence Service in the East: A Network Beyond Colonial Medicine

Edgar Sydenstricker's initiatives at the LNHO mainly reached statisticians from European countries. Other parts of the world were mostly excluded, as the great distances involved prevented them from sending their officials to the Health Committee or exchange programs.[76]

---

[72] Léon Bernard, "C.H. 455. Note by Professor Léon Bernard, Concerning the Procedure Which Should Be Adopted for the Revisions of the International List of Causes of Death," April 1926, 12B/51488/22685/R842/1926, League of Nations Archives.

[73] Moriyama et al., *History of the Statistical Classification of Diseases and Causes of Death*, 15.

[74] Gear, Biraud, and Swaroop, *International Work in Health Statistics, 1948–1958, 8*.

[75] League of Nations, "The League of Nations Health Committee Minutes of the 29th Session," October 12, 1938, 39, C. H./29th Session/Revised Minutes, League of Nations Archives.

[76] This did not mean that there was no prior international health collaboration in the region. As Tomoko Akami's research demonstrates, the Far Eastern Association of Tropical Medicine, established in 1908, comprised an inter-colonial and national network of public health experts. Akami further shows that the LNHO's subsequent actions in the region made use of the Association's network (Tomoko

Moreover, colonialism in the Far East meant that polities had varying levels of sovereignty, which presented a challenge to the LNHO's position as an international organization.[77] The organization's ambition to become the leading international health authority through its statistical reporting network came up against the colonial system in the region. The LNHO therefore had to adopt a different strategy from that used in Europe to include the Far East in the sphere of its statistical reporting.

One significant exception was Japan, which played no small part in the LNHO's drive to extend its scope to East Asia. Before the Manchurian Incident of 1931 (which led Japan to withdraw from the League of Nations in 1933), the Japanese government considered the League of Nations as an interface through which it could convince other powers to recognize Japan as the regional power in East Asia.[78] Japanese high officials of all types took active part in the League's policy-making. As Tomoko Akami has chronicled, Mikinosuke Miyajima, a pathologist and member of the Health Committee, stated during a session of the Committee in 1922 that the people of the Far East suspected the League of Nations of being focused solely on European affairs. Miyajima invited the League to "give concrete proof" that this was not the case.[79]

Miyajima's invitation was well received by Rajchman and other members of the Health Committee, who were eager to promote the standing of the LNHO.[80] By collecting statistics from different continents, the LNHO could justifiably claim to be a truly global health organization, not merely a European one. Given the high cost of travel to Asia, exchanging statistical information was also a more economical way for the LNHO to expand its sphere of influence.

By the end of 1922, Rajchman sent Norman White – a LNHO staff member, and former assistant to the director of the Indian Medical Service, who had worked with the LNHO to collect epidemiological data in Eastern Europe – on an expedition to Asia to investigate public health organizations in the region.[81] From late 1922 to July 1923,

Akami, "Imperial Polities, Intercolonialism, and the Shaping of Global Governing Norms: Public Health Expert Networks in Asia and the League of Nations Health Organization, 1908–37," *Journal of Global History* 12, no. 1 (2017): 4–25).

[77] Akami has demonstrated the different "layers" of international health governance that the LNHO was forced to navigate. Akami, "A Quest to be Global"; Akami, "Imperial Polities, Intercolonialism, and the Shaping of Global Governing Norms."

[78] Thomas W. Burkman, *Japan and the League of Nations* (Honolulu, HI: University of Hawai'i Press, 2008), 16.

[79] League of Nations, "Minutes of the Fourth Session Held at Geneva, August 14th to 21st, 1922.," quoted in: Akami, "A Quest to be Global," 1.

[80] League of Nations, "Minutes of the Fourth Session Held at Geneva, August 14th to 21st, 1922.," cited in: Borowy, *Coming to Terms with World Health*, 108.

[81] Ludwik Rajchman, "Norman White C. V.," February 10, 1923, 12B/24282/23230/ R843/1922, League of Nations Archives.

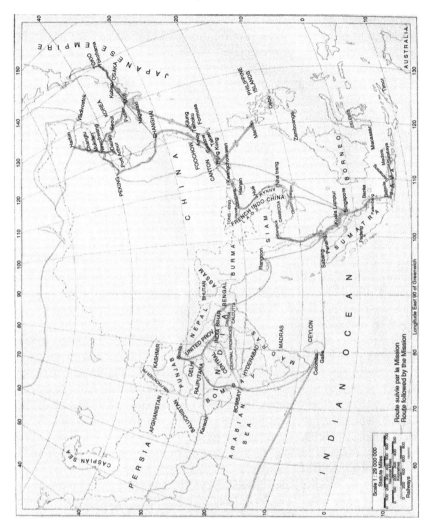

Figure 3.1 Norman White's route to the Far East.
Norman White, "The Prevalence of Epidemic Disease and Port Health Organization and Procedure in the Far East," 1923, 12B/31957/23230/R843/1923, League of Nations Archives. Courtesy of United Nations Archives at Geneva.

White traveled from India to Japan, conferring with local authorities and collecting government-recorded epidemic statistics along the way (see Figure 3.1). With White's expedition, key ports of Asia appeared on the LNHO's radar of epidemiological intelligence.

White's expedition is illustrative of how the LNHO's attempt to expand its network of epidemiological intelligence meant negotiating with colonial powers. The colonial system undermined the LNHO's work in Asia, as the organization's ties to imperial powers inevitably affected indigenous governments' willingness to share information. Chinese officials, for example, were reluctant to host an expert of Japanese nationality, fearing the information would be used in an invasion of China.[82] Rajchman made deliberate efforts to avoid being seen as an ally of colonial powers. Likely because he himself came from a country (Poland) that had been occupied by foreign powers, he understood local governments' reticence. He insisted that nationality should be taken into account when choosing the envoy, citing Chinese reluctance to collaborate with a Japanese envoy.[83] Rajchman initially hoped to send Josephus Jitta, since he considered Jitta's native Netherlands to be too small a power to arouse suspicion, unlike the United Kingdom, France, or Japan.[84] But the Netherlands, though small in area, had a colony in Indonesia and was, in fact, a colonial power in Asia; the archives contain no clues as to whether Rajchman's reasoning was simply flawed or whether he had some other agenda. In the end, Jitta turned down the invitation because his government refused to grant him six months' leave. White, by that time already employed by the LNHO, had to sail alone.

On his expedition, White sought to go beyond the existing colonial networks and create a new channel of communication that included all Asian territories, colonies or not, for the exchange of epidemic statistics. As White indicated in a letter to W. R. Edwards, the director-general of the Indian Medical Service, the LNHO planned to go further than the OIHP, which was focused on protecting Europe from epidemics. White wrote that the LNHO would aim to have "the ports in the Far East ... protecting themselves against the importation of infection from elsewhere."[85] Specifically, the OIHP's core mission was to collect statistics for the timely implementation of quarantine measures, as decreed by the International Sanitary Convention, in order to stop epidemics from spreading to Europe. White described the OIHP as an international organization whose activities resembled "colonial medicine," a term coined by historians for the medical systems established in colonial settings that prioritized the colonial

---

[82] Ludwik Rajchman, "Personnel of Epidemiological Commission to be Dispatched to the Far East," September 22, 1922, 12B/24282/23230/R843/1922, League of Nations Archives.

[83] Ibid.

[84] Ibid.

[85] Norman White, "To Major General Sir W. R. Edwards, Director General of Indian Medical Service," October 28, 1922, 3, 12B/25734/23230/R843/1922, League of Nations Archives.

power's commercial benefit over the local population's well-being.[86] European empires used the OIHP to protect their own interests while ignoring the local population's health. Positioning the LNHO in opposition to the OIHP, White stressed that the LNHO hoped to empower local governments to protect their populations' health. This ideal, however, came up against the existing colonial channels for epidemiological information. The Indian Medical Service was one of the first to protest: at first, it even refused to let White visit, stating that all epidemiological reports were sent through British official channels and that, according to Edwards, "it [was] not possible for an outsider to settle this question."[87] Although it is not clear why Edwards' attitude eventually softened, in the end White's visit was permitted.

Upon his return from months of traveling, White prepared a report recommending the establishment of a new bureau within the epidemiological intelligence service to serve the Far East. In 1924, the Health Committee endorsed his proposal and devised the Eastern Bureau, located in Singapore, to serve as a branch of the service's headquarters in Geneva.[88] The LNHO thus gained a means of strengthening its presence in East Asia, which was essentially achieved through the collection and exchange of statistics. With financial backing to the tune of $155,000 provided by the Rockefeller Foundation IHB between 1924 and 1929, along with contributions from the Japanese and Indian governments, the Eastern Bureau was responsible for collecting epidemic statistics for the Geneva office and the OIHP and distributing the LNHO's epidemiological reports to authorities in the region.[89] The Bureau also collected statistics on vaccine field trials and conducted epidemiological investigations at the request of the authorities.[90] Ports in the region, such as those in China, Japan, and the Dutch East Indies, proved more willing to send their information to Singapore than to Geneva as the telegraph fees were significantly cheaper.[91] Until it was forced to close due to the Japanese

---

[86] Further discussion of colonial medical systems can be found in: Shula Marks, "What is Colonial about Colonial Medicine? And What has Happened to Imperialism and Health?" *Social History of Medicine* 10, no. 2 (1997): 205–19.

[87] Norman White, "To Major General Sir W. R. Edwards, Director General of Indian Medical Service," December 27, 1922, 12B/25734/23230/R843/1922, League of Nations Archives.

[88] LNHO, "Minutes of the Health Committee First Session," 11.

[89] LNHO, 12–13; International Health Board, "League of Nations – Pledge," January 3, 1929, 29042, RF/1.1/100/20/164, Rockefeller Archive Center.

[90] Norman White, "The Prevalence of Epidemic Disease and Port Health Organization and Procedure in the Far East," 43; LNHO, "Health Committee Ninth Session," 75–7.

[91] Norman White, "The Prevalence of Epidemic Disease and Port Health Organization and Procedure in the Far East," 43.

occupation of Singapore in 1942, the Eastern Bureau exchanged epidemiological information with 137 ports across the Indian Ocean and Western Pacific, including ports in Africa, Asia, and Australasia.[92] Just as at the Geneva office, the Eastern Bureau's responsibilities eventually extended to training public health workers through exchanges, organizing study groups, and sponsoring and participating in scientific conferences.[93] Though in the beginning it was focused solely on collecting epidemic statistics, the LNHO gradually became an indispensable stakeholder on health matters in Asia. White's hopes, as expressed during his expedition, partly came true: the Eastern Bureau pushed the LNHO's work in the Far East beyond that of the OIHP and brought more technical support and information to local governments. However, the Bureau's mission to become a node of epidemiological information was only made possible because colonial powers agreed to share the information infrastructure they had already put in place.[94]

### The LNHO: The Only Suitable Partner for Chinese Maritime Quarantine Reform

Despite finding an intermediary in the form of the Eastern Bureau, countries made their own decisions regarding how to react to the LNHO's epidemiological intelligence reporting system. The case of China, as one of the rare uncolonized nations in the region, offers insights into Asian governments' reasons for adhering to the LNHO system.

Although China was one of the founding members of the League of Nations, it was not an active member of the Health Committee. When Norman White visited China in 1923 during his Far East expedition, power was divided among warlords, and the Beiyang government (the central government in Beijing) had very limited control over the country. White ended up meeting with the foreign powers in control of treaty ports and officers of the Central Epidemic Prevention Bureau, which was supported by the Beiyang government. Despite the many complaints he received from China-based institutions, White did not propose any reforms to address the patchwork of quarantine systems. In hindsight, the main function of White's visit was to make the LNHO and the Chinese government aware of each other: the LNHO acquired basic

---

[92] LNHO, "Health Committee Eleventh Session," October 1927, 54, C. 579. M. 205.1927. III, League of Nations Archives; Borowy, *Coming to Terms with World Health*, 146.

[93] Manderson, "Wireless War in the Eastern Arena," 109. For more on the LNHO's involvement in the Far East, see e.g.: Akami, "A Quest to be Global."

[94] Tworek, "Communicable Disease," 830.

information on the Chinese health system, and treaty ports in China and the Central Epidemic Prevention Bureau began to share their epidemic statistics with the LNHO.[95]

The relationship deepened in 1925, when the Beiyang government invited Rajchman to visit China on his way to Japan and organized a committee to accompany him on visits to treaty ports. These visits were indirectly linked to the statistical reporting system: Rajchman offered advice on treaty-port health and helped create a design for a Chinese national quarantine service, which would serve as the administrative basis for the epidemiological intelligence reporting system.

The Rockefeller public health network in China played no small part in Rajchman's visit. Specifically, contact was initiated by John B. Grant, director of the Rockefeller-funded PUMC Department of Public Health. Grant first wrote to New York requesting IHB authorization to tackle Chinese quarantine reform. Victor Heiser, an IHB officer, turned down Grant's request, as quarantine organization was considered a sovereignty issue; Heiser advised that the Rockefeller Foundation could not enter such troubled political waters and should leave the matter to the League of Nations, the impartiality of which would facilitate reform without causing a backlash.[96]

Indeed, the quarantine system in Chinese ports was an extremely delicate issue in terms of sovereignty, as it involved several different authorities: foreign powers exercised extraterritorial power in their respective treaty ports, and the Chinese Maritime Customs Service had been under the control of British officers since its founding in the mid-nineteenth century.[97] The only paid position related to quarantine measures within

---

[95] LNHO, "Health Committee Ninth Session," 32; "Health Committee: Minutes of the Sixth Session," May 1926, 19, C.252,M.96,1926, III., League of Nations Archives.

[96] Oral History Research Department, Columbia University, "Reminiscences of Dr. John B. Grant (Vol. 2)," 248–9.

[97] The Chinese Maritime Customs Service was established by the British at the request of the Qing administration. From that point on, all its directors were British, and it was not until the 1940s that the service had its first American director. Despite the nationality of its directors and the clear British influence, the Service was part of the Chinese government. Recent scholarly works have pointed out that the Service enjoyed a degree of independence from British imperial interests, especially during the Nanjing Decade (Hans Van de Ven, *Breaking with the Past: The Maritime Customs Service and the Global Origins of Modernity in China* [New York: Columbia University Press, 2014]; Felix Boecking, *No Great Wall: Trade, Tariffs and Nationalism in Republican China, 1927–1945* [Cambridge, MA: Harvard University Asia Center, 2017]). For medical officers' accounts within the Service, see: Li Shang-Jen, "Shijiu shiji Zhongguo tongshang gangbu de weisheng zhuangkuang: haiguan yiguan de guandian" ["Health Conditions of Treaty Ports in China during 19th Century: From the Perspective of Customs Medical Officer]," in *Jiankang yu shehui: Huaren weisheng xinshi [Health and Society: The New History of Chinese Hygiene]*, ed. Chu Ping-Yi (Taipei: Linking Books, 2013), 69–93.

the Chinese government was that of medical officer within the China Maritime Customs Service, subordinated to the Ministry of Finance. These medical officers were either British or American nationals who were private practitioners and worked only part-time in the customs service.[98] The complex nature of treaty-port sovereignty made it impossible for any one country to intervene. Moreover, quarantine measures involved detaining infected boats and personnel, which required forceful legal backing. The League of Nations, as an intergovernmental organization, seemed to be the only actor capable of providing a solution.

Rajchman's 1925 visit proceeded much as Grant and Heiser had hoped: Rajchman decided that Chinese port health reform would be the *raison d'être* of his young health organization. To the LNHO Health Committee, Rajchman argued that the LNHO's involvement in Chinese quarantine reform would not be charity, as it would have a profound impact on maritime commerce worldwide.[99] He went on to note that the Chinese quarantine service was an international health issue that only the LNHO could take on,[100] and that the LNHO's involvement in establishing a modern quarantine service in China might even justify the organization's very existence: "[I]f the task of facilitating the application of modern medicine into a country of four hundred million inhabitants could be undertaken, such a work would in itself justify the existence of an international public health administration."[101] Many committee members were in favor of the LNHO's involvement in Chinese quarantine reform. Although no official agreement was signed, Rajchman and Chinese public health officers arrived at a mutual understanding: Rajchman learned about Chinese public health organizations, and the Chinese officers came to trust that the LNHO was not working for any imperial power.

The third contact between the LNHO and the Chinese government confirmed the organization's leading role in constructing the Chinese national health system, including statistical reporting. The fact that the LNHO was an international organization and thus geopolitically impartial was the decisive factor in favor of this collaboration. In 1928, the Nationalist government, led by Chiang Kai-Shek, gained control of the majority of Chinese territory by unseating warlords in several regions. Riding a wave of mounting nationalism, Chiang's priority was to undo the unequal treaties that had been in force since 1842. The ROC

---

[98] Ludwik Rajchman, "Report to the League of Nations," *National Medical Journal of China (Shanghai)* 13, no. 3 (1927): 288–92.
[99] LNHO, "Health Committee: Minutes of the Sixth Session," 20.
[100] Ibid., 20.
[101] Ibid., 20.

government's collaboration with the League of Nations can be understood as a way of counterbalancing the influence of foreign powers in China. Major imperial powers, including the United Kingdom, Japan, Russia, and France, had carefully carved out spheres of influence in China, and if any were to work with the ROC government, it ran the risk of offending the others. This division of power existed not only in treaty-port management, but also in the provision of health and medical services. Medical doctors in China, whatever their nationality, were divided into three camps: those who had received German or Japanese training and were largely employed by health organizations; those who had been trained in the British or American system, which included Grant and his students; and those, a small group, who had received French or Belgian training. Doctors from the different camps competed for influence vis-à-vis the Chinese Ministry of Health (reorganized into the National Health Administration [NHA] in 1931).[102] Each doctor hired was interpreted as a gain or loss of power, depending on the new employee's camp. As Grant recalled, "I myself belonged to what was called an Anglo-American group, regardless of what I tried to dub myself."[103]

Given the competition among the imperial powers in China, the LNHO's impartiality presented a unique opportunity for the NHA to reform the quarantine system while sidestepping doctors' rivalries. As Grant wrote in a letter to Heiser, "It is possible the League may be the best mechanism through which such technical help may be secured. Going through the League, provided the League did its job well, would or should have the advantage of impartiality."[104] In addition, as the LNHO represented its member states as a whole, the ROC could take back quarantine authority in every treaty port at once without negotiating with individual foreign powers. The political ramifications were significant. Tellingly, it was the ROC Ministry of Foreign Affairs, not the Ministry of Health, that wrote to Rajchman inviting him to carry out a "sanitary mission" in China.[105]

---

[102] Xi Gao, "Foreign Models of Medicine in Twentieth-Century China," in *Medical Transitions in Twentieth-Century China*, eds. Mary Brown Bullock and Bridie Andrews (Bloomington, IN: Indiana University Press, 2014), 173–211. In 1931, the Ministry of Health was reorganized as the National Health Administration and made part of the Ministry of the Interior.

[103] Oral History Research Department, Columbia University, "Reminiscences of Dr. John B. Grant (Vol. 2)," 250.

[104] John B. Grant, "To Victor Heiser (Personal)," March 30, 1931, RF/2,1931/601/61/501, Rockefeller Archive Center.

[105] Ka-Che Yip, *Health and National Reconstruction in Nationalist China: The Development of Modern Health Services, 1928–1937* (Ann Arbor, MI: Association for Asian Studies Incorporated, 1995), 116.

Chinese health officials, in addition to diplomats, also considered quarantine responsibilities to be an important sovereignty issue. In 1929, *Public Health Monthly* published an appeal to the Chinese minister of health, the authors of which were not named, demanding an official protest against the United States government's policy of sending its own medical officers to Shanghai to conduct quarantine meningitis controls on Chinese citizens departing for the United States. The appeal noted that the measure was "violating our country's sovereignty and harming our country's international reputation."[106] The authors of the appeal further requested the establishment of a quarantine service and improved public health infrastructure to eliminate any excuse the United States government might have for such an intervention. To the authors, public health infrastructure was a key way to recover the nation's sovereignty.

In 1929, Rajchman visited China again, this time to investigate the customs situation. He brought along his assistant, Frank Boudreau, an American statistician-epidemiologist.[107] Rajchman and Boudreau reviewed the health conditions in Shanghai and agreed to send experts to study the cholera epidemics there along with related quarantine regulations.[108] The LNHO then sent C. L. Park, chief of the quarantine division of the Australian Health Service,[109] to visit China on his way to Singapore, where he was to assume directorship of the Eastern Bureau. Park visited Chinese treaty ports in 1930 and proposed establishing a national quarantine service to facilitate the implementation of the 1926 International Sanitary Regulations.[110] Park also discovered during his visit that shipping companies were willing to contribute to medical investigations, and that the lack of port health officers in China needed to be remedied by sending officers on fellowships to European and North American ports.[111]

---

[106] Weisheng yuekan, "Wei qing xing wen kangyi Meiguo zhengfu weipai yiguan zai hu jianyi bing ken sushe haigang jianyi jiguan chen gaijin weisheng jianshe yi du jiekou you [Plea for Protest Against the US Government's Appointment of Medical Officers in Shanghai for Quarantine and for the Prompt Establishment of a Maritime Quarantine Authority to Improve Public Health Infrastructure so as to Eliminate Justifications]," *Weisheng yuekan [Health Monthly]* 2, no.7 (1929):32.

[107] ROC, "Proposals of the National Government of the Republic of China for Collaboration with the League of Nations on Health Matters," February 12, 1930, 7, C.118.M.38.1930.III, League of Nations Archives.

[108] Watt, *Saving Lives in Wartime China*, 43.

[109] Yip, *Health and National Reconstruction in Nationalist China*, 116.

[110] ROC, "Proposals of the National Government of the Republic of China for Collaboration with the League of Nations on Health Matters," 7.

[111] LNHO, "Health Committee: Minutes of the Seventeenth Session," August 1931, 14, C.398,M.160,1931, III., League of Nations Archives.

The same year, the Chinese ministries of finance and health and the Maritime Customs Service conferred and decided that the ROC government would establish the National Quarantine Service to take over the quarantine responsibilities that had previously been under the auspices of the Maritime Customs Service.[112] The new Service was put under the directorship of Wu Liande (Wu Lien-Teh), who had worked on controlling the 1910 plague epidemics in northern Manchuria and was a Chinese delegate to the LNHO. That same year, the LNHO paid for Edward B. Young (Yang Tingguang, also known as Yang Ting-Kwong), a graduate of the Detroit College of Medicine and Surgery and vice-superintendent of the quarantine hospital in Niuzhuang (Newchwang), to tour ports in Hamburg, Bremen, Amsterdam, London, Liverpool, New York, Baltimore, and New Orleans.[113] Young prepared lengthy reports on the quarantine measures of each port he had visited.[114] Upon returning to China, he took on the position of senior quarantine officer with the National Quarantine Service in Shanghai's Wusong (Woosung) port district.[115] Young's return to China coincided with the ROC gradually reclaiming quarantine responsibilities in treaty ports from foreign powers.[116] Moreover, the LNHO must have considered Young's tour successful as, in 1932, it organized eleven fellowships of three to six months for Chinese doctors to study abroad on subjects ranging from shipping fumigation to quarantine stations.[117]

Despite the conspicuous political motivations behind China's acceptance of the LNHO's involvement, their collaboration on quarantine reform itself was intended to be purely technical and administrative. Collecting statistics as a way of implementing quarantine measures fell perfectly into the category of technical collaboration, as statistics had the image of being indisputably factual. Through Park, Rajchman, and Boudreau's visits to China – and through Chinese doctors' fellowships in

---

[112] Song Zhiai and Jin Naiyi, "Woguo haigang jianyi shiwu yange [History of our country's maritime quarantine affairs]," *Zhonghua yixue zazhi [National Medical Journal of China (Shanghai)]* 25, no. 12 (1939): 1072.

[113] *The League from Year to Year, October 1st, 1929–September 30th, 1930* (Geneva: League of Nations Information Section, 1931), 109.

[114] Edward B. Young, "Individual Study of Port Medical Sanitation in Ports in Germany and Holland," 1930, R5906/8A/18366/10595, League of Nations Archives.

[115] The China Weekly Review, "Chinese Take Over Shanghai Quarantine Service," September 20, 1930, Millard Publishing House.

[116] Shanghai in 1930; Xiamen, Shantou, Yingkou, Andong, Wuhan in 1931; Tianjin, Tanggu, Dagu, Qinhuangdao in 1932; Guangzhou in 1936 (Song and Jin, "Woguo haigang jianyi shiwu yange [History of our country's maritime quarantine affairs]," 1072–1074).

[117] League of Nations Secretariat Information Section, *The League from Year to Year, October 1st, 1929–September 30th, 1930*, 132.

Europe – Chinese officials became familiar with the quarantine measures used in European ports and worked to maintain a similar standard. The National Quarantine Service implemented quarantine measures and collected related numbers on plague, cholera, smallpox, yellow fever, and typhus: the diseases specified in the 1926 International Sanitary Regulations. Keeping up with international standards also served as a counterargument to domestic resistance. In his speech celebrating the fourth anniversary of the National Quarantine Service, Wu Liande defended it against mounting doubts, especially those of transportation companies, by saying that "our Service does not take on any new policies, but merely complies with international regulations."[118] Through quarantine reform, Chinese ports were linked to the Eastern Bureau by cable and integrated into the network of the epidemiological intelligence service, where it was noted that "the gap which still existed in respect of information from China ha[d] been filled" and the ROC National Quarantine Service was "in a position to supply the Eastern Bureau with information."[119]

The LNHO's involvement in Chinese quarantine reform was an attempt to make the ROC health administration conform to LNHO standards, which was in line with Sydenstricker's plan to unify health administrations throughout the world so as to collect comparable statistics. Seeking to take back custom-tariff autonomy and gain control of its ports, the ROC government collaborated with the LNHO to devise a national epidemiological information system that served to communicate epidemic data among ports, national health administrations, and international organizations such as the LNHO and the OIHP. For the ROC, constructing such a system was a way to appear modern and present itself as a reliable partner to foreign powers so as to regain a level of sovereignty over its ports, which was the regime's top diplomatic priority. That strategy worked: between 1930 and 1932, most foreign powers ceded quarantine authority to the ROC's newly established National Quarantine Service.

The ROC government generally considered its partnership with the LNHO on quarantine reform to be successful. Telling proof was that the government again sought the League of Nations' support for general economic reconstruction. As a government representative wrote in a letter to the League of Nations in 1930:

---

[118] Wu Liande, "Haigang jianyi guanlichu di si nian zhi gongzuo [The Fourth Year of Work of the National Quarantine Service]," *Zhonghua yixue zazhi [National Medical Journal of China (Shanghai)]* 20 (1934): 131.

[119] Ibid., 136.

The Chinese government is impressed with the value of expert and disinterested service which the League had rendered in many parts of the World, and wishes to enlist its assistance in the immense task of Reconstruction [sic] in China. Conscious of the debt which the Chinese people already owes to the League of Nations for the advice of the Director and other officers of the Health Organisation, my Government believes that the time has come to seek the co-operation of other section[s] of the League.[120]

Nevertheless, there were lingering political sensitivities even in this type of technical collaboration, and both sides made efforts to avoid political interference that might affect their partnership. For instance, before taking on a position as a League correspondent in China, Robert Haas made a detour to Japan in 1935 to explain to the Japanese government that the League's collaboration with China was purely technical in nature.[121]

*

The construction of the LNHO's international epidemiological intelligence network illustrates the mechanism and process through which public health administration became globalized. And yet, as this chapter has illustrated, it was not simply a matter of handing down directives from the League's Geneva headquarters to the rest of world; rather, it was a patchwork resulting from negotiations between organizations and exchanges among tiered circles of experts with varying levels of capacity when it came to statistical collection. Public health officials had to travel to the places in question before epidemic statistics could circulate. Some of these officials were involved in drafting statistical standards, others took part in exchange programs, and some (Chinese) officials toured North Atlantic ports to learn about their health systems.

This patchwork also involved polities with different levels of sovereignty in an era of colonization. Public health officers working for the LNHO and the Rockefeller Foundation – such as Rajchman, White, Grant, and Heiser – contributed to carving out a space for epidemiological intelligence exchanges without directly touching upon sensitive geopolitics. In East Asia, the LNHO presented its epidemiological intelligence service as an alternative to the OIHP, distancing itself from the latter's focus on protecting Europe from imported epidemics. The relationship between the LNHO and the Chinese government epitomizes

---

[120] ROC, "To the League of Nations," August 2, 1930, 11-11-01-06-005, Archives of Ministry of Foreign Affairs of the Republic of China, Academia Sinica.
[121] Robert Haas, "Press Comments on the Arrival of M. Haas at Yokohama En Route to China," 1935, R5682/15062/980, League of Nations Archives.

how an international epidemic statistics exchange network came to be established against a backdrop of geopolitical tensions. The impartial nature of the League of Nations provided a unique solution for interwar China, which was seeking to free itself from the unequal treaties forced upon it by foreign powers. The Chinese government went along with the LNHO's plan, using the organization's resources to establish a national quarantine system not only to contain epidemics but also to comply with international standards so as to recover partial sovereignty. With the inauguration of the Chinese National Quarantine Service in 1930, collecting statistics and communicating them with the LNHO became routine work in Chinese ports, strengthening the LNHO–China statistical information network.

# 4  The Language of Policy-Making
Research and Advocacy through
Health Demonstrations

> The reduction of the death rate is the principal statistical expression and
> index of human and social progress. It means the saving and lengthen-
> ing of the lives of thousands of citizens, the extension of the vigorous
> working period well into old age, and the prevention of inefficiency,
> misery and suffering. These advances can be made by organized social
> effort. Public health is purchasable.[1]

The above passage is excerpted from an editorial in the *Monthly Bulletin of the Department of Health of the City of New York,* published in
July 1911. The author of the editorial (presumably Hermann Biggs, the
department's general medical officer)[2] calls for an organized effort to
improve public health and asserts that the death rate could serve as the
index of that improvement. As part of his effort to increase the budget
for health within the department, Biggs coined one of the most famous
adages in public health policy: "Public health is purchasable."[3]

This chapter traces how Biggs' motto was put into practice, from New
York State to China in the interwar years. In particular, it justified the
incorporation of vital and health statistics into budget calculations in
order to rationalize public health programs. To show that health was

---

[1] Department of Health, "Monthly Bulletin of the Department of Health of the City of
New York," October 1911 (New York: The Department of Health 1911), 226, https://
babel.hathitrust.org/cgi/pt?id=hvd.32044103093621;view=1up;seq=93.
[2] The phrase "health is purchasable" is commonly attributed to Hermann Biggs.
Nevertheless, the text that I read bore no trace of the author of the editorial.
[3] The famous phrase has had enduring appeal. It has often been cited by public health
experts from the time it was written to today. As recorded in the Milbank Memorial
Fund archives, the phrase "health is purchasable" was widely quoted in various speeches
from the 1910s to the 1940s. C. E. A. Winslow used it in his speech entitled "The
Economic Values of Preventive Medicine," given to the WHO's Fifth World Health
Assembly Technical Discussion in 1952. And public health publications of all sorts
continue to use it in their introductions (C. E. A. Winslow and Gunnar Myrdal, "The
Economic Values of Preventive Medicine [Fifth World Health Assembly Technical
Discussion]," Geneva: WHO, 1952. apps.who.int/iris/handle/10665/101988.)

"purchasable," Biggs persuaded the Milbank Memorial Fund to establish public health demonstrations in New York State: these were demarcated zones where a range of health services were implemented and their impact measured. The demonstrations included statistical collection and budget reporting, with the aim of proving not only that health was purchasable, but that investing in health was economically advantageous for local authorities. The demonstrations were therefore more than just a test-run for health services: they were small-scale health systems in which policies were integrated into a system whose financing and health outcomes were quantified and measured, as research by Martin Gorsky and Christopher Sirrs has defined.[4] The episodes related in this chapter can be considered early prototypes of the type of health system metrics that Gorsky and Sirrs describe.[5] I expand on their research by showing how the Milbank health demonstrations were transplanted to rural China, first by the Chinese National Association of the Mass Education Movement (MEM), and later emulated by the central government of the Republic of China in its public health research institute.

Drawing on archives from three continents, this chapter reveals the interwar transnational connections in the use of statistics in health system policy-making, both in terms of individual initiatives and the connection between them; these had previously sunk into historical obscurity.[6]

[4] Gorsky and Sirrs use the term "health system" to refer to a comprehensive structure in which all health-related items – including services, financing, and outcomes – are interconnected (Gorsky and Sirrs, "World Health by Place," 362–3.).

[5] The authors mention the United States Committee on the Costs of Medical Care (CCMC) as one of the potential forerunners of health system metrics (ibid.). Notably, the CCMC and the New York State demonstrations had several key actors in common, including Edgar Sydenstricker and the Milbank Memorial Fund itself.

[6] For accounts of the Milbank demonstrations, see, e.g.: Elizabeth Toon, "Selling the Public on Public Health: The Commonwealth and Milbank Health Demonstrations and the Meaning of Community Health Education," in *Philanthropic Foundations: New Scholarship, New Possibilities*, ed. Ellen Condliffe Lagemann (Bloomington and Indianapolis, IN: Indiana University Press, 1999), 119–30; Daniel M. Fox, "The Significance of the Milbank Memorial Fund for Policy: An Assessment at its Centennial," *The Milbank Quarterly* 84, no. 1 (2006): 5–36. Some rare exceptions on the Chinese end were: Iris Borowy, "Thinking Big – League of Nations Efforts Towards a Reformed National Health System in China," in *Uneasy Encounters: The Politics of Medicine and Health in China 1900–1937*, ed. Iris Borowy (Frankfurt am Main: Peter Lang, 2009), 205–28; Yi-Tang Lin, "Waiguo weisheng zuzhi yu Minguo huangjin shinian de gonggong weisheng shiyan: Dingxian xiangcun baojian xi tong yu zhongyang weisheng sheshi shiyanchu de Jiangning shiyanxian (1928–1937)" ["Foreign Health Organizations and Public Health Experiments during the Nanjing Decade: Ting Hsien Rural Health Experiment System and the Central Field Health Station's Jiangning County Experiment (1928–1937)"], *Yiliao shehuishi yanjiu [Journal of Social History of Medicine]* 3, no. 1 (2017a): 156–75.

I detail the implementation and appropriation of the health demonstration method in New York State, Ding Xian (or Ding County, historically known as Ting Hsien), and eventually other places in China, under the auspices of the Central Field Health Station (CFHS) – the research institute of the Chinese national health system – in collaboration with the League of Nations Health Organization (LNHO).

In the circuit of transference of health demonstrations and related statistical practices, experts who had been trained at the public health schools discussed in Chapter 2, and the LNHO officers introduced in Chapter 3, again took center stage. When LNHO statistician Edgar Sydenstricker returned to the United States from Geneva in 1924, he contributed statistical work to all three Milbank demonstrations and later used his Chinese connection to transplant Milbank's methods to the MEM's rural reconstruction program in Ding Xian, some 200 kilometers southwest of Beijing. Alumni of the Peking Union Medical College were eventually put in charge of reporting statistics from Ding Xian to their funding organizations in New York – first Milbank, and later the Rockefeller Foundation.

In both New York State and Ding Xian, public health staff working at different levels collected and communicated statistics to their partners and funding organizations. Both groups encountered similar difficulties and opted for comparable strategies when promoting their programs using statistics. There were discrepancies in both places as to whether such programs should be considered laboratories or demonstrations. The programs' founders first framed them as laboratories, since they were designed to test and tailor a financially feasible public health service for wider application; statistical reporting and budgeting were therefore at the core of the programs. Nevertheless, in both New York and Ding Xian, authoritative experts played salient advocacy roles while the numbers were still insufficient to make a strong case. Although a statistical collection system was considered indispensable when designing demonstrations, it was not indispensable for policy advocacy. In that regard, expert authority still held considerable sway. Experts from both programs were not ignorant users of statistics but were able to decide the extent to which they used statistics when advocating for their preferred policies. When the numbers did not support what their knowledge of public health work made them consider to be true, experts instead used their field knowledge to promote the demonstrations.

The final section of this chapter focuses on the CFHS and its demonstration areas. By collecting numbers, the CFHS generated an extensive array of quantified knowledge on public health, from chemical composition in nutrition to the cost of public health administration in

impoverished regions. And, yet again, CFHS officers wielded the authority to decide if the numbers collected in their demonstrations were applicable to real-world situations.

### "Health is Purchasable": The Background
### of the Milbank Demonstrations

When Albert Milbank took the helm of the 16-year-old Memorial Fund
from his cousin in 1921, the organization was a purely grant-giving one,
having contributed $2 million between 1905 and 1921 to other associa-
tions working in aid relief, public health, and education.[7] Albert Milbank
was more ambitious, adding his family name to the foundation's title and
appointing John Kingsbury to be its first full-time chief executive.[8]

Kingsbury was part of an inner circle of American progressive reformers. He was the director of the Association for Improving the Condition
of the Poor and was associated with the Charity Association Society,
the American Association for Labor Legislation and *Russell's Survey*
magazine.[9] When he started at the Milbank Memorial Fund, Kingsbury
brought with him both the core concerns and campaign methods of his
previous work, namely: the impact of medical costs on wage-earners'
family finances and advocacy that used statistical data to promote the
need for compulsory health insurance.[10] Under Kingsbury's directorship,
the Milbank Memorial Fund became a pioneer in the use of vital and
health statistical analysis (including the enumeration of births, deaths,
and disease cases, and the cost of health services) as a means of evaluating
the public health programs it funded. Unlike its contemporaries during
the 1920s – the Rockefeller Foundation, the biostatistics department of
the Johns Hopkins School of Public Health, and the LNHO – all of which
analyzed vital and health statistics to observe the evolution of a specific
epidemic or to research the efficacy of a public health technology (such
as vaccines),[11] the Milbank Memorial Fund was among the first to focus
on studying the costs of health and to research the complex social environment in which community health administrations had been operat-
ing since the early 1920s. It was not until the Great Depression that the
Fund's contemporaries likewise shifted focus partly to community health.

---

[7]  Milbank Memorial Fund, "Twenty-Five Years of Philanthropy," 1930, 1–2, IV/32/2
     Historical records, twenty-fifth anniversary: charts and tables, Milbank Memorial
     Fund Archives, University of Yale.
[8]  Fox, "The Significance of the Milbank Memorial Fund for Policy," 6.
[9]  Hoffman, *The Wages of Sickness*, 35–6.
[10]  Ibid., 39–41.
[11]  See Chapters 2 and 3 for statistical practices of the International Health Board and
     the LNHO.

Milbank and Kingsbury drew inspiration from the health demonstration in Framingham, Massachusetts, which was co-sponsored by the Fund and the Metropolitan Life Insurance Company.[12] Metropolitan Insurance's statistician, Dr. Lee K. Frankel, set up the Framingham demonstration in 1917, probably with an eye to designing health insurance policies, with support from the National Tuberculosis Association. The goal was to determine the possibility of lowering the number of tuberculosis cases through organized public health campaigns.[13] The Framingham demonstration was successful in delivering favorable statistics, as the tuberculosis death rate in the district declined from 121 cases per 100,000 inhabitants in 1909 to only 38 per 100,000 in 1916.[14]

Framingham's success laid the foundation for New York State Commissioner of Health Hermann Biggs to develop a comprehensive public health administration that would decrease the death rate not only from tuberculosis but from all causes. Biggs was a firm believer in the significant role of economic investment in improving health conditions. He contended that, as the tuberculosis mortality rate was declining both within and outside the United States, it would be difficult to achieve a result that could justify such expenditure based on tuberculosis case rates alone. Speaking in front of the Milbank Memorial Fund's advisory council, Biggs put the issue in financial terms:

[I]t is quite evident, I think, that we would not think of going into a community of 100,000 and spending $100,000 or $125,000 or $150,000 a year to reduce deaths from tuberculosis which amounted to only 75 or 100 a year; it is quite evident on the face of it that there is no reason to assume that in four or five years we could accomplish anything which would justify the expenditure of such sums as this.[15]

Biggs further added that a general health demonstration would help to determine the cost of sound public health administration in rural areas.[16]

---

[12] Armstrong, "The Framingham Health Tuberculosis Demonstration," 319.

[13] Michael E. Teller, *The Tuberculosis Movement: A Public Health Campaign in the Progressive Era*, Contributions in Medical Studies 22 (New York: Greenwood Press, 1988), 124. The Framingham demonstration included four major initiatives: i) X-ray screening for tuberculosis cases; ii) hospitals for conducting surveillance and managing tuberculosis patients; iii) visits by public health workers to schools and factories to examine sanitary conditions; and iv) community health education (John A. Kingsbury, "The Effect of the Anti-Tuberculosis Campaign," *The World's Health Monthly Review of the League of Red Cross Society* 6, no. 2 (1925): 63–70). The article is found in II/24/10 Kingsbury, John A. Speeches/ 1898-1925, Milbank Memorial Fund Archives, University of Yale.

[14] Teller, *The Tuberculosis Movement*, 124.

[15] Milbank Memorial Fund, "Minutes of Meeting of the Milbank Memorial Fund Advisory Council," November 16, 1922, 6, I/1/1 advisory council: minutes, proceedings and guests list, 1922 nov 16, Milbank Memorial Fund Archives, University of Yale.

[16] Ibid., 5–7.

His unspoken motivation was his pursuit of financial support for public health work. As the State Commissioner of Health Biggs was constantly troubled by the government's lack of financial support for health.[17] In 1920, his call for the creation of mobile units that would bring consultation services to rural parts of the state was turned down by the state legislature, which drove him to seek support from the Milbank Memorial Fund.[18]

In response to Biggs' appeal, the Fund launched health demonstrations in three areas in New York State.[19] The official principle of the demonstrations was to invest $2 million over five years to determine an appropriate means of advancing disease prevention and health conservation.[20] Kingsbury's speech during the Fund's fourth annual meeting in 1923 sheds light on the Fund's motivation for embarking on the health demonstration project:

If I were asked to indicate how this demonstration may be distinguished from others, I should be inclined to say by its *universality*. It deals with larger groups of population than other demonstrations, the character of the population is more varied. It has a greater diversity of population and environmental conditions. ... [T]hey deal with health not in its narrowest sense, but rather in its *broadest* social setting and social implication. The demonstration of the Milbank Fund may be called efforts at social control of physical and mental welfare.[21]

Although neither Biggs nor Kingsbury mentioned it explicitly, the capacity of statistics to aggregate different aspects under a single scale was key to realizing Biggs' goal of determining the financial needs for health,[22] as well as to Kingsbury's universalist vision that sought to comprehend health in its environment. By quantifying health status and social conditions and calculating them in terms of budget numbers, the Milbank demonstrations would be able to showcase a community health policy that was transferrable to other communities. It is thus unsurprising that statistics were at the center of discussions from day one of the demonstrations.

[17] Ibid.
[18] John M. Eyler, *Sir Arthur Newsholme and State Medicine, 1885–1935* (Cambridge: Cambridge University Press, 1997), 358.
[19] The fund selected three districts – Cattaraugus County, the City of Syracuse, and Bellevue-Yorkville – to serve as laboratories of public health administration in a rural county, an industrial city, and a metropolitan area, respectively.
[20] Milbank Memorial Fund, "Minutes of Meeting of the Milbank Memorial Fund Advisory Council," 5–7.
[21] Emphasis mine. John A. Kingsbury, "Progress in the Health Demonstration of the Milbank Memorial Fund," May 17, 1923, II/24/10 Kingsbury, John A. Speeches/ 1898–1925, Milbank Memorial Fund Archives, University of Yale.
[22] Espeland and Stevens, "A Sociology of Quantification," 408.

## Demonstrations or Laboratories?

The Milbank demonstrations were closely based on that in Framingham but attempted to correct one of the latter's flaws: a lack of statistical significance in its results. Although the tuberculosis mortality rate dropped over the course of the Framingham demonstration, Kingsbury informed the Fund's advisory committee that the small number of beneficiaries made it impossible to prove that it was the demonstration that had reduced the tuberculosis mortality rate.[23] Without explicitly citing him, Kingsbury was implicitly referring to the concept of statistical significance that originated in Karl Pearson's mathematical statistics. Pearson argued that, based on probability theory, any difference observed in a sampled population could be due to a sampling error. To determine if such a difference was "factual," he developed the chi-squared test method of statistical hypothesis testing.

The designers of the Milbank Fund's health demonstrations therefore selected areas with no fewer than 75,000 inhabitants, so that each was at least four times the size of Framingham.[24] The total population covered by the three demonstrations added up to half a million.[25] Site selection was critical, since the core principle of the demonstrations was to produce statistically significant results. The advisory committee eliminated nine potential test areas either because their populations were too small, their tuberculosis cases too few, or because hospitals were lacking.[26] Eventually, the committee selected Cattaraugus County as the rural health demonstration site. The tuberculosis mortality rate there had been more or less flat over the past ten years, which made it ideal for proving the effectiveness of the action undertaken. The population size was also ideal: large enough for achieving statistical significance without being too large for the available budget.[27]

Despite the supposed focus on statistical significance and determining the cost of public health administration, in its first two years, the Cattaraugus demonstration served merely to collect basic vital information

---

[23] John A. Kingsbury, "Executive Session Advisory Council of the Milbank Memorial Fund," March 13, 1929, 2, II/24/13 Kingsbury, John A. Speeches, 1928–1932, Milbank Memorial Fund Archives, University of Yale.

[24] Kingsbury, "The Effect of the Anti-Tuberculosis Campaign," 69–70.

[25] John A. Kingsbury, "Demonstrations and Official Agencies: An Address on the Upbuilding of Official Agencies in the Tuberculosis Campaign," June 22, 1923, 7, II/24/10 Kingsbury, John A. Speeches/ 1898–1925, Milbank Memorial Fund Archives, University of Yale.

[26] Milbank Memorial Fund, "Minutes of Meeting of the Milbank Memorial Fund Advisory Council," 10.

[27] Ibid., 11.

without any statistical research being conducted. When the demonstration was launched in 1923, statistics collection was placed under the responsibility of the tuberculosis bureau. It was not until the end of 1924 that the advisory committee recruited a full-time statistician to compile statistical data.[28] Prior to that, the Milbank Memorial Fund had relied on Otto R. Eichel, the head statistician at the New York State health department and an LNHO statistical veteran, to organize statistics collection at the demonstration sites.

Eichel subsequently called for all vital statistics collection to be put under the responsibility of a single director who would collaborate with the health department and the demonstration staff.[29] The recruitment process is a striking example of statisticians' low level of professionalization at the time.[30] Though the advisory committee agreed to hire a statistician, that did not mean a statistician with research skills; they saw the job as being one for a secretary familiar with bookkeeping techniques. They even proposed hiring someone who would split their time, working as both a secretary and a statistician. The Fund eventually hired a woman referred to in the minutes simply as "Miss Whitney" to compile vital records collected from the local authorities.[31] Although her job title was "statistician," Whitney's work was very close to bookkeeping, as she was also put in charge of correcting and arranging disease case files by age group.[32]

In 1926, Kingsbury delivered a speech at a health education conference that provided insights into how he navigated this fundamental discrepancy in the health demonstrations: they had been promoted as laboratories for determining the cost of public health services, but their statistical practices were only loosely organized. In his speech, Kingsbury explained that he preferred not to provide any statistics rather than give out faulty numbers. He stopped claiming that the Milbank

[28] C. E. A. Winslow, *Health on the Farm and in the Village: A Review and Evaluation of the Cattaraugus County Health Demonstration* (New York: The Macmillan Company, 1931), 2.
[29] Milbank Memorial Fund, "Minutes of Meeting of the Milbank Memorial Fund Advisory Council," 38.
[30] See, e.g.: Delphine Gardey, *Écrire, calculer, classer: comment une révolution de papier a transformé les sociétés contemporaines, 1800–1940* (Paris: Éd. La Découverte, 2008).
[31] Milbank Memorial Fund, "Memorandum of Matters Taken Up at a Meeting Between Dr. Williams, Mr. Folks, and Mr. Kingsbury at One O'clock on Monday, November 3, 1924, At Fraunces," November 3, 1924, 1, I/10/75 Technical Board minutes books 1924, Milbank Memorial Fund Archives, University of Yale.
[32] Milbank Memorial Fund, "Minutes of the Meeting of the Technical Board of the Milbank Memorial Fund," June 16, 1927, 398, I/10/77 Technical Board minutes books 1–4, pp. 303–636, 1926–1928, Milbank Memorial Fund Archives, University of Yale.

demonstrations were laboratories and instead referred to them as "demonstrations" in the true sense of the word, in that they served to illustrate the effectiveness of public health administration to county governments. He contended that, as the Fund had designed its demonstrations based on the Framingham demonstration, it was already certain that they were effective in reducing disease and death rates; their main purpose was actually to inspire similar policies in other places.[33] Indeed, probably thanks to Kingsbury's speeches and articles published in the *Milbank Quarterly Bulletin* – which had readers throughout the world – 266 public health workers came to visit the Cattaraugus demonstration in 1929. Among the visitors, 217 were from the United States, while forty-nine came from other twenty-one countries, including Australia, Siam, Spain, China, and Japan, to name a few.[34]

Biggs' successor as New York State Commissioner of Health, Matthias Nicoll, Jr., held the same view that the function of the demonstrations was not to determine a model through trial and error but to serve as a showcase of public health administration. As Nicoll observed:

The statistics don't demonstrate. ... It does not have any effect at all when it comes to a consideration of what it means to the average man in taxes, and until we demonstrate to that man that he is going to get benefit from these things to himself, not to his community or city so much, I think he is going to look on the tax bill and take his chance on death.[35]

Nicoll thus understood the importance of demonstrating the concrete benefit of a public health system to his constituents.

Kingsbury's change in discourse and Nicoll's testimony reveal that the Milbank demonstrations were driven by two contradictory rationales: one laboratorial and one demonstrative. The first was aimed at scientific discovery; the second valued political impact. At the discursive level, Kingsbury and Biggs stood firmly behind the former stance at first, describing health demonstrations as laboratories for determining financially feasible public health administrations. However, when

[33] John A. Kingsbury, "Fostering a Wider Application by Other Communities of the Methods and Practices Developed in the New York Health Demonstrations," April 9, 1926, 6, II/24/10 Kingsbury, John A. Speeches/1898–1925, Milbank Memorial Fund Archives, University of Yale.

[34] The twenty-one countries are Australia, Austria, Bulgaria, Canada, Ceylon, China, Denmark, England, France, Holland, Hungary, India, Italy, Japan, Jugo-Slavia, Mexico, Norway, Poland, Serbia, Siam and Spain. (Milbank Memorial Fund, "The Minutes of the Technical Board," February 14, 1929, 646, I/11/78 Technical Board minutes books 1–4, pp. 637–908, 1929–1931, Milbank Memorial Fund Archives, University of Yale.)

[35] Milbank Memorial Fund, "Verbatim Report of Speeches at Dinner Meeting of Advisory Council of the Milbank Memorial Fund," November 20, 1924, 26, I/1/5 Advisory council: dinner meeting transcripts extracts 1924 nov 20, Milbank Memorial Fund Archives, University of Yale.

statistical data remained insufficient over the first five years of the demonstrations, Kingsbury, as well as Nicoll, shifted to publicizing the demonstrations as awareness-raising tools for local authorities and residents. Despite this change in public discourse, in private Kingsbury did not abandon his belief in statistical analysis, and hired former LNHO statistician Edgar Sydenstricker first to tackle statistical analysis for the demonstrations and later to lead the Fund's research activities.

## Health Demonstrations as Social Experiments

The situation changed when the Milbank Memorial Fund partnered with Edgar Sydenstricker – at that time still a statistician with the USPHS – to analyze the statistical data produced by the health demonstrations. Sydenstricker was rigorous about using statistical analysis to support his arguments. He made the demonstrations' scientific value a priority over efforts to increase their political visibility.[36]

Sydenstricker aspired to transform social experiments into a fully-fledged branch of science. Blaming the scientific community's aversion to them on a lack of scientific rigor in such experiments, he strove to apply strict statistical methodology when analyzing social experiments himself. He embraced the idea that through meticulous statistical practices, the Milbank Fund's demonstrations could contribute to advancing the science of public health, writing:

Science too long has been ignorant in the field of social experiments, not because it can learn nothing, but because of a reluctance to regard the evaluation of the results of such experiments as essentially a part of the experimental method. In other words, we have not gone about the task in a scientific way.[37]

Sydenstricker thought principles drawn from laboratory experiments should be applied to the health demonstrations and presented various

[36] Sydenstricker was also concerned about the rapid rise in health care costs in the United States; he was one of the fourteen founding members of the CCMC, and also the person who brought the Milbank Memorial Fund's attention to the CCMC in the first place. Likely considering that it was the CCMC's responsibility, not the Fund's, to gather information about health care costs, Sydenstricker separated the Milbank health demonstrations from related policy campaigns and focused his statistical analysis on each public health action implemented in the demonstrations (Jonathan Engel, *Doctors and Reformers: Discussion and Debate over Health Policy, 1925–1950*, Social Problems and Social Issues [Columbia, SC: University of South Carolina Press, 2002], 21–2).

[37] Edgar Sydenstricker, "The Statistical Evaluation of the Results of Social Experiments in Public Health," *Journal of the American Statistical Association* 23, no. 161 (1928a): 156.

means of achieving that goal. According to Sydenstricker, a demonstration could not be regarded as a single experiment but as a group of experiments, and the results of each public health action should be measured separately.[38] He also suggested setting up control groups, either by measuring outcomes in other areas with similar populations and socioeconomic conditions, or in the demonstration areas after a certain time interval had passed.[39]

Sydenstricker's conviction that social experiments should follow a laboratorial model explains why he was reluctant to use existing statistics from the health demonstrations when he first began to work with the Milbank Memorial Fund. He did not consider bookkeeping to be scientific and disparaged Eichel and Whitney's work, contending that the Fund should have included a statistical service within its demonstrations from the outset.[40] On several occasions, Sydenstricker contended that more time was needed for the Cattaraugus demonstration to accumulate statistical data and obtain demonstrable results. During a technical board meeting in 1929, six years after the health demonstrations began, Sydenstricker insisted that he still did not think it was possible to make an appraisal from a statistical point of view and that such an appraisal could only be made after several years.[41] He stood firm on his principle of setting up control groups and insisted that the decreasing mortality rate did not prove the efficacy of the demonstrations in and of itself but was merely reference data that needed to be compared against future years.[42]

Despite Sydenstricker's reservations, the Fund's advisory committee was impatient to obtain an expert endorsement that would confirm the demonstrations' achievements. And so, just as Kingsbury had promoted their demonstrative value while statistics were still being collected, the Fund looked to another authority to validate its demonstrations – an established public health researcher. In 1929, the Fund paid

[38] Edgar Sydenstricker, "The Measurement of Results of Public Health Work: An Introductory Discussion," in *The Challenge of Facts: Selected Public Health Papers of Edgar Sydenstricker*, ed. Richard V. Kasius (New York: Prodist, 1974), 47–8.
[39] Ibid., 53.
[40] Milbank Memorial Fund, "Minutes of the Meeting of the Technical Board of the Milbank Memorial Fund," December 18, 1930, 822, I/10/78 Technical Board minutes books 1–4, pp. 637–908, 1929–1931, Milbank Memorial Fund Archives, University of Yale.
[41] Milbank Memorial Fund, "Minutes of the Meeting of the Technical Board of the Milbank Memorial Fund," May 28, 1929, 691, I/10/78 Technical Board minutes books 1–4, pp. 637–908, 1929–1931, Milbank Memorial Fund Archives, University of Yale.
[42] Milbank Memorial Fund, "Minutes of the Meeting of the Technical Board of the Milbank Memorial Fund," June 16, 1927, 397–8.

Charles-Edward A. Winslow, a distinguished professor and the founder of Yale University's department of public health, to conduct research on the three demonstrations.[43] Winslow accepted, though he stated openly that his research would be nothing more than a historical study that sought to make "an administrative, social appraisal of the undertaking."[44] Two years later, Winslow published a 400-page monograph on the Cattaraugus County demonstration that presented in detail its principles, programs, and budget. In the monograph, Winslow defended the substantial expansion of the demonstration's budget, which had been considered inappropriate given that financial feasibility was one of the demonstration's priorities. Winslow, however, decided that the high cost of the demonstration was standard for a rural health program, and that it showed that increased funding for rural health should be a top priority in public health work.[45] With an expert as distinguished as Winslow as its author, the monograph was an ideal piece of advertising for the Cattaraugus demonstration.

Sydenstricker eventually used Pearson's chi-squared test to demonstrate that the decline in the mortality rate in Cattaraugus County between 1925 and 1927 was not a mere sampling error. Applying the principle of control groups, Sydenstricker compared Cattaraugus' 1925–1927 data with data from three other counties with populations of roughly 50,000 that had set up tuberculosis sanitaria between 1900 and 1927; he also compared Cattaraugus' 1925–1927 data with its tuberculosis mortality rate between 1900 and 1922.[46] All statistical tests indicated that the drop in Cattaraugus' tuberculosis mortality rate during the demonstration (compared to the control groups) was statistically significant.[47] The Fund's demonstrations had finally obtained the type of results that Kingsbury had hoped for in 1922.

Kingsbury attached great value to Sydenstricker's dedication to statistics, likely more than he valued health demonstrations. In 1928, Kingsbury announced that the Fund would gradually withdraw from health demonstrations to concentrate on projects "which might have more

[43] Winslow originally asked for $25,000, which the Fund sought to reduce to $20,000. It is unclear how much the Fund eventually paid (Milbank Memorial Fund, "Minutes of the Meeting of the Technical Board of the Milbank Memorial Fund," October 7, 1929, 707–10, I/10/78 Technical Board minutes books 1–4, pp. 637–908, 1929–1931, Milbank Memorial Fund Archives, University of Yale).
[44] Ibid., 708.
[45] Winslow, *Health on the Farm and in the Village*, 231.
[46] Edgar Sydenstricker, "The Decline in the Tuberculosis Death Rate in Cattaraugus County," in *The Challenge of Facts: Selected Public Health Papers of Edgar Sydenstricker*, ed. Richard V. Kasius (New York: Prodist, 1974a), 376.
[47] Ibid., 373.

bearing on problems of wider territorial scope."[48] The Fund then created a research division with Sydenstricker at the helm. As head of the division, Sydenstricker's research had a dual focus: first, improving the quality of vital statistics and how public health activities were measured; and second, studying factors with a potential impact on mortality and morbidity rates, such as nursing services, maternal hygiene campaigns, and economic conditions.[49] He abandoned the demonstrations' original aim of evaluating health system as a whole and instead sought to evaluate individual public health actions.

## The Creation of a Chinese Public Health Laboratory

Coincidentally, the same year that Edgar Sydenstricker and the Milbank Memorial Fund shifted away from health demonstrations in New York, the seed was sown for a Cattaraugus-style demonstration in China. James Yen, founder of the Chinese National Association of the MEM, was traveling in the United States in 1928 in search of financial support for his association's rural reconstruction program in the county of Ding Xian. He considered the county to be a typical Chinese rural area and called the program a rural reconstruction laboratory that would be applied countrywide once proven effective. Swayed by John Dewey's theory that knowledge could be generated and tested only through experiments, Yen contended that, like a laboratory experiment, Ding Xian's rural reconstruction measures would produce data that would help in later efforts.[50] The county's entire population would be test subjects, and rural reconstruction efforts – including cultural programs, the introduction of

[48] Milbank Memorial Fund, "Minutes of the Meeting of the Technical Board of the Milbank Memorial Fund," December 20, 1928, 629, I/10/77 Technical Board minutes books 1–4, pp. 303–636, 1926–1928, Milbank Memorial Fund Archives, University of Yale.

[49] Sydenstricker listed the division's projects as follows: "1. Studies in the measurement of results of public health activities, to find out how successful certain public health activities or programs actually are. Not only in accomplishing their specific purposes, but in improving the health of the population; 2. Studies in vital statistics: to indicate and to collect statistical data for use in studying the results of public health activities in specific localities; 3. Nursing service; 4. Epidemiological field studies in Cattaraugus and Syracuse; 5. General survey in rural health 6. Disease and impairment of human life; 7. Population studies." (Milbank Memorial Fund, "Minutes of the Meeting of the Technical Board of the Milbank Memorial Fund," February 20, 1930, 750, I/10/78 Technical Board minutes books 1–4, pp. 637–908, 1929–1931, Milbank Memorial Fund Archives, University of Yale.)

[50] Barry Keenan, *The Dewey Experiment in China: Educational Reform and Political Power in the Early Republic* (Cambridge, MA: Council on East Asian Studies, Harvard University, 1977), 90.

advanced agricultural techniques, public health campaigns, and political education – would be experimental trials aimed at tackling poverty, ignorance, physical weakness, and civic disintegration, the four key problems faced by inhabitants of rural China, according to Yen.

Yen's idea of referring to Ding Xian as a laboratory of rural reconstruction bore an uncanny resemblance to the rhetoric used in the Milbank health demonstrations, which had also called its health demonstrations "laboratories" for determining the cost of health. Although there is no source proving that Yen's laboratory idea came directly from the Milbank Memorial Fund, it is undeniable that the Fund was one of the earliest sponsors of the Ding Xian health program. Specifically, Sydenstricker was probably the key person behind Milbank's support of the Ding Xian experiment. Sydenstricker had a special connection to China: he had been born into an American missionary family in China, and his sister, the writer Pearl S. Buck, had remained there. He and Yen had both attended Yale University, and the two men had probably crossed paths during Yen's 1928 fundraising tour in the United States. Another trace of the connection between the Milbank demonstrations and the Ding Xian program lies in the fact that the Fund referred to the latter as the "Chinese Cattaraugus," in reference to its health demonstration in Cattaraugus County.[51] Indeed, because the Ding Xian program involved designating a specific area for various rural reconstruction campaigns, it provided the ideal setting to implement a Milbank-style health demonstration in China, which would also test the feasibility of public health administration in a predetermined area before it was applied to other areas with similar conditions.

In the beginning, statistical collection in Ding Xian encountered a similar problem to the New York health demonstrations: a lack of administrative capacity on the ground. Sydenstricker arrived in Ding Xian in March 1930, six months after the official launch of the program, and his visit led the Milbank Memorial Fund to change its original plan. Sydenstricker had been planning to conduct a comprehensive statistical survey and tailor the Cattaraugus demonstration to China. But after conferring with staff in Ding Xian, he learned that the selection of the experimental site had been more or less random and that the statistical data produced was not trustworthy, let alone comparable to what had been collected prior to the MEM.[52] Although village elders regularly reported births

[51] Charles Wishart Hayford, *To the People: James Yen and Village China* (New York: Columbia University Press, 1990), 132.
[52] Edgar Sydenstricker, *The Proposed Public Health Program for Ting Hsien, China, of the Chinese National Association of the Mass Education Movement in Collaboration with the Milbank Memorial Fund* (New York: Milbank Memorial Fund, 1930), 28.

and deaths to the local government, they had not been trained to report comprehensively. It was extremely difficult to collect vital statistics for the health actions in Ding Xian.[53]

Not only did this situation disappoint the statistically-minded Sydenstricker, the overall situation in China made him realize that it would be impossible to construct a vital and health statistics apparatus there. Prior to Sydenstricker's trip, Victor Heiser of the Rockefeller Foundation had entrusted him with inquiring into the possibility of developing a practical, fit-for-purpose system for vital statistics collection in China.[54] Sydenstricker visited the Central Statistics Bureau and the National Health Administration (NHA) in Nanjing and eventually came to a pessimistic conclusion. In a memo to Heiser, he listed three essential conditions for the development of vital and health statistics: first, the government must be functional and provide support to collection staff; second, vital statistics must be seen as an essential government function; and third, statistics must be regarded as a social institution and a custom.[55] None of these conditions had been met in China at the time. Sydenstricker told Heiser that even if vital statistics collection gradually developed in China, it would not be well established for many years.[56]

Given these difficulties, Sydenstricker abandoned his efforts to implement systematic statistical collection in Ding Xian and gave up on the idea of transplanting the Cattaraugus demonstration to China.[57] He redirected the Milbank Memorial Fund's $10,000 donation to hospital construction in Ding Xian and adopted a more conservative goal, writing: "Proper provision should be made for measuring the results of the experiment" and adding, "It should be fully realized that these results cannot be attained in a few years."[58]

### Affordable Statistical Practices Through Local Connections

Despite Sydenstricker's decision to give up leading Ding Xian's statistical practices, the idea of making Ding Xian a "health demonstration"

---

[53] Victor Heiser, "Memo on the Conference with Sydenstricker," October 7, 1930, RF/2,1930/601/46/379, Rockefeller Archive Center.
[54] Victor Heiser, "A Letter to Sydenstricker," January 31, 1930, RF/2,1930/601/46/379, Rockefeller Archives Center.
[55] Edgar Sydenstricker, "Memo on Vital Statistics in China," October 21, 1930, RF/2,1930/601/46/379, Rockefeller Archive Center.
[56] Ibid.
[57] Heiser, "Memo on the Conference with Sydenstricker."
[58] Sydenstricker, The Proposed Public Health Program for Ting Hsien, China, 44.

area remained, at least nominally. When Chen Zhiqian (Ch'en Chih-Ch'ien, commonly known as C. C. Ch'en) – a former student of John B. Grant at the Peking Union Medical College – took over health work and related statistical practices in Ding Xian in 1931, he continued to claim to his sponsors in New York (i.e. the Milbank Memorial Fund and, later, the Rockefeller Foundation) that the Ding Xian rural reconstruction project was a "laboratory."

On a practical level, the Ding Xian project had evolved. Chen no longer aspired to collect statistics that would make Ding Xian a universally applicable model; instead, the program used statistics only to grasp the preliminary outcomes of public health work in the county. Chen came to prioritize financial feasibility in his statistical collection, and no emphasis was placed on setting up a collection model for other rural reconstruction programs.

Chen relied on Li Jinghan (Lee Ching-Han), the head of the MEM's survey department, to obtain information about household incomes and medical practices in Ding Xian. Li reported that the average family of five spent $1.50 per year on medical treatment, basically the cost of herbal medicine.[59] That put the average household budget for health care at only $0.30 per person annually; Chen therefore argued that people in Ding Xian could not afford a "modern" doctor.[60] And as relatively few people lived in the county seat, only a small percentage of inhabitants could take advantage of health services offered at the district- or subdistrict-level.[61]

Taking into account the socioeconomic and health conditions in Ding Xian, Chen came up with four ground-rules for a new system that would provide affordable health services to the community: "[The new health system] must be grounded in the village – the basic administrative unit of the districts; cost must be in accordance with the economic resources of the village; its basic personnel must come from the village; its proper functioning must be the responsibility of the village leadership."[62]

Chen also applied the above rules to his statistical practices. In order to keep costs low, he trained laymen to become village health workers and provide simple first-aid care to their fellow villagers as well as collect vital statistics. Though modestly paid, most of these workers were highly

---

[59] James Y. C. Yen, "Chinese Mass Education Movement, a Summary," 1934, RF/1/601/8/78, Rockefeller Archive Center.
[60] A "modern doctor" being one trained in Western medicine, as opposed to a practitioner of traditional Chinese medicine.
[61] C. C. Ch'en and Frederica M. Bunge, *Medicine in Rural China: A Personal Account* (Berkeley, CA: University of California Press, 1989), 76.
[62] Ibid., 76.

motivated and regarded the job as a great honor. Moreover, because they served in their own villages, their fellow villagers were more likely to accept their care and answer surveys. The simple first-aid care provided by village health workers was the first modern health care in the area.[63] Using village health workers not only solved economic difficulties, it also improved rural inhabitants' access to health care and understanding of scientific medicine. In the *Chinese Medical Journal*, Chen explained the principle upon which he had based his idea:

Recent public health administration has placed emphasis on expertise, and so people think vital statistics can only be entrusted to statistical experts, and school health education can only be undertaken by school health education experts. ... Since experts are expensive, the local society and economy cannot afford them, making such activities unsustainable. I therefore believe that rural health in Chinese conditions cannot be overly reliant on experts.[64]

Chen was a pragmatist: he preferred to channel all available resources – which were scarce – into actions themselves rather than collect statistics for research purposes. Statistical collection was thus of secondary importance to him. In an article written in Chinese, he insisted that collecting vital statistics would exhaust Ding Xian's limited resources.[65] Moreover, collecting reliable statistics required a well-designed system, which Ding Xian did not have. In a document prepared for the Rockefeller Foundation, Chen wrote:

It is true that we cannot be too ambitious about getting reliable figures in such a place where the statistical idea has never been developed in the minds of the people, and it is perhaps useless for us to devote too much time and energy to secure figures which may be of no practical importance.[66]

Chen may have accorded only secondary importance to statistical practices, but he did not hesitate to use terms like "research" and "science" in the English-language articles he wrote for the *Milbank Memorial Fund Quarterly*. In one, he stressed the experimental nature of the program, portraying it as being aimed at devising a public health system that was well adapted to rural China. He contended that "it would be a great contribution to the application of science in the whole country if

---

[63] Bullock, *An American Transplant*, 167.

[64] Translated from: Chen Zhiqian, "Hebei Dingxian shiyan xiangcun weisheng [Experimental Rural Health Program in Ding County, Hebei]," *Zhonghua yixue zazhi [National Medical Journal of China (Shanghai)]* 20, no. 9 (1934a): 1125.

[65] Chen Zhiqian, "Dingxian shehui gaizao shiye zhong zhi nongcun weisheng shiyan [Reform of the Rural Health Experiment in Ding County]," *Weisheng yuekan [Health Monthly]* 4 (1934b): 6.

[66] C. C. Ch'en, "Implanting Rural Health by the Mass Education Movement," n.d., 12, RF/1/601/7/69, Rockefeller Archive Center.

we could in the two years or so work out an adequate system of medical relief for the Chinese rural people."[67] In another article published in the same journal, Chen used death and birth rates to compare the health situation in rural China with that in the United Kingdom and the United States, countries that the Chinese authorities considered advanced. This led Chen to shift his focus from lowering death rates to lowering birth rates:

The average death rate is about twice that of England or the United States, but the birth rate is even higher. On the top of the already over-populated condition, there is still such an excessive number of births! For improvement of public health and of general socio-economic conditions, the reduction of birth rate is perhaps just as important in this country as the reduction of death rate, if not more so.[68]

Statistical reasoning led Chen's actions in this sense, as he understood vital statistics to be key indicators of the health conditions of a given population. Just as his teacher, Grant, had sought to lower death rates through public health actions, Chen attempted to lower birth rates through birth control education. Although the issues that Chen and Grant identified as the source of Chinese "backwardness" were different, the ways in which they used vital statistics to represent a given population's health and determine the most efficient way to improve it were extremely similar, if not identical.

One statistical calculation used by Chen that did not come from Grant's work at the Peking First Health Station (PFHS) was health cost per capita, which Chen calculated by taking the total expenses of health administration and dividing it by the number of local inhabitants. Chen's focus on health cost per capita reflected Milbank's work in Cattaraugus. Chen concluded that the per-capita cost of the Ding Xian program was even lower than the villagers' former annual spending on traditional health care; the program came to be known as the cheapest public health system of its time.[69] Chen's calculations were nonetheless controversial; Grant reflected that the low number might be due to a significant portion of the population never having obtained health services through the program.[70]

Despite Grant's reservations, the Ding Xian program became famous among its contemporaries thanks in part to Chen's low estimation of

[67] Ibid., 9.
[68] C. C. Ch'en, "Public Health in Rural Reconstruction at Ting Hsien," April 13, 1934, 6, RF/1/601/8/77, Rockefeller Archive Center.
[69] Ibid., 39.
[70] Oral History Research Department, Columbia University, "Reminiscences of Dr. John B. Grant (Vol. 3)," 1961, 132, RF/13/2/3, Rockefeller Archive Center.

its cost per capita. Chen's design for collecting vital statistics inspired several similar registration systems in China. Specifically, his method shifted the focus away from the use of a central statistical authority with specialized inspectors that aimed to collect statistics throughout its jurisdiction, and toward the reinforcement of local organizations of all grades that relied solely on health care providers and laymen's reporting.[71] In so doing, Chen renounced any claim to scientific rigor in his statistical practices, instead making use of local social connections. Xu Shijin (Hsu Shih-Chin), another of Grant's students and a vital statistician who organized statistics collection in various localities from the 1930s, also agreed on the importance of local connections. As he noted when he visited Ding Xian and other experimental collection sites: "with well-organized local organizations, vital statistical collection is not very difficult."[72]

## Statistics as Fundraising Jargon: Yen and Chen's Uses of Statistics

Perhaps equally as impactful as Chen Zhiqian's use of village health workers in the Ding Xian program was James Yen's fundraising rhetoric. In every report and speech to his philanthropic sponsors, Yen consistently described Ding Xian as a laboratory for studying rural China. Calling it a "typical Chinese rural area," Yen claimed the results achieved at Ding Xian would help tailor reconstruction measures to rural China while also serving as model for similar areas elsewhere.[73] By using the term "laboratory," Yen contended that the numbers collected at Ding Xian gave the project with universal implications. He used statistical analysis to bolster his claim that the MEM's rural reconstruction measures were feasible throughout rural China; moreover, with statistical backing, the model tested in Ding Xian was expected to provide a relevant model for rural reconstruction work throughout the world.

Chen's use of statistics in his English-language reports and articles, as presented in the previous section, resonated with Yen's discourse. Although Chen was aware that the statistics collected in Ding Xian were of questionable quality, he did not hesitate to cite them in his reports to various sponsors, including the Milbank Memorial Fund and the

---

[71] This was a counterexample to I. C. Yuan's design for the PFHS.
[72] Translated from: Xu Shijin, "Wo ruhe banli weisheng tongji [How I Implemented Public Health Statistics Collection]," *Fuwu yuekan [Service Monthly]* 2, no. 3–4 (1929): 18.
[73] Yen, "Chinese Mass Education Movement, a Summary"; Pearl S. Buck, "Tell the People: Mass Education in China" (American Council Institute of Pacific Relations, 1945), Family/2.OMR/G/3/16, Rockefeller Archive Center.

Rockefeller Foundation.[74] This optimistic vision contrasted, however, with the blunt observations of a health worker charged with collecting statistics, which were published in a Chinese public health journal:

People thought the world was going to the dogs again. They thought the government was either enlisting young men or increasing taxes as in the past. They could not imagine any other reason why the authorities would want to know how many people were in their families, and how many were male or female. ... In reaction, they either responded that there was no one at home, or locked their doors and left their houses through the back door; those who could not manage to escape would simply respond to questions with ambiguous answers. When they responded, health workers had to treat their brush-offs as scientific material, how ridiculous is that?[75]

Furthermore, despite Yen's assertion that Ding Xian represented a "typical Chinese rural area," in reality the MEM's choice of rural reconstruction site was essentially random and based on local connections.[76] In a report submitted to the Rockefeller Foundation, Yen contended that Ding Xian had been chosen based on a social survey that had concluded the county to be a "typical" rural area with a population size well suited to such an experiment.[77] In fact, no preliminary study had been made when the MEM moved into Ding Xian in 1926. Moreover, when the MEM launched its integrated rural reconstruction actions in 1929, only one study had been conducted in the area, covering only 400 families, or approximately 0.5% of the county's population.[78] How could the MEM have concluded that Ding Xian was "typical"? Yen spoke frankly in an interview with Pearl S. Buck in 1945: "One other reason why we went to Ting Hsien [Ding Xian] was that there was a famous old civil-service examination hall of Sung architecture. The gentry told us that if we

---

[74] C. C. Ch'en, "Scientific Medicine as Applied in Ting Hsien: Third Annual Report of the Rural Public Health Experiment in China," *The Milbank Memorial Fund Quarterly Bulletin* 11, no. 2 (1933): 97–129; "Public Health in Rural Reconstruction at Ting Hsien: Fourth Annual Report of the Rural Public Health Experiment in China," *The Milbank Memorial Fund Quarterly* 12, no. 4 (1934): 370–8; "The Rural Public Health Experiment in Ting Hsien, China," *The Milbank Memorial Fund Quarterly* 14, no. 1 (1936): 66–80; "Ting Hsien and the Public Health Movement in China," *The Milbank Memorial Fund Quarterly* 15, no. 4 (1937): 380–90.
[75] Translated from: Wu Zhengji, "Dao min jian qu! Banli xiangcun weisheng de kunnan [Go to the People! The Difficulties in Implementing Rural Health Programs]," *Weisheng yuekan [Health Monthly]* 1–2 (1935): 109.
[76] Buck, "Tell the People: Mass Education in China," 15.
[77] Yen, "Chinese Mass Education Movement, a Summary."
[78] The study was conducted by Sidney Gamble (1890–1968), the grandson of one of the founders of Procter & Gamble and a graduate of Princeton who was involved in the YMCA's social work in China (Sidney David Gamble, *Ting Hsien: A North China Rural Community* [New York: Institute of Pacific Relations, 1954], 23).

would come to Ting Hsien they would give us that hall for our headquarters. I could not resist it."[79] Yen had never mentioned this fact during the interwar years, when the project was still ongoing. To his sponsors, Yen always advertised it as a scientific endeavor. Even though the Ding Xian experiment was largely dependent on personal connections and local networks, these were seldom mentioned in progress reports submitted to the Rockefeller Foundation.

As with the Milbank health demonstrations, no matter how much effort was put into presenting Ding Xian as a laboratory, the project became famous largely because of Yen's eloquence, which charmed the program's sponsors. Statistical data eventually became of secondary importance. From the outset, the Ding Xian demonstration had never lacked attention; it was "swamped with visitors" from both within and outside China.[80]

### The CFHS: Statistics for Chinese National Health Research

The Ding Xian demonstration and its statistical practices left their mark on the Chinese national health system. One concrete result was the creation of the CFHS by the NHA. The CFHS was China's first national health research institute, with demonstration areas for testing the economic feasibility of different policies. Statistical practices at the CFHS served for more than just demonstration, however. Thanks to the financial and technical support of the LNHO, the Station had the expertise and facilities to collect all sorts of quantified data, on everything from bacteria to social levels, in order to establish a picture of public health in China.

The work of the CFHS is representative of the process by which actors with different aims came together, with their visions crystallizing into distinctly different statistical practices within the Chinese national health system. The Station's principal designer was Liu Ruiheng (J. Heng Liu), the director of the NHA. In a draft submitted to the League of Nations Health Committee, Liu envisioned the CFHS as the nucleus of Chinese public health administration and policy.[81] Its work would include social hygiene and bacteriological research; it would be composed of ten departments,

---

[79] Buck, "Tell the People: Mass Education in China," 26.
[80] G. E. Hodgmen, "To M. Beard," June 13, 1931, RF/1/601/7/70, Rockefeller Archive Center.
[81] LNHO, "Health Committee: Minutes of the Sixteenth Session," December 1930, C.627,M.248,1930, III., League of Nations Archives, 58.

ranging from sanitary engineering to health education and vital statistics; and it would run experiments in three areas with varying levels of urbanization where it could test the outcomes of public health actions.

Liu was pragmatic when it came to geographic scope. He argued that the NHA could not establish an institution in charge of public health research and actions covering the entire Chinese territory right away; instead, he supported concentrating research and policies on a given area in China. The CFHS would work with local authorities to devise its three experimental areas: a rural area (Tangshan), an urban area (a district of Nanjing), and the entirety of Jiangning County.[82] Much like the New York and Ding Xian demonstrations, the CFHS demonstrations would involve public health campaigns and investigations in the experimental areas to gather facts, based on which the CFHS would "furnish the central authorities with the data on which to base the future health policy for the country."[83] The NHA hoped that, after some years of work, the Station could be reorganized into a national field health service and be put in charge of setting public health policy for all of China.[84] After organizing a consultation with participants in the Conferences of Directors of Schools of Hygiene, mostly based in Europe,[85] the LNHO agreed on a total budget of $514,640 for the first three years, of which $138,000 was allocated annually to each of the three experimental areas.[86] Director-General Ludwik Rajchman gave a speech during his 1930 visit to China in which he explained why the LNHO was backing the CFHS:

[I]t would be doubtful wisdom to elaborate a general scheme of sanitary reconstruction for the whole country in the absence of reliable data as a basis. Accurate information must be sought by means of exploration and surveys, while a tentative application of preliminary schemes in selected localities should reveal appropriate measures of solving numerous health problems.[87]

---

[82] Ibid., 91.
[83] Republic of China, "Proposals of the National Government of the Republic of China for Collaboration with the League of Nations on Health Matters," 44.
[84] LNHO, "Annual Report of the Health Organisation for 1929," July 1930, 15–16, A.9.1930.III, League of Nations Archives.
[85] There are no direct sources indicating which countries participated in the 1930 conference. However, the conference report includes work from public health schools in seven European countries: Czechoslovakia, France, Germany, Great Britain, Hungary, Poland, and Yugoslavia (LNHO, "Report on the Work of the Conferences of Directors of Schools of Hygiene, Held in Paris, May 20th to 23rd, 1930; and in Dresden, July 14th to 17th, 1930," 1930, C.H. 888, League of Nations Archives).
[86] John B. Grant, "To Victor Heiser: Three Year Plans for the Chinese National Health Service," April 25, 1931, RF/2,1931/601/61/501, Rockefeller Archive Center.
[87] Ludwik Rajchman, "Proposals of the National Government of the Republic of China for Collaboration with the League of Nations on Health Matters – Secretary General Speech," February 13, 1930, 10, R5906/8A/18022/10595, League of Nations Archives.

Combining laboratory research and social surveys, the CFHS was designed to further science and take concrete action at the same time. However, it remained unclear how those two goals were to be balanced, even to public health workers at the time. The confusion surrounding the name of the Station is a case in point: whereas the LNHO was satisfied with the name "Central Field Health Station," the Rockefeller Foundation officers usually referred to it as the "National Institute of Health," and its Chinese name, literally translated, was the "Central Bureau of Experiments on Public Health Measures."[88] This is indicative of the different ways that these different entities understood the Station. The LNHO's name stressed the importance of public health actions in the field; the Chinese name focused on the experimental element, which included both action and science; and the Rockefeller Foundation's radically different wording suggests that they saw it primarily as a research institute. Experts were aware of the confusion surrounding the name. Marshall Balfour, a Rockefeller officer in China, once complained bitterly that "Central Field Health Station" was another League of Nations misnomer, since the Station actually acted as the technical branch of the NHA, similar to the United States National Institute of Health vis-à-vis the United States Public Health Service.[89]

Balfour's understanding was not entirely correct, as he was unaware of the Eastern European social medicine tradition that had inspired the CFHS, which would explain the use of "Field Health" in the name.[90] The CFHS was clearly based on the Institute of Social Medicine in Zagreb; Berislav Borčić, the LNHO expert involved in designing the CFHS, had once worked for the Zagreb institute and had experience implementing rural health services focused on empowering local communities in Croatia.[91] Borčić arrived in China in 1930 and visited Ding Xian, Beijing, and Tianjin to familiarize himself with the country's situation.[92] Riding

---

[88] In Chinese: 中央衛生實驗院, Zhongyang weisheng shiyanyuan.
[89] Marshall Balfour, "Marshall C. Balfour's Diary," May 22, 1939, RF/12 Officers' Diaries/12/23, Rockefeller Archive Center.
[90] For more on Eastern European social medicine, see, e.g.: Lion Murard, "Designs within Disorder: International Conferences on Rural Health Care and the Art of the Local, 1931–1939," in *Shifting Boundaries of Public Health: Europe in the Twentieth Century*, 141–173.
[91] B. Johan, "To Boudreau," March 6, 1930, R5906/8A/18366/10595, League of Nations Archives. It is interesting to note that the LNHO sent the Institute's founder and one of its doctors (Andrija Štampar and Berislav Borčić) to oversee the LNHO's involvement in Chinese public health. Štampar was tasked with establishing basic health structures in the northwestern and southern provinces, Borčić with setting up the CFHS (Ludwik Rajchman, "To Borcic," May 22, 1930, R5906/8A/18807/10595, League of Nations Archives; LNHO, "Report to the Council on the Work of the Twenty-First Session of the Health Committee," 16).
[92] LNHO, "Health Committee: Minutes of the Sixteenth Session."

the wave of the MEM's rural reconstruction efforts, the Zagreb model, which correlated public health with living standards while emphasizing local communities' participation, was well received by Chinese experts. The convergence of the Eastern European tradition and the Chinese rural reconstruction movement popularized the concept of a public health framework that aimed to mobilize local communities.

The CFHS was established in September 1932. In the end, Borčić's design did not differ from Liu's original proposal: the CFHS was to conduct a wide range of activities, such as collecting vital statistics, controlling epidemics, conducting chemical analysis on food and pharmaceutical substances, building sanitary engineering infrastructure, training public health workers, and improving local health services. Its three experimental health areas would serve as the testing grounds for these functions.[93]

Collection of quantified facts was at the center of these disparate activities. The CFHS relied on statistics for its core missions to: 1) gain an understanding of the health situation and lifestyles in its experimental areas; 2) document its activities; 3) assess the results and financial feasibility of public health services; and 4) document the laboratorial results. A table from the Station's 1936 annual report (see Table 4.1) shows these four categories of statistics and gives a general picture of how each CFHS department used them and which types of content were presented in quantified language.

The first core mission (collecting statistics to grasp health situations) resembled Grant's work at the PFHS, presented in Chapter 2. Specifically, the CFHS vital statistics department was responsible for collecting statistics from hospitals and health units and analyzing them using machines (see Figure 4.1). The presentation of vital and health statistics was very much in line with the standards of the time, e.g. birth and death rates categorized by common criteria such as sex, age, and cause of death. Xu Shijin, the head of the department during its first five years, had received a standard education in vital and health statistics: he had been trained by Grant at the PFHS from 1926 to 1929, during which time he was associated with the compilation of the Chinese International Classification of Diseases, and subsequently spent one year at the Johns Hopkins School of Public Health in 1929. Before joining the CFHS, he was in charge of statistics collection at the Shanghai Municipal Health Bureau, from 1930 to 1932.[94] Xu designed initiatives for collecting data on the numbers of births, deaths, and patients with communicable

---

[93] J. Heng Liu and P. Z. King, "Annual Report of the Central Field Health Station: For the Year Ending December 31, 1936" (National Economic Council, 1937), R5682/50/19116/980, League of Nations Archives.

[94] Ibid., 60.

Table 4.1 *Categories of statistics presented in the annual report of the CFHS\* for the year ending December 31, 1936\*\**

| Department | Categories of statistics | Items |
|---|---|---|
| Vital statistics service | Vital and health statistics; lifestyle | • Notifiable disease cases<br>• Age group of communicable disease cases among hospital patients<br>• Birth and death numbers/rates<br>• Death rates by sex/age group<br>• Death rates by cause<br>• Death rates by age group<br>• Maternal deaths<br>• Blindness<br>• Medical expenses |
| | CFHS activity numbers | • Hospital reports received<br>• Hospital inpatient and outpatient cards<br>• Health records of school children received<br>• Questionnaires received regarding maternal deaths |
| | Health service costs | • Registration cost per capita |
| Prevention and control of epidemic diseases | CFHS activity numbers | • Door-to-door fumigation campaign (burrows, rooms, communicating holes)<br>• Rat-proofed food containers and food shops<br>• People vaccinated<br>• Plague investigation stations established<br>• Counties receiving vaccination training<br>• Calf lymph doses<br>• Strain numbers of *B. typhosus* under study<br>• Samples of sputum collected<br>• Bacteriological and parasitological examinations |
| | Laboratory results | • Rat index<br>• *Clonorchis sinensis* infections among freshwater fish<br>• Tuberculosis positivity rate<br>• Serological examination results |
| Investigation and control of parasitological diseases | CFHS activity numbers | • Free kala-azar treatments provided<br>• Quinine tablets distributed<br>• Villages covered by sandfly distribution survey<br>• Malaria epidemic areas visited<br>• Children examined for spleen and parasite indices<br>• Mosquito breeding places (number, surface area) under control<br>• Patient visits to clinics<br>• Stool specimens under examination<br>• Snails killed |

Table 4.1 (*cont.*)

| Department | Categories of statistics | Items |
|---|---|---|
| | Laboratory results | • Kala-azar infection rate for three species of sandflies<br>• Spleen indices, parasite indices<br>• Percentage of positive schistosome ova of examined stool specimens<br>• Kala-azar infected villages and infection rate |
| Drug studies, manufacture, and control | Vital and health statistics; lifestyle | • Pharmaceutical products sold |
| | CFHS activity numbers | • Foods and drinks under review<br>• Total samples of native common salts<br>• Samples received for chemical examination |
| | Laboratory results | • Percentage of drugs and patented medicines meeting pharmacopeia standards<br>• Chemical examination results<br>• Source and fluorine contents of common salt samples |
| Sanitary engineering and environmental sanitation | Vital and health statistics; lifestyle | • Percentage of huts built from earth and straw |
| | CFHS activity numbers | • Latrines constructed and holes dug<br>• Houses improved (plastering or whitewashing, skylights, ventilation)<br>• Experimental wells<br>• New refuse containers<br>• Wells and latrines examined<br>• Water and sewage analyses conducted<br>• Shops inspected<br>• Equipment manufactured (surgical instruments, full and partial leg prostheses for crippled soldiers) |
| | Health service costs | • Construction cost of bore-hole latrines<br>• Construction cost of reinforced mud walls (0.5 m thick and 1.5 m high)<br>• Housing improvement costs |
| | Laboratory results | • Parasitological survey results<br>• Percentage of ascariasis and hookworm infection among children<br>• Percentage of helminthological infestation (any type) among children |
| Promotion of school health | CFHS activity numbers | • Participants in national school health conference<br>• Staff sent to schools; students covered<br>• National Boy Scout camps<br>• First-aid kits distributed to students |

| Department | Categories of statistics | Items |
|---|---|---|
| Popular health education and preparation of teaching materials | CFHS activity numbers | • Total materials distributed (posters, charts, models, molds, specimens, slogans, photos)<br>• Specimens produced<br>• Summary of publications<br>• Public health education and propaganda produced (radio shows, news items, visitor groups, exhibitions, health talks, lantern-slide and movie shows) |
| Industrial health | CFHS activity numbers | • Reports on factory provision of health care<br>• Analysis of attendance numbers: Yungli Ammonia and Acid Plant health service |
| Training of health personnel* | CFHS activity numbers | • Publications in the library<br>• Summary of training courses given<br>• Fellowships awarded |
| Promotion of health service | CFHS activity numbers<br><br>Laboratory results | • Counties with new health organizations<br><br>• Results of examination of stool and blood samples collected from army hospitals and field clinics |

*Source:* J. Heng Liu and P. Z. King, "Annual Report of the Central Field Health Station: For the Year Ending December 31, 1936" (National Economic Council, 1937), R5682/50/19116/980, League of Nations Archives
* The numbers regarding other organizations that partnered with the CFHS have been excluded from this table.
** Some item names have been edited for clarity.

diseases in the experimental areas. Much as Grant had done at the PFHS, the police, medical practitioners, and midwives were put in charge of reporting births, deaths, and cases of communicable diseases in Jiangning County. To ensure the quality of the data collected, these individuals were given statistical training.[95] In its 1936 annual report, the CFHS proudly described the reporting system it had constructed: some 1,000 hospitals regularly submitted patient numbers for nine notifiable diseases, 204 of which also sent in numbers on nineteen communicable diseases.[96] Quantified data on inhabitants' lifestyles – such as the quantity of pharmaceutical products sold and the percentage of habitations consisting of straw-and-mud huts – were also collected by other departments.

In addition to the routine collection system, Xu calculated birth and death statistics that reflected the socioeconomic context. The NHA, for

[95] Ibid., 1.
[96] Ibid.

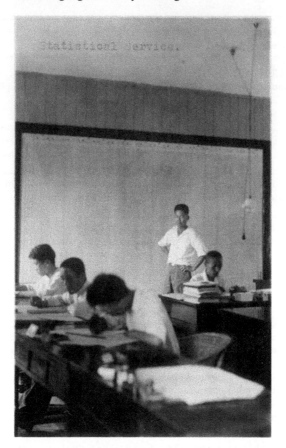

Figure 4.1 Statistical service of the Central Field Health Station. "Photo of Statistical Service," n.d., CMB.Inc/1048/25/302, Rockefeller Archive Center. Courtesy of Rockefeller Archive Center.

instance, conducted an infant mortality investigation in Nanjing by visiting families with babies born in the past year.[97] The report used pivot tables that showed how infant mortality varied depending on the parents' occupations, the monthly household revenue, and the newborn's birth order.[98] These pivot tables were purely descriptive, as Xu did not conduct mathematical tests to gauge the sampling error. Presenting his

[97] Xu Shijin and Wang Zuxiang, "Nanjing shi yinger siwanglu diaocha [Infantile Mortality Investigation in Nanjing City]," *Gonggong weisheng yuekan [Public Health Monthly]*, no. 4 (1935): 23–7.
[98] Ibid.

statistics as facts, Xu relied on his knowledge of infant care to make sense of the differences in numbers. His arguments included: families with higher incomes had the benefit of specialized facilities for infant care; the first two children born suffered from the mother's lack of experience and thus had a higher mortality rate; and heightened mortality rates for children born fifth or later were due to the mother being unable to take care of so many children. Sometimes Xu simply let the statistics stand: "it is not easy to explain why the infant mortality rate [for children with parents working] in the transportation sector was only 106.2 per thousand."[99]

Almost all CFHS departments used numbers to show the scope of their activities. The statistics were so diverse, and sometimes focused on such minor aspects of the Station's activities, that it is difficult to list them all succinctly (see Table 4.1). Some of the information was of the type commonly reported for public health actions at the time, including vaccination numbers, number of facilities and other infrastructure constructed, number of schools, children, samples, shops and factories surveyed, as well as the number of samples of salts, food, and food smears collected. But numbers were also collected on the materials used in public health work, which was less common. In a section entitled "Popular Health Education and Preparation of Teaching Materials," the 1935–6 report chronicles the number of posters, charts, models, molds, specimens, posters, slogans, photographs, etc. that had been produced and distributed.[100]

The third type of statistical practices employed at the CFHS were for evaluating the results and economic feasibility of public health services, including health administration structures, vital statistic registration, and sanitary infrastructure. In terms of health administration, this strongly resembled the Ding Xian program. Although no source indicates a direct connection between Ding Xian and the CFHS, it is worth noting that Xu and Chen were both students of Grant at almost the same time, and it is certain that they knew each other and were informed of each other's work. Specifically, the CFHS copied Ding Xian's three-tiered public health model for its Jiangning demonstration area, and Xu was tasked with designing statistical investigations to gauge the model's feasibility. He concluded that public health administration in Jiangning was economically feasible, given that health expenses per capita were only $0.10 and were paid by the local population and the

[99] Ibid., 25.
[100] Liu and King, "Annual Report of the Central Field Health Station: For the Year Ending December 31, 1936," 33–7.

county government.[101] Xu conducted the same investigation in Tang-shan, the CFHS's rural experimental area. Having obtained favorable results, the CFHS promoted the three-tiered model to provincial governments.[102] It should be noted that favorable statistical results did not directly translate into concrete action. CFHS officers were aware of the significant difference in administrative capacity between the demonstration areas and the other places, and that the Tangshan experiment's success was thanks to the additional administrative capacity that most provincial governments did not have. They thus did not insist on the tiered system being fully implemented in other provinces, only the aspect of using county hospitals as local health centers. By 1934, the CFHS had set up health centers at thirty-five locations in eight provinces.[103]

Just as in Ding Xian, vital statistics investigation was itself the subject of financial examination by the CFHS. In 1934, the CFHS hired eighteen investigators to collect vital statistics in Jurong, a small county near Nanjing. With the help of local gentry, the investigators concluded after one month that Jurong had 280,000 inhabitants, and that the cost of investigation per capita was 0.005 Chinese silver dollars.[104] Starting in 1935, Xu was also mandated to devise a vital statistics collection system in the city of Nanjing. He devised a system with nine statistical investigators acting as intermediaries between the police in charge of civil registration and health service providers; these investigators were responsible for verifying and synchronizing the reports sent in by health service providers that had municipal civil registration records. Xu's collection system cost the government 5,040 silver dollars annually, with each birth or death reported costing 0.12 silver dollars.[105] After carrying out vital statistics collection in Nanjing, Jurong, and other counties, Xu concluded that the key to successful collection was to mobilize communities. When the local community was involved, vital statistics collection was not particularly difficult.[106] Xu thus reached a similar conclusion to

[101] Berislav Borcic, "Public Health Activities in China From 1929–1935," November 23, 1935, 16–17, r/5711/50/21438/6501, League of Nations Archives.
[102] Ibid., 17.
[103] Yip, *Health and National Reconstruction in Nationalist China*, 57.
[104] Xu Shijin, "Shiban Jurong xian shengming tongji ernian lai gaikuang [Two Years after Implementing Vital Statistics Collection System in Jurong]," *Gonggong weisheng yuekan [Public Health Monthly]* 1–6 (1936): 153.
[105] Xu Shijin, "Nanjing shi shengming tongji lianhe banshichu diernian gongzuo baogao [The Second Annual Report of the United Vital Statistical Office of Nanjing City]," October 1936, 10, Shanghai Library.
[106] Xu Shijin, "Wo ruhe banli weisheng tongji [How I Implemented Public Health Statistics Collection]," 18.

Chen's in Ding Xian, where village health workers were used instead of highly trained experts.

Xu's method had a limited impact, as the Second Sino-Japanese War broke out shortly afterward. A report published in 1937 by Jin Baoshan and Xu himself found that funding for vital statistics in provincial capitals and special municipalities represented a mere 0.6–2.0 percent of their total budgets.[107] Lin Jingcheng, a public health officer, wrote in an article that "[m]any thought vital statistical work was not worth the money, because it was difficult for everyday people to understand its value."[108] Lin's observation shows that, unlike public health services that directly improved the health conditions of local people, the collection of statistical data to evaluate and design public health actions remained an abstract, insignificant endeavor in the eyes of the public.[109]

Sanitary infrastructure faced the same scrutiny. The CFHS also estimated the cost – and thus the economic feasibility – of improving sanitary infrastructure in its experimental areas. Following a general sanitation and water survey, forty-one latrines, two experimental wells, and seventy-eight new refuse containers were constructed in three districts of Jiangning County. The CFHS concluded in its 1936 annual report that the experiment was successful because it was inexpensive, and that the local residents were willing to pay for the material cost of the improvements.[110] Similar reconstruction work was done to improve housing in the county. The CFHS led initiatives to plaster or whitewash walls, open glass skylights, add ventilation holes, and repair leaky straw roofs.[111] A total of 152 houses were improved with financial contributions from villagers; those who could not contribute money contributed labor. The reported numbers were straightforward, enumerating the average cost of improving one room, one house, one ventilation hole, etc.[112] These

---

[107] Jin Baoshan and Xu Shijin, "Geshengshi xianyou gonggong weisheng sheshi zhi gaikuang [The Current Conditions of Public Health Services in Provinces and Municipalities]," *Zhonghua yixue zazhi [National Medical Journal of China (Shanghai)]* 23, no. 11 (1937): 1246.

[108] Translated from: Lin Jingcheng, "Zhongguo gonggong weisheng hangzheng zhi zhengjie [The Problems of Chinese Public Health Administrations]," *Zhonghua yixue zazhi [National Medical Journal of China (Beijing)]* 22, no.10 (1936): 966.

[109] Despite local people's indifference, Xu's expertise in vital statistics registration survived the Second Sino-Japanese War (1937–1945) and the Chinese Civil War. After the People's Republic of China was founded in 1949, the government mandated Xu to devise vital statistics collection systems in 73 localities across China (see Chapter 7).

[110] Liu and King, "Annual Report of the Central Field Health Station: For the Year Ending December 31, 1936," 25.

[111] Ibid.

[112] Ibid., 27–8.

examples demonstrate the spirit of social experimentation behind the CFHS's initiatives: the Station would start by conducting field surveys in order to understand villagers' living conditions; then, public health initiatives were specifically designed for each experimental area to test their financial feasibility and gauge social reaction. Just as in Ding Xian, the CFHS made public health actions commensurate to their cost, and mobilized the local community to reduce the latter.

Lastly, the CFHS's also relied on quantified data to document its laboratory results, ranging from bacteriological and parasitological tests on people and animals to tests of chemical ingredients in food and drugs (see Table 4.1). The CFHS laboratory collected human biological samples to gauge the prevalence of various bacteria and parasites. Animals were also put under microscopic scrutiny. Rats, fish, and sandflies were collected to check the prevalence of parasites. Every year, the CFHS also conducted hundreds of tests on the components in substances ranging from patented drugs to salt collected throughout China.[113] By analyzing component statistics, the CFHS gained an understanding of the Chinese population's pharmaceutical and nutritional habits. This food and drug research continued to gain importance during the Second Sino-Japanese War, when lack of food and resources spurred the NHA to seek nutritional substitutes.

Since its establishment, the CFHS had an overall plan for conducting experiments related to public health services, vital statistics collection, housing, water supply systems, and substance analysis. As in Ding Xian, the CFHS designated geographic areas that were considered representative of Chinese urban and rural environments. The statistical practices of the CFHS reveal its diverse goals: it was not focused solely on public health actions but also aimed to build an overall understanding of the Chinese population's health and related behavior. However, despite an apparent dedication to quantification, the CFHS officers still relied considerably on non-quantified information, using their knowledge of Chinese society to explain differences in vital statistics in their reports. In addition, although the demonstrations were presented as laboratories in which Chinese health policies could be tested, the CFHS officers were themselves aware that the quantified data collected from the demonstration areas was not directly applicable to the real world, given that the demonstration areas had greater administrative capacity than any other

---

[113] The results of these examinations showed that most of the patented drugs used in China did not adhere to international pharmaceutical regulations, and that the salt did not have any nutritional value (ibid., 18).

province in China. Their knowledge of the local conditions therefore continued to be crucial in policy-making.

*

From New York to Ding Xian to Nanjing, the circuit of health demonstrations and related statistical practices is illustrative of efforts to test public health policies in their socioeconomic context. Although there were some differences in the way statistics were collected and analyzed in the three places, it cannot be denied that statistical collection and analysis had become an integral part of health system programming. Experts in all three places used similar rhetoric to frame health demonstrations as laboratories, at least at the beginning. By implying that the results from demonstration areas could be applied to other places, statistical collection was a way to abstract local realities and give them universal implications.

What exactly, then, were these "laboratories" supposed to be testing? In line with Hermann Biggs' famous motto, "health is purchasable," the financial aspect was a key part of public health campaigns in New York, Ding Xian, and Nanjing alike. In all three places, vital and health statistics were calculated against budget numbers to estimate the price of health. However, despite the clear lineage and connections uniting them, Cattaraugus and its sister demonstrations in China positioned themselves differently when it came to the cost of public health work. The Cattaraugus experts put less emphasis on making health affordable and instead aimed to show that the rate of return would nonetheless be high enough to benefit local economies, so that the local authorities would agree to spend more on health. In Ding Xian and at the CFHS, however, the impoverished state of rural China and the financial constraints faced by local governments were key factors. The Chinese experts therefore aimed to make their actions as affordable as possible, mobilizing the local population to compensate for budgetary constraints.

Armed with their knowledge of public health conditions, experts in all three places were able to choose whether or not they used the numbers they collected, the extent to which those numbers were indispensable in promoting their demonstration areas, with whom they shared the numbers, and whether their numbers could be applied to the real world outside of the demonstration area. In both Cattaraugus and Ding Xian, the experts adjusted their rhetoric based on their policy advocacy needs. Having incomplete statistics did not prevent them from selling their programs to a larger audience, nor did it impede the effectiveness of their salesmanship. In New York, Kingsbury promoted his program by framing the demonstrations as an awareness-raising tool and resorted to the authority of public health researcher C. E. A. Winslow to promote them. Sydenstricker's mathematical statistical analysis was produced only later. In Ding Xian, James Yen used laboratory rhetoric, whereas Chen Zhiqian used orthodox vital and health statistical analysis in papers published in the United States, while downplaying the unscientific manner in which the site had been selected and the statistics reported. In contrast to New York and Ding Xian, favorable data that came out of the CFHS experimental areas were not used to promote policies to provincial governments, as the CFHS officers were well aware of the difference between their demonstrations and the real-world administrations.

The demonstration method, like other interwar circuits through which statistical practices were transferred, was eventually doomed to peter out. Growing hostility and outright war between countries prevented the exchange of epidemiological information as public health work in warzones such as China came to focus on emergency relief. It was not until World War II began to come to an end that the LNHO, alongside the newly founded United Nations Relief and Rehabilitation Administration (UNRRA), and eventually the WHO, revived the international epidemiological intelligence network that had lain dormant during the war. In the following chapter, I investigate the renaissance of international epidemiological intelligence as well as the WHO's design for an all-encompassing statistical system. Chapter 6 focuses on the WHO's communicable disease control campaigns, in which the laboratory/demonstration discourse re-emerged.

# 5  Popularization at a Global Scale
## The WHO and the Postwar Health
## Statistics Reporting System[1]

> The great wars of history have been accompanied and followed by sweeping epidemics, usually directly related to the devastation and hardship. In the recent World War, since the destruction was more widespread than ever before, the greatest catastrophes were to be expected. Multitudes of people were being driven from place to place. Thousands were crowding into makeshift dwellings. Scarcity of food, clothing, medical care, and even of pure drinking water was almost universal. And most of the health departments that had survived the war had been completely disrupted and so largely deprived of necessary personnel and supplies that they were quite ineffectual.[2]

The quotation from Wilbur Sawyer, a former officer at the Rockefeller Foundation's International Health Division (IHD) and director of health at the United Nations Relief and Rehabilitation Administration (UNRRA), vividly illustrates the international health backdrop as Word War II was coming to an end. In the same article, Sawyer went on to analyze how the existing international health organizations, such as the Office international d'hygiène publique (OIHP) and the League of Nations Health Organization (LNHO), had been weakened and were unable to provide countries with the guidance needed to tackle latent health crises. Under these circumstances, the UNRRA established a health division with a budget of approximately $82 million, far surpassing that of its forebears, to fill gaps in international health governance and epidemic prevention.[3] The UNRRA health division took on several functions that

---

[1] Parts of this chapter were previously published in *Monde(s)*. I am grateful for the feedback that I received during the journal's peer-review process. See Yi-Tang Lin, "Making Standards to Quantify All Health Matters: The World Health Organization's Statistical Practices (1946–1960)," *Monde(s)*, no. 11 (2017b): 247–66.
[2] Wilbur A. Sawyer, "Achievements of UNRRA as an International Health Organization," *American Journal of Public Health and the Nations Health* 37, no. 1 (1947): 46.
[3] Ibid., 41–2.

had previously belonged to its predecessors: it provided national governments with medical facilities, oversaw the care of displaced persons, and provided training to government staff.[4] Some of these functions were taken over by the World Health Organization Interim Commission (WHOIC) in 1946 and 1947. As Sawyer aptly put it in his article, the UNRRA "bridged the war-caused gap in the evolution of international health organization."[5]

That is why this chapter, in which I focus on the statistics reporting system of the World Health Organization (WHO), begins in 1943: the year the UNRRA's health division was launched. The pressing need for relief in warzones led the UNRRA to collect vital and health statistics in order to plan its relief activities. As Jessica Reinisch has argued, the UNRRA came into existence at the crossroads of international collaboration inspired by the aftermath of World War II and the beginning of the Cold War mindset;[6] this context makes the UNRRA's health statistics reporting system an apt case study for grasping how the international epidemiological network was forged ahead of the postwar years.

This chapter covers the postwar revival of a global network for the exchange of epidemiological intelligence and cause-of-death data. Notably, the American philanthropic foundations that had been the driving force behind statistical work during the interwar years ceded center stage to the United Nations system during this period, as the extensive membership of the latter allowed for broader implementation of statistical standards.[7] The LNHO had been obliged to engage in extensive negotiations in order to become the center of a network for the exchange of epidemic statistics information and thereby establish itself as an authority in international health collaboration. The UNRRA's task, however, was less complicated, as it took over the LNHO's functions with backing from the Allied countries. This was indispensable to maintaining an epidemic reporting system, as governments would send their statistics only to an organization they felt they could trust. Under the United Nations framework, the transfer of the statistical reporting system to the WHO was largely administrative in nature and did not spark competition or

[4] Ibid., 45.
[5] Ibid., 45.
[6] Jessica Reinisch, "'Auntie UNRRA' at the Crossroads," *Past & Present* 218, suppl. 8 (2013): 71.
[7] Marcos Cueto, "International Health, the Early Cold War and Latin America," *Canadian Bulletin of Medical History* 25, no. 1 (2008), 29–30. The Rockefeller Foundation nevertheless remained influential in WHO policy-making. See, e.g.: Anne-Emanuelle Birn, "Backstage: The Relationship between the Rockefeller Foundation and the World Health Organization, Part I: 1940s–1960s," *Public Health* 128, no. 2 (2014): 129–40.

conflict. To again cite Theodore Porter's landmark thesis that statistics bolster trust in groups of experts in need of authority,[8] the history of the international epidemic reporting system demonstrates that statistical collection also hinged upon the organization's political authority. Trust in numbers and trust in organizations were symbiotic.

In this chapter, I also recount the visions and actions of WHO experts regarding statistics. When the WHO officially opened its doors in 1948, the organization positioned itself as a clearinghouse for the world's vital and health statistics. Influenced by their experiences during the interwar period and motivated by scientific developments during World War II, the WHO's founders aimed for it to do more than merely maintain an epidemiological intelligence network; it would also collect all types of health-related statistics from its member states. The goal was to erase the boundaries separating research, administration, and policy-making, in the hope that the numbers collected in one context would serve to inform the others.

As in the previous chapters, I will seek to describe how statistical practices were transferred between the North Atlantic world and China, and then implemented on the ground. Like the LNHO statistical network presented in Chapter 3, the WHO's network was multi-tiered, with statisticians from different regions occupying different positions of standard-making. Because the WHO member states had different levels of administrative capacity, WHO statisticians designed the system to be adapted to different regional and national contexts. To ensure that the network was international, they were willing to integrate local knowledge on statistical reporting into their standard-making processes.[9] The history of epidemiological intelligence during the 1940s – from the era of the UNRRA to the beginning of the WHO – includes two different epidemic statistics transfer circuits: one at the international level and one on the ground. Though attempts were made to systematize statistical reporting to the headquarters of international organizations, collection on the ground was makeshift.

The final section of this chapter focuses on the Republic of China (ROC) – which became embroiled in a civil war after 1945 and whose government was eventually exiled to Taiwan in 1949 – and its reaction to the WHO's statistical initiatives. Despite constant attempts by WHO

---

[8] Porter, *Trust in Numbers*, 8.

[9] It is probable that these processes eventually came to discredit local knowledge, as many quantification researchers have rightly indicated. (See, e.g.: ibid., 93; Sally Engle Merry, *The Seductions of Quantification: Measuring Human Rights, Gender Violence, and Sex Trafficking* [Chicago, IL: University of Chicago Press, 2016], 6–7.)

experts to depoliticize public health matters, the government's Cold War strategy was the principal lens through which it viewed the organization and its statistical reporting system.

## Transfer of the LNHO's Epidemiological Intelligence Service to the UNRRA and the WHO

In 1943, forty-four countries, led by the World War II Allies, signed an agreement establishing the UNRRA, an organization tasked with rehabilitating territories ravaged by war and repatriating displaced people. With a total budget of $3 billion (70 percent of which came from the United States government), the UNRRA dispatched material and financial aid, as well as technical support, mostly to territories in Europe, but also to some parts of Asia and northern Africa.[10] As epidemics constituted a major menace in warzones, and with huge groups of displaced people on the move after the war, public health was one of the core missions taken up by the UNRRA.

The new organization relied on the expertise of the LNHO to design its health programs. Ludwik Rajchman, who had by that time stepped down as the LNHO's director-general, prepared a report for the UNRRA on how to control epidemics in warzones. In his report, Rajchman envisaged an organization that fully encompassed the LNHO's missions, from epidemiological intelligence to public health research, with an emphasis on the health issues of displaced people in European warzones.[11] The UNRRA's staff considered Rajchman's proposal too ambitious, given that the agency was focused on relief programs, not health administration reform. The leadership therefore accepted only one of Rajchman's suggestions: that the UNRRA should take over the LNHO's epidemiological intelligence service, as this would have the quickest and most direct effect on relief efforts.[12]

Why, then, did the LNHO agree to transfer its only remaining function, the epidemiological intelligence service, to the UNRRA? The answer speaks volumes about the international collaborative authority that the LNHO's founders sought to establish and its symbiotic relationship with

---

[10] David Ekbladh, *The Great American Mission: Modernization and the Construction of an American World Order* (Princeton, NJ: Princeton University Press, 2011), 87. The UNRRA shipped five times more goods to Europe than to the rest of the world taken together. (Reinisch, "'Auntie UNRRA' at the Crossroads," 73.)

[11] Ludwik Rajchman, "Report on UNRRA Health Functions," March 29, 1944, S-1533-0000-0015, United Nations Archives.

[12] Harold E. Caustin, "Memo on the Report on UNRRA Functions by Dr. Rajchman," December 30, 1946, S-1533-0000-0015, United Nations Archives.

statistical collection. The wartime hostilities among the LNHO's member states had called its authority into question. Without that authority, the statistical reporting system had run into difficulties. Countries on both sides of the conflict, including the United States, stopped sending their epidemiological reports to the LNHO, as such information was considered an important stake in military strategy.[13] Transferring the epidemiological intelligence service to the UNRRA was a last-ditch effort to save the system. The UNRRA, thanks to its close relationship to the Allied countries, had stronger authority to implement the International Sanitary Convention and collect epidemiological reports from various territories.[14]

What remained of LNHO's staff were well aware that the UNRRA's authority was crucial to the survival of its epidemiological intelligence service. Tellingly, Raymond Gautier, the director-general of the LNHO, did not seek to retain the service, only to keep it in Geneva, and sent two LNHO statisticians to work at the UNRRA's Washington, DC, office as epidemiological researchers.[15] For Gautier, it was important to keep the service in Geneva as Switzerland's neutral status facilitated the acquisition of epidemiological reports from countries in different geopolitical spheres. He also stressed that the LNHO statisticians' analytical techniques for processing raw epidemic numbers were "necessary for planning, or appreciating anti-epidemic campaigns projected by national services."[16]

The UNRRA visibly had the upper hand in negotiations with the LNHO, and Gautier's appeal was only partly successful. In 1944, the UNRRA created its own Epidemiological Information Bureau in Washington, DC, to take over administration of the International Sanitary Convention, which had been transferred from the OIHP and absorbed into the LNHO epidemiological intelligence service.[17] In line with Gautier's proposal, the UNRRA did, however, hire Knud Stowman to act as the Bureau's chief.[18] Stowman was a former LNHO statistician

[13] Iris Borowy, "Maneuvering for Space: International Health Work of the League of Nations during World War II," in *Shifting Boundaries of Public Health: Europe in the Twentieth Century*, 87–113.
[14] Rajchman, "Report on UNRRA Health Functions," 22.
[15] Raymond Gautier, "On Medical, Epidemiological and Public Health Intelligence and the Collaboration with the League of Nation's Health Organization," March 1, 1944, 3, S-1533-0000-0015, United Nations Archives.
[16] Ibid., 3.
[17] Andrija Štampar, "Suggestions Relating to the Constitution of an International Health Organization," in *Minutes of the Technical Preparatory Committee for the International Health Conference*, WHO Official Records 1 (Geneva: United Nations World Health Organization Interim Commission, 1947), 54–61.
[18] Stowman changed the spelling of his name from Stouman when he immigrated to the United States.

who had been charged by Jacques Bertillon with continuing to revise the classification of causes of death after Bertillon's death. At the UNRRA, Stowman was responsible for compiling data sent in by governments and analyzing the epidemiological situation in each beneficiary country.

Ultimately, the UNRRA's epidemiological intelligence service functioned for less than three years. In the October 1946, the newly established WHOIC began the process of taking over the service and bringing it back to Geneva.[19] WHOIC officials conferred several times with counterparts at the UNRRA to arrange the transfer of functions. Again, in discussions on which functions should be transferred, the epidemiological intelligence service was not even a subject of debate. From the beginning, it seems, the WHOIC and the UNRRA agreed that the service should be transferred to the WHO. Wilbur Sawyer, director of the UNRRA's medical mission, put forward a proposal recommending that the WHOIC also take on fellowship training, a mission in Ethiopia, tuberculosis and malaria control, and expert missions in fourteen countries.[20] Knowing that the UNRRA did not have a separate budget line for public health activities, Sawyer conservatively budgeted $2,025,000 for those five functions.[21] To Sawyer's disappointment, the WHOIC did not accept his proposal, considering the budget to be too limited, and granted the WHOIC only partial access to the UNRRA's responsibilities and financial resources.[22] The WHOIC, after all, wanted to distinguish itself – and the future WHO – from the UNRRA. Because it had chosen to focus on health, not relief, the WHOIC refused to take over responsibility for distributing medical supplies, even when put under pressure

[19] The establishment of the WHO was not a historical inevitability but rather the work of a cohort of public health experts. Unlike the UNRRA, which recognized the central importance of public health from the beginning, it was not immediately clear that the United Nations would create a health organization. In 1945, delegates from fifty countries gathered in San Francisco to discuss forms of international alliance after World War II, during which they endorsed a Chinese–Brazilian resolution to establish a health organization within the United Nations framework, leading to the creation of the WHO. Support for creating a United Nations health organization was deeply rooted in the public health programs of the interwar years. Tellingly, Brazil and China, the two sponsors of the resolution, were the two major beneficiaries of public health programs financed by the Rockefeller Foundation during the interwar years. (For more on this episode, see, e.g.: Szeming Sze, "The Birth of WHO: Interview [with] Dr Szeming Sze," *World Health*, May 1989, http://apps.who.int//iris/handle/10665/45224; Cueto, Brown, and Fee, *The World Health Organization*, 37–9.)
[20] W. A. Sawyer, "Functions to be Transferred to the Interim Commission of the World Health Organisation," October 7, 1946, S-1536-0000-0631, United Nations Archives.
[21] "Minutes of the Meeting of the Joint UNRRA Interim Commission of the WHO Subcommittee," October 16, 1946, 3, S-1536-0000-0631, United Nations Archives.
[22] "Authority of UNRRA and World Health Organisation in Relation to Transfer of Functions," 1946, S-1536-0000-0631, United Nations Archives.

by the UNRRA's staff.[23] After much heated debate, the transfer of the International Sanitary Convention from the UNRRA to the WHOIC was dropped from the discussion. The minutes of the WHOIC–UN–UNRRA meetings do not mention the International Sanitary Convention once, and yet its transfer, along with the affiliated epidemiological intelligence service, appears in the final decision of the second session of the WHOIC.[24]

That final decision, made during the WHOIC's second session in November 1946, did not differ much from Sawyer's original proposal, only with a 25 percent smaller budget. The WHO would take on epidemiological intelligence, medical fellowships, the health training program in Ethiopia, technical assistance in tuberculosis and malaria control, and expert missions with special relation to China.[25] In the end, the UNRRA provided only funding to cover certain field workers' salaries, fellowships, and office materials for these functions.[26]

Once the transfer of the epidemiological intelligence service was decided, the question became: where was the ideal place to host such a service? It was already certain that the United Nations would have its headquarters in New York; the question was therefore whether the epidemiological intelligence service should be transferred to New York as well. That idea was rejected by the UNRRA's staff. Dr. N. M. Goodman, the director of health at the UNRRA's European regional office, pointed out that a transfer to New York, which had never hosted any epidemiological information mechanism, would cause a "deplorable gap."[27] The UNRRA and the WHOIC were to move the International Sanitary Convention and its reporting system to Geneva, where the former LNHO's epidemiological intelligence service had been located. In late November 1946, the UNRRA prepared to send statisticians to Geneva, while the UNRRA regional offices requested governments to send their information to Geneva instead of Washington, DC.[28] The WHOIC officially took control in January 1947.

Compared to its predecessors (the OIHP and the LNHO), the WHOIC faced less political interference regarding statistical reporting and quarantine measures. The outbreak of a cholera epidemic in Egypt

---

[23] Glen E. Edgerton, "Note to Colonel F.D. Harris," January 3, 1947, S-0528-0008-0008, United Nations Archives.
[24] Neville M. Goodman, "Report on Second Session of the Interim Commission of the World Health Organization," November 1946, S-1536-0000-0631, United Nations Archives.
[25] Ibid., 1.
[26] Ibid.
[27] Ibid.
[28] Ibid.

in 1947 also helped the WHOIC to convince the authorities there and in neighboring countries to adhere to the International Sanitary Convention.[29] In Geneva, the Convention and its reporting system were no longer a major political battlefield. It is illuminating that the United States and the Netherlands originally turned down seats on the WHO Committee on Epidemiology and Quarantine. Representatives of the two countries stated that their governments would be willing to provide expertise but were more interested in sitting on other WHOIC committees.[30] At the insistence of Brazilian and Chinese representatives, who argued that a wider geographical basis would make it easier to establish an effective reporting system, the committee in question was eventually composed of representatives from nine countries, including the major postwar powers: the United States, the United Kingdom, the Soviet Union, China, and France, as well as countries where quarantine measures were essential, such as Egypt and India.[31] With this carefully selected membership, the WHO aimed to ensure that its decisions regarding quarantine measures were implemented across a broad geographical area.

Although public health experts eventually secured the structure for a global epidemiological intelligence network based on both sides of Atlantic, the level of implementation of that network remained doubtful, as it faced administrative failures and national authorities' strategic positioning vis-à-vis international health organizations. I will return to these issues of implementation later in the chapter. First, let us consider the WHO's strategy regarding vital and health statistics collection.

## The WHO Centralizes All Categories of Statistical Practices

The microbe was no longer the main enemy: science was sufficiently advanced to be able to cope with it admirably, if it were not for such barriers as superstition, ignorance, religious intolerance, misery and poverty.[32]

[29] Chiffoleau, *Genèse de la santé publique internationale.*
[30] WHOIC, *Minutes of the Technical Preparatory Committee for the International Health Conference*, WHO Official Records 1 (Geneva: World Health Organization Interim Commission, 1947). WHO, "Committee Structure of Interim Commission World Health Organization," November 1946, S-1536-0000-0631, United Nations Archives.
[31] Nine countries were represented in total: Brazil, China, Egypt, France, India, the Netherlands, the United Kingdom, the United States, and the Soviet Union (WHO, "Committee Structure of Interim Commission World Health Organization").
[32] WHO Interim Commission, *Minutes of the Technical Preparatory Committee for the International Health Conference*, 13.

The quotation from Brock Chisholm, the Canadian representative to the WHOIC at the time and soon to become the WHO's first director-general, effectively captures the WHO founders' optimistic faith in science. As many historians have observed from various perspectives, during the organization's formative years its staff were committed believers in technological advancement and its potential for improving health conditions across the world.[33] Statistics, with their supposed objectivity, were used by WHO staff not only for epidemiological intelligence – the function inherited from forerunner organizations – but also as a central element in planning epidemic control campaigns, administrating fieldwork, and conducting research on public health measures.

The decision to devise an all-encompassing statistical system within the WHO was made by participants in the technical preparatory committee (March–April, 1946), the International Health Conference (June–July, 1946), and the WHOIC (November 1946–April 1948). During these meetings, veterans of the LNHO, the UNRRA, and the OIHP, as well as officers of the Pan American Sanitary Bureau and health officials sent by national governments,[34] agreed that the future WHO should collect all types of statistics, including those related to epidemic control campaigns, epidemiological patterns of various diseases, and the health expenditure of WHO member states. Statistical practices played an essential role at the WHO from day one. When the organization officially opened its doors in 1948, it included a statistics division with sections for morbidity statistics, statistical studies, and revisions to the International List of Causes of Death (ICD).[35] The WHO's statistics division went beyond the collection of raw data on epidemics and deaths; the plan was to compile and analyze statistics of all sorts.

[33] Niels Brimnes, "BCG Vaccination and WHO's Global Strategy for Tuberculosis Control 1948–1983," *Social Science & Medicine* 67, no. 5 (2008): 863–73; Bhattacharya, "International Health and the Limits of its Global Influence"; Birn, "Backstage: The Relationship between the Rockefeller Foundation and the World Health Organization, Part I: 1940s–1960s."

[34] The minutes of the technical preparatory committee lists observers from the LNHO, the UNRRA, the Pan American Health Organization (PAHO), and the OIHP, as well as representatives from sixteen countries: Argentina, Belgium, Brazil, Canada, China, Czechoslovakia, Egypt, France, Greece, India, Norway, Mexico, Poland, the United Kingdom, the United States, and Yugoslavia. As for the WHOIC, its eighteen members came from the following countries and territories: Australia, Brazil, Canada, China, Egypt, France, India, Liberia, Mexico, the Netherlands, Norway, Peru, the United Kingdom, Ukrainian Soviet Socialist Republic, the United States, the Soviet Union, Venezuela, and Yugoslavia (WHO, "Minutes of the First Session of the Interim Commission," July 1946, Official Record 03, WHO Library).

[35] WHO, "The Organizational Structure of the World Health Organization (1948–1974) Vol. II," 1974, 26, WHO Library.

There were two forces underpinning trust in statistics and the central role they were to play within the WHO: a continued faith in transnational health cooperation carried over from the interwar period, and a general scientific optimism inspired by World War II.[36] Having either sat on committees at the LNHO or the OIHP, or been associated with the Rockefeller Foundation's public health programs, the experts who participated in the technical preparatory committee and the WHOIC had inherited the visions of those organizations. Like Ludwik Rajchman (see Chapter 3), these experts were advocates – and sometimes enactors – of "health internationalism": the idea that health crises could best be solved through the pooling of resources and transnational cooperation.[37] Moreover, these experts were persuaded that scientific advancements could improve health conditions throughout the world, having witnessed the revolutionary disease control technologies developed during World War II. A quotation from Gregorio Bermann, a former professor at the University of Córdoba in Argentina, sums up what took place in the committee. Bermann begins by observing that discussions revolved around the question of the new organization's scope, and goes on to express his faith in the scientific advancements achieved during World War II, which to his mind justified the new organization taking on broader responsibilities than its predecessors:

The world was in a period of medical reform, and the Organization should face new needs and even anticipate events. ... No better occasion for the success of an international health organization could be envisaged; for the war had shown to everyone the important role played by science.[38]

The WHO planners embraced the idea that health science should be introduced all over the world.[39] Statistics were the ideal medium for implementing health-related research worldwide for, as historians and sociologists have demonstrated, numbers were easily transferable, which allowed for instantaneous comparison across territories.[40] Moreover, the expansion

---

[36] The WHO's uptake of the spirit of interwar health internationalism is covered in a wealth of historical accounts. See, e.g.: Birn, Pillay, and Holtz, *Textbook of Global Health*; Cueto, Brown, and Fee, *The World Health Organization*.

[37] Here I use the definition from: Akira Iriye, *Global Community: The Role of International Organizations in the Making of the Contemporary World* (Berkeley, CA: University of California Press, 2004), 9–10.

[38] WHO Interim Commission, *Minutes of the Technical Preparatory Committee for the International Health Conference*, 12.

[39] Sunil Amrith, *Decolonizing International Health: India and Southeast Asia, 1930–65* (New York: Palgrave Macmillan, 2006), 2.

[40] See, e.g.: Kevin Davis, Agelina Fisher, Benedict Kingsbury, and Sally Engle Merry, eds., *Governance by Indicators: Global Power through Quantification and Rankings* (Oxford: Oxford University Press, 2012); Merry, *The Seductions of Quantification*.

of mathematical statistics into different domains had led statistics to be considered an objective means of subjecting local conditions to scientific scrutiny.[41] This objective quality persuaded committee members to endorse an all-encompassing statistical system within the new health organization.

Notably, United States government support was also decisive for this new system. It was first proposed in a draft submitted to the technical preparatory committee on behalf of the United States by Thomas Parran, then surgeon general of the United States Public Health Service (USPHS). Among the four drafts submitted (by the United Kingdom, France, Yugoslavia, and the United States), Parran's was the only proposal to include a more comprehensive function for the WHO when it came to statistics. He suggested that the WHO should "[e]stablish and maintain an epidemiological and statistical service for the collection, analysis, interpretation and dissemination of information pertaining to health, medicine, and related subjects."[42] The three other drafts, in contrast, envisioned the new health organization merely as a clearinghouse for vital and health statistics, much like its predecessors.

The American draft was in line with wartime public health efforts in the United States; the government had relied heavily on statistics to plan health programs and research during the war, and a bill had been passed requiring comprehensive nationwide health surveys aimed at collecting statistics in order to better organize public health matters at the national level.[43] The USPHS also collaborated with the biostatistics department at the Johns Hopkins School of Public Health (JHSPH) to devise random-sampled trials for penicillin (used to treat syphilis) and streptomycin (for tuberculosis control).[44] Such work was not limited to the United States, as the government also exported its programs on syphilis, polio, and malaria control to warzones in other parts of the world.[45]

Because the American proposal resonated with the prevailing spirit of health internationalism and scientific optimism, and given that the United States government had contributed the lion's share of the WHO's funding, the experts involved in establishing the new organization had no reason to go against it. Yves Biraud – a former LNHO statistician educated at the JHSPH – was also on the committee, doubtless contributing

---

[41] Porter, *The Rise of Statistical Thinking*; *Trust in Numbers*.
[42] Thomas Parran, "Proposals for the Establishment of An International Health Organization," in *Minutes of the Technical Preparatory Committee for the International Health Conference*, WHO Official Records 1 (Geneva: United Nations World Health Organization Interim Commission, 1947), 46.
[43] Thomas, *Health and Humanity*, 71.
[44] Ibid., 44.
[45] Ibid., 27.

to the WHOIC's adoption of the American draft and, with it, the principle that statistics were the ideal medium for informing public health programs. As stipulated in the proposal, the WHO's statistical practices from 1948 to 1960 were all-encompassing and included: consolidating data, developing member states' national health statistics services, surveying statistical collection in member states so as to provide long-term assistance, securing a sound statistical method, processing statistical data, and revising the ICD.[46]

This vision of the organization as a center for all-encompassing health-related statistical practices was undermined from the beginning, however. The seemingly objective action of collecting statistics ended up touching a political nerve. In 1948, the WHO outsourced the collection of vital statistics to the United Nations Statistical Office; the WHO's director-general, Brock Chisholm, had realized that vital statistics might become problematic for the WHO owing to their uncomfortable association with eugenics and birth control. In a letter to his assistant director-general, Chisholm wrote that all demographic statistics should be handled by the UN so that the WHO's director consultant on health statistics could "be protected from any of the criticism which might attend his close collaboration with the [UN] Population Division or the Population Commission and which might seriously impede his work in stimulating governments in the development and improvement of their health statistics."[47] Even though vital and health statistics were often collected together, the WHO and the UN processed them separately.

## Accounting for Local Variation: Revisions to the ICD

The ICD revisions are illustrative of the WHO's strategy when it came to devising a global health statistical network and endeavoring to extend its reach. In contrast to the LNHO, which had focused on creating a single standard through consistent exchange with specialists from its member states, the WHO opted for a different strategy, offering different standards to countries with different levels of administrative capacity in order to extend the coverage of its statistical system within the ever-expanding UN membership.

In 1947, when the WHO had yet to be officially founded, the WHOIC took over revisions to the ICD from the United States government, which had been put in charge of the process while World War II made it

---

[46] Gear, Biraud, and Swaroop, *International Work in Health Statistics, 1948–1958*.
[47] Brock Chisholm, "To Assistant Director-General," December 18, 1952, VH2, World Health Organization Archives.

impossible for the LNHO to prepare the sixth revision. In 1948, the year of the WHO's founding, the French government (in association with the WHO), convened the Sixth Revision Conference; representatives from twenty-nine countries participated. The conference endorsed the inclusion of approximately 800 new rubrics (which included injuries and morbidities, in addition to causes of death), which were to be integrated into the previous version of the ICD.

A few months later, the First World Health Assembly adopted the ICD-6, giving the ICD binding legal status in all WHO member states. Member states that had not made an explicit objection were automatically obligated to apply the death certificate form promulgated by the ICD-6 as their official form for recording causes of death.[48] The legally binding nature of the ICD-6 did not lead to its full implementation, however. As with the International Sanitary Convention, it was always local administrative capacity (political considerations aside) that determined whether statistical practices would actually be used. For instance, a letter from the ROC's Ministry of Foreign Affairs simply stated: "The current situation in China does not allow for implementing the ICD-6."[49]

The WHO statisticians were aware of these difficulties. Yves Biraud, the WHO's founding statistician, rolled out several measures to promote implementation. After the ICD-6 passed in 1948, Biraud and his fellow statisticians at the WHO invited chief medical statisticians, mostly from Western countries, to participate in the Expert Committee on Health Statistics and define a variety of vital situations.[50] This measure was very similar to Sydenstricker's work in the 1920s, which brought statisticians from Western Europe and North America into extensive discussions of the LNHO's statistical measures. From the first (1949) to the sixth (1958) sessions of the Expert Committee, most of the discussion was dedicated to defining concepts such as stillbirth, abortion, cancer, and morbidity, along with their registration methods.[51]

Biraud and his colleagues also standardized statistical practices in a such a way that they could be adopted by member countries with

---

[48] Gear, Biraud, and Swaroop, *International Work in Health Statistics, 1948–1958*, 18.

[49] Waijiao bu [Minister of Foreign Affairs], "Neizheng bu gongjian [To the Ministry of the Interior]," April 25, 1950, 02800000221a, Academia Historica.

[50] With exception of the Venezuelan statistician Darío Curiel, the first two sessions of the Expert Committee included only statisticians from France, the United Kingdom, and the United States (WHO, "Expert Committee on Health Statistics: Report on the First Session," Geneva: WHO, 1950; "Expert Committee on Health Statistics: Report on the Second Session," Geneva: WHO, 1950).

[51] WHO, "Expert Committee on Health Statistics: Report on the First Session."

different levels of administrative capacity. Unlike Sydenstricker, who worked mainly with European countries, the WHO statistics staff had to deal with a larger and more diverse membership: at the end of 1949, fifty countries on five continents were members of the UN; in a decade, the number of member states would grow to eighty-six. Biraud and his colleagues adopted strategies to make statistical practices more accessible for countries with no or little health administration, systematically encouraging countries with varying levels of administrative capacity to implement the ICD. Methods of ICD registration in less developed regions were repeatedly discussed in sessions of the Expert Committee on Health Statistics. During the first session, the Expert Committee suggested that the WHO conduct research on available methods for measuring the state of health in less developed territories.[52] At the third session, the Expert Committee took the important step of categorizing member states according to their existing public health services and proposing specific suggestions on the collection of morbidity statistics for each category.[53] They also provided suggestions on which morbidity statistics to collect, which populations to survey, and how to use the statistics collected for each category.[54]

The WHO's strategy in promoting the ICD was thus to take local differences into account. By allowing countries with limited administrative capacity to collect some types of statistics only in a sample area, Biraud and his colleagues tailored the standard for countries with less capable health administrations to adopt the ICD-6. They believed that statistics could be easily converted into comparable numbers so long as the survey methods were well documented. This emphasis on documenting survey methods recalled the LNHO's efforts to compile a statistical manual for its member countries. Nevertheless, unlike the LNHO, which published a handbook only for selected "significant" countries (see Chapter 3), the WHO tailored its statistical standards to take all member states into account. Moreover, in order to systematically account for the local variation that was undermining its implementation, the WHO established the WHO Centre of ICD within the United Kingdom General Register Office in London to provide guidance to national statisticians on ICD-related challenges and to collect feedback from member states.[55]

In 1955, the strategy of making the ICD accessible in as many territories as possible – regardless of their level of administrative capacity – was

[52] Ibid.
[53] WHO, "Expert Committee on Health Statistics Third Report," 1952.
[54] Ibid., 6–8.
[55] Gear, Biraud, and Swaroop, *International Work in Health Statistics, 1948–1958*, 20.

made official with the ICD-7, which allowed non-professionals to record causes of death. In defense of this strategy, Biraud argued that causes of death in a given region were often recurrent, especially in less developed countries, where over half of deaths were from early childhood diseases. In such cases, the child's mother, for example, would be qualified to distinguish the cause of death.[56] The decision to adopt the ICD-7 was evidence of the WHO's increasing emphasis on local conditions when devising how statistical data should be collected. For instance, when two statistical advisers from the Eastern Mediterranean Regional Office and the Regional Office for the Americas attended the fifth session of the Expert Committee on Health Statistics in 1956, committee members were impressed by their contributions and recommended that every WHO regional office should employ a statistical adviser, arguing it was "only through the knowledge of local conditions prevailing in different areas of the world that the most constructive statistical advice can be given."[57] The WHO thus added two additional ICD centers to cater to regional needs: one for Latin America, in Caracas (1955); and one for South-East Asia, in New Delhi (1958).[58]

The sixth and seventh revisions of the ICD proved to be of historical significance. The sixth was the first to gain legally binding status, making the ICD applicable worldwide for the very first time. However, the inclusion of so many countries proved problematic: it required health administration structures and qualified medical workers that were absent in most places. To remedy this problem, WHO statisticians adopted several strategies for making statistical collection possible in most countries: the Expert Committee on Health Statistics tailored its suggestions to take local variation into account; among other measures, ICD centers were equipped to serve as helpdesks for national statisticians. As opposed to the LNHO, which had revised the ICD without tailoring implementation guidelines to countries with less organized health administrations, the WHO's statistical standardization efforts were not about creating and imposing a single standard, but rather about adapting standards to local conditions. In 1955, the ICD-7 included the compromise of granting non-professionals the right to register causes of death, in the hope of encouraging more countries to implement the ICD. Along with this significant amendment, the Expert Committee placed increasing value

[56] Moriyama et al., *History of the Statistical Classification of Diseases and Causes of Death*, 35.
[57] WHO, "Expert Committee on Health Statistics Fifth Report," 1957, 11.
[58] Gear, Biraud, and Swaroop, *International Work in Health Statistics, 1948–1958* 22–23.

on statistical practices in territories without advanced health administrations, and invited statisticians who practiced statistics in such countries to participate in the creation of statistical standards.

## A Tiered Network of Statisticians for Spreading WHO Statistical Standards

The WHO's ICD strategy of accounting for local variation also translated into a three-tiered network of statisticians tasked with sharing standardized statistical practices among member states. The choice of a tiered network resembled Sydenstricker's strategy at the LNHO. However, the WHO had a group of JHSPH-trained staff who acted directly as the top tier and engaged in standard-making. The middle tier was made up of a network of statisticians at the WHO regional offices, who organized training sessions and participated in expert committees. Their role was not only to pass down standards created at headquarters to the regions, but also to integrate local variation into policy-making in Geneva.[59] The bottom tier included vital and health statisticians working in member states, who mostly received and implemented statistical standards from headquarters. In the following paragraphs, I will discuss each tier in turn (see Table 5.1).

The top tier was made up of statisticians who had been trained at the JHSPH. These statisticians shared a faith in numbers and statistical practices. Yves Biraud, who had previously worked at the LNHO and the WHOIC, played a significant role in shaping the WHO's statistical programs. He was the director of the WHOIC Division of Epidemiology and Health Statistics. As Biraud was fully in charge of the WHOIC's statistical work, it is probable that Marie Cakrtova, Satya Swaroop, and Marcelino Pascua – all graduates of the JHSPH biostatistics department – were hired at his recommendation. All four belonged to a group of health statisticians who were educated during the interwar years and who directed different sections of the health statistics division. Biraud, Cakrtova, and Pascua had studied at the JHSPH biostatistics department on Rockefeller Foundation fellowships, while Swaroop had worked at the All India Institute, another Rockefeller-funded public

---

[59] The WHO's regional tier was made more official thanks to the existence of the regional offices. The establishment of these offices was the result of lengthy negotiations and regional political struggles. Historians have shown that the design and structure of the regional offices was inspired by the integration of the PAHO into the WHO. For more on the WHO's regional offices, see, e.g.: Marcos Cueto, *The Value of Health: A History of the Pan American Health Organization* (Rochester, NY: University of Rochester Press, 2007); Pearson, *The Colonial Politics of Global Health*.

Table 5.1 *WHO tiered network of statistical standard-setting*

|  | First tier | Second tier | Third tier |
|---|---|---|---|
| Composition | • WHO statisticians | • WHO regional office statisticians | • Member state statisticians |
| Contribution to WHO activities | • Drafted standards<br>• Organized expert committees on health statistics | • Supervised statistical production and monitored WHO-supported projects<br>• Participated in expert committees<br>• Organized regional statistical training centers<br>• Granted fellowships to national statisticians for short-term training | • Carried out fellowships and short-term training<br>• Worked with the second tier to improve statistics |

health institution, and joined the biostatistics department after World War II.[60] All were directly associated with the Rockefeller Foundation's public health programs, and had been supervised by Lowell J. Reed, a mathematician and the director of the biostatistics department until the 1950s (see Chapter 2).

The middle tier comprised statisticians at the WHO's six regional offices. In line with the suggestion of the Fifth Expert Committee on Health Statistics, in which two regional statisticians participated, the WHO created the position of regional statistician in every regional office. Regional statisticians were put in charge of supervising the production of statistics within all WHO-supported public health projects in their regions. They were also responsible for organizing regional statistical training centers and offering fellowships to member states' health statisticians.[61] On some occasions, they acted as evaluators of other WHO programs.[62] Notably, this regional tier of the WHO network partly overlapped with the network of JHSPH alumni. For example, Ruth Rice Puffer, a JHSPH biostatistics graduate, directed the statistics department at the PAHO from 1953

[60] See: "Fellowship Card: Yves Biraud"; "Fellowship Card: Marie Cakrtova"; "Fellowship Card: Marcelino Pascua"; "Fellowship Card: Satya Swaroop."

[61] Apart from these common tasks, responsibilities differed depending on the regional office. Details as to the activities of each regional office's statistician can be found in the WHO archives under the series number S5/418/3.

[62] One example was statistician S. K. Quo's evaluation of WHO fellowships, in which he was credited as "Programme Evaluator" (S. K. Quo, "Analysis of WHO Fellowships Awarded during the Period 1957–1963 and Evaluation of Those Awarded during the Period 1955–1961," May 25, 1964, S5/418/3, World Health Organization Archives).

to 1970 and was also in charge of scaling up ICD implementation in Brazil.[63] A second example is Guo Songgen (Quo Sung-Ken, commonly known as S. K. Quo), another JHSPH biostatistics graduate who served as the statistician of the WHO Western Pacific Regional Office. During his service, Guo traveled from country to country to work with officials on various aspects of implementing the ICD (e.g. death certificate design and legislation regarding death and birth certificates), fieldwork statistics, and hospital records. Guo was also in charge of briefing field workers before they reported for duty in the region.[64]

The third and bottom tier consisted of national statisticians, who were generally excluded from standard-making procedures but had various opportunities to become familiar with statistical standards. The WHO provided fellowships for short-term training, either in regional training centers or at institutions that were known for their statistical practices. From 1946 to 1958, the WHO awarded 365 health statistics fellowships throughout its six regions and organized seven regional training centers and seminars on health statistics.[65] The fellowships and regional training centers taught bottom-tier statisticians how to register and analyze statistics on births, deaths, and medical conditions. In addition, member states could also file requests to consult with regional statisticians.

The WHO's use of exchanges, fellowships, and expert committees was very similar to Sydenstricker's at the LNHO. This was no coincidence, as Biraud had worked for the LNHO since the mid-1920s and was familiar with its statistical initiatives. Nevertheless, Biraud and his colleagues at the WHO had a larger and more diverse group of countries to deal with than Sydenstricker had. In order for the WHO's network to cover a larger area and more diverse statistical practices, regional statisticians served as intermediaries between WHO headquarters and member states. Though the WHO engaged actively with local knowledge, the statistical reporting system remained highly susceptible to geopolitics and administrative failures, as will become clear in the following sections.

## Separate Circuits of Epidemiological Information

The epidemiological intelligence services of the UNRRA and the WHO faced failures on the ground that were similar, if not identical, to those

---

[63] Thomas, *Health and Humanity*, 33.
[64] Sung-Ken Quo, "Activity Reports by the WPRO Regional Adviser on Health Statistics," 1962, S5/418/3, World Health Organization Archives.
[65] Specifically: the Interamerican Seminar (1950) and the International Training Centers for South-East Asia (1951, 1958), the Eastern Mediterranean (1951, 1954), the Western Pacific (1952), and Africa (1956) (ibid., 26–7).

of their interwar counterparts. That is, the limited administrative capacity of their member states made it impossible to report epidemic cases in time. This eventually became emblematic of the two organizations' weak governance. Indeed, the archives contain two very different visions of the epidemiological situation around the world during this period. Reports published in Washington, DC, or Geneva and distributed to governments gave the impression that the international organizations were overseeing the epidemiological situation in their member states.[66] Public health workers on the ground, however, based their daily decisions on their first-hand observation of patients admitted to nearby hospitals and health stations; they did not use the organizations' reports to plan their day-to-day work. The situation in China is a case in point.

At the end of World War II, the Chinese government had very limited capacity to collect epidemic statistics through its National Health Administration (NHA). For example, in 1945, Leland E. Powers, the chief medical officer of the UNRRA's China Office, complained to the Washington, DC, office that epidemiological intelligence reports from China had stopped being delivered because the Chinese epidemiology expert had left the country for the United States.[67] The expert in question was Rong Qirong (historically known as Winston Yung), a port health specialist trained by the LNHO who later became a statistician at the NHA. Powers' complaint shows how the China's epidemic reporting system depended on a single individual, and the absence of one expert could easily cause the breakdown of the entire system. Powers eventually learned about an ongoing epidemic in Chongqing from Jin Baoshan, the head of the NHA. Jin's information was based only on vague impressions, however. According to Powers, Jin admitted in a personal letter to him that his account of the "epidemiological situation" was based purely on the number of patients admitted to hospitals each day.[68] In spite of the malfunctions mentioned above, the NHA routinely sent its statistics to the China Office and the Epidemiological Information Bureau in Washington, DC, for further analysis.[69] Moreover, there is nothing in the archives to suggest that the NHA made use of the UNRRA's epidemiological reports when planning relief actions.

[66] Jessica Reinisch, "Introduction: Relief in the Aftermath of War," *Journal of Contemporary History* 43, no. 3 (2008): 375–8.
[67] Leland E. Powers, "To Dr. Szeming Sze," July 26, 1945, S-1303-0000-2157, United Nations Archives.
[68] Ibid.
[69] Szeming Sze, "Letter to Dr. Powers," March 28, 1945, S-1303-0000-2156, United Nations Archives. Leland E. Powers, "Weekly Report for Week Ending May 26, 1945," May 1945, 3, S-1303-0000-2157, United Nations Archives; Leland E. Powers, "Suggested Organisation and Plans for the Medical Division of the China Area Office," May 29, 1945, S-1303-0000-2157, United Nations Archives.

This episode is illustrative of how a weak link at the national level cut the circulation of statistics into two separate circuits of information: first, there was an UNRRA–NHA circuit, through which the two organizations shared epidemiological information among themselves; second, there was a local circuit, through which the number of patients admitted to local health services was communicated among staff who made day-to-day decisions but never reported to the UNRRA. The local circuit and the UNRRA–NHA circuit rarely communicated with each other. Local aid workers did not always report their statistics to the NHA, and they did not use the statistical analysis provided by the UNRRA to plan their public health relief on the ground. In a report summarizing the UNRRA's medical mission in China, for example, the author mentions only one of Knud Stowman's reports and refers to its categorization of two cholera epidemics in China according to different mortality rates, without referencing any of the UNRRA's other epidemiological publications.[70]

UNRRA officers stationed in China did, however, use statistics as a rhetorical device in the reports they presented to other international organizations. A telling episode took place at an UNRRA meeting on public health work in China in 1946. Dr. Berislav Borčić, a founding staff member of the Central Field Health Station and the medical director of the UNRRA's China Office, rejected the validity of the available statistics but nonetheless held them up as evidence of China's generally poor health situation:

Health statistics are extremely poor and unreliable. China, however, is known to have all types of diseases except yellow fever. The death rate of 30 per thousand a year is very high as compared with other countries. Smallpox represents 500–700,000 cases per year, typhus 500–700,000 cases per year; typhoid 500–700,000 cases per year; 2 million have Kala-Azar; 6–10 million have dysentery; some 10 million have hook-worm.[71]

For these statistics, all of which Borčić described as rough estimates, no trace can be found in the archives as to how they were collected and the basic assumptions underlying them. Borčić's way of citing statistics demonstrates their forceful persuasive power at the time. Though transparent as to their lack of reliability, Borčić nonetheless relied on statistics to draw a general picture of the Chinese public health situation for his colleagues at the UNRRA.

---

[70] W. S. Fu, "The UNRRA Medical Mission in China," N/A, 6, S-1547-0000-0033, United Nations Archives.
[71] UNRRA, "Health Program. Chairman: Dr. Borcic," September 3, 1946, 1, S-1121-0000-0136, United Nations Archives.

In the end, the UNRRA Epidemiological Information Bureau never had time to resolve the difficulties it faced in China. Starting in 1946, a mere two years after its founding, it was transferred to the newly established WHOIC, where the implementation of epidemiological intelligence at regional and national levels would be just as crude. The Eastern Bureau provides a case in point. From 1946 (when the WHO Committee on Epidemiology and Quarantine took over the Eastern Bureau) until December 1947, Lucius Nicholls of the British military in South-East Asia was in charge of administering the Bureau part-time. Nicholls proudly described to Yves Biraud, who oversaw epidemiological intelligence at the WHOIC, how he had reduced telegram fees from £2,000 per month to £1,000 by decreasing the number of words used and ignoring telegrams that were too out of date upon arrival.[72] The anecdote is telling: the reporting system immediately after the war was not aimed at sharing precise and reliable statistics, but rather at promptly announcing the outbreak of epidemics.

At the national level, too, the WHO faced a situation similar to that of its interwar predecessors, with local administrative failures nullifying the effects of the international epidemiological framework. When the UNRRA ended its missions in China in April 1947, the WHOIC took over its remaining fellowship programs, foreign consultants, and the China Office along with its director, Borčić.[73] The partnership between the WHO and the ROC got off to a rough start: when the WHOIC took over the UNRRA's office in Shanghai, the Chinese mainland was being wracked by armed clashes between the ROC and Communist forces. The validity of the entire framework was doubtful, as national health authorities were too poorly organized to report precise epidemic statistics to the WHO promptly. Monthly reports by the Eastern Bureau noted that some Chinese ports sent their reports up to three months late, some sent in reports at irregular intervals, and some had never sent anything to the Bureau.[74] P. H. Deng, a port officer in Hong Kong, also recorded the complete failure of quarantine measures and epidemic information collection in southeast China. Returning from a visit to the ports there, Deng wrote a report to the WHO enumerating the malfunctions he had observed: officials had boarded an arriving ship before the medical inspectors (these being mostly local sages with little medical

[72] Lucius Nicholls, "To Dr. Biraud," March 31, 1947, 452-6-1, WHO Archives.
[73] W. S. Fu, "The UNRRA Medical Mission in China," 19–20. For more on Borčić's work before and during his stay in China, see Chapter 2.
[74] "Epidemiological Information: Singapore Epidemiological Intelligence Station, Reports on Activities," 1948, 452-6-13, World Health Organization Archives.

training); tourism agencies were willing to issue false immunization certificates to facilitate their customers' travel; doctors were reluctant to report cholera cases, knowing it would disrupt maritime commerce; and a lack of refrigeration had damaged smallpox vaccine stocks.[75]

Epidemiological intelligence under the ROC regime did not improve after the regime lost the civil war against the Communists and retreated to Taiwan. The ROC government continued to represent China within the WHO and considered Taiwan to be a temporary military base for reconquering the mainland. National planning – including for health – was not a priority. Against this backdrop, the implementation of the visions and practices of WHO statisticians was very limited in Taiwan.

### Caught Up in the Cold War: The ROC's Strategies and the WHO's Statistical Reporting System

To comprehend how the WHO reporting systems came to be implemented after the ROC government settled in Taiwan in 1949, it is first necessary to discuss the relationship between the WHO and the ROC. The ROC's reaction to WHO statistical initiatives was, after all, largely conditioned by the general relationship between them. The ROC played various different roles over the course of the relationship. First, as an important member of the World War II Allies, the ROC government was a major player in the United Nations Conference on International Organization (also known as the San Francisco Conference) that led to the establishment of the WHO.[76] But at the domestic level, the ROC's struggling health administration (which was further undermined by the Second Sino-Japanese War and the Chinese Civil War) made it a passive partner in the WHO's reporting systems for epidemics and deaths. Lastly, the failures of the ROC health administration ironically made it the source of much-needed manpower for the newly established WHO, as several ROC statisticians, including Guo Songgen, Rong Qirong, and Yuan Yijin, all eventually left Taiwan to work for the WHO until their retirement.

The latter two roles – those of passive implementer and source of WHO statisticians – were closely related to the failures of the WHO's reporting systems in Taiwan. These failures were due to three separate but interrelated causes: the ROC government's Cold War mindset; an inadequate

---

[75] P. H. Teng, "A Short Visit to the Ports of Swatow, Amoy and Poochow," April 28, 1947, 452-6-6, World Health Organization Archives.

[76] Mitter, "Imperialism, Transnationalism, and the Reconstruction of Post-War China."

national health administration; and the brain drain of ROC statisticians. These three dynamics created a vicious circle, with each impacting the others. I will elaborate on all three over the following paragraphs.

The first cause of failure was the general mindset in the ROC government during the Cold War. Not only was the government's reasoning affected by this mentality, but WHO policy was also impacted by the Cold War rivalry, despite the fact that its staff constantly insisted on the organization's purely technical nature.[77] From its founding in 1948, WHO staff found themselves trapped in the oppressive atmosphere of the conflict. Yves Biraud, the WHO's founding statistician, who had been responsible for epidemic statistics since the WHOIC years, complained in a letter to the chief of the Eastern Bureau, P. M. Kual, about the withdrawal of the Soviet Union from the WHO:

Morally, this withdrawal is a blow to WHO which had tended towards, and claimed, world-wide membership. Materially and technically, however, it has no significance, since the Soviets had never contributed a single expert to our committees, a single specialist to our staff, nor a single figure or piece of information to our epidemiological, legal or other services.[78]

As the quotation indicates, WHO staff members were resentful of the Soviet Union's boycott. Moreover, the WHO inevitably sided with the Western bloc because of the United States government's generous financial support. That support was based on the Truman Doctrine, under which the United States government made a strong commitment to assist other countries with science and technology. Expecting to benefit from this political promise and budgetary engagement, Biraud, in the same letter to Kual, explained that the WHO had even organized its budget so as to follow the Truman Doctrine: the regular budget was to remain "comparatively stable and small," as specified by the United States Congress when it ratified the WHO's Constitution, while the expenditure envisaged in the supplemental budget was to be borne by

---

[77] For more on the Cold War's impact on specific instances of WHO policy-making, see: John Farley, *Brock Chisholm, the World Health Organization, and the Cold War* (Vancouver: University of British Columbia Press, 2009); Erez Manela, "A Pox on Your Narrative: Writing Disease Control into Cold War History," *Diplomatic History* 34, no. 2 (2010): 299–323; Anne-Emanuelle Birn and Nikolai Krementsov, "'Socialising' Primary Care? The Soviet Union, WHO and the 1978 Alma-Ata Conference," *BMJ Global Health* 3, suppl. 3 (2018): 1–15.

[78] Biraud also complained that the main difficulty during the first World Health Assembly was that member state representatives were reluctant to approve the WHO's budget (Yves Biraud, "To Dr. P. M. Kual," March 11, 1949, 452-6-3, World Health Organization Archives).

voluntary contributions from governments, of which the United States government was naturally expected to provide a "fair share."[79] With the United States as the WHO's main financial backer, the organization tended to focus on the Western bloc's preoccupations when devising public health programs. The focus on malaria control during the 1950s and 1960s was one result of the WHO's close ties to the West,[80] ties that led the socialist countries to withdraw from the WHO in the 1950s.[81]

The Cold War backdrop, compounded by budgetary deficits, catalyzed the ROC's exit from the WHO. The ROC had defaulted on its mandatory contributions to the WHO for the years 1948 and 1949; its defeat in the Chinese Civil War in 1949 – and its expectation that it would one day reconquer the mainland – led to constant increases in its military expenditure. In this context, membership in various international organizations was seen as an unnecessary financial burden. The ROC Ministry of Foreign Affairs prepared a list with a specific strategy for every international organization, in which it noted that as the ROC had already defaulted on two years of dues to the WHO, its rights as a member had already been suspended. Re-entering the WHO would therefore be costly.[82] The ROC therefore left the WHO in 1950. The ROC was far from alone in balking at the cost of WHO membership, however: it was a common issue at the WHO during its early years. Many member state representatives were troubled by the high cost of membership and were unsure if their governments would provide budget authorization.[83]

Another illuminating anecdote can be found in the reaction of the ROC minister of foreign affairs to the WHO's invitation to rejoin, which again demonstrates the Cold War mindset that reigned at the time. The minister examined the invitation in terms of the Soviet bloc's relations with the WHO. In a letter to the minister of interior, he described the invitation as merely a routine encouragement to join the organization, given that the WHO had also sent such an invitation to the Soviets. Moreover, he stated that since Communist China had not received an

[79] Yves Biraud, "To Dr. P. M. Kual," March 11, 1949.
[80] See, e.g.: Packard, *The Making of a Tropical Disease.*
[81] There is an emerging group of literature covering the socialist countries' varying attitudes towards the WHO. See, e.g.: Xun Zhou, "From China's 'Barefoot Doctor' to Alma Ata: The Primary Health Care Movement in the Long 1970s," in *China, Hong Kong, and the Long 1970s: Global Perspectives*, eds. Priscilla Roberts and Odd Arne Westad (New York: Palgrave Macmillan, 2017), 135–57; Vargha, *Polio Across the Iron Curtain*; Birn and Krementsov, "'Socialising' Primary Care?"
[82] Waijiao bu [Minister of Foreign Affairs], "Guanyu woguo yingfou jiaru shijie weisheng zuzhi shi [On Whether Our Country Should Join the World Health Organization]," July 11, 1950, 028000002213A, Academia Historica.
[83] Yves Biraud, "To Dr. P. M. Kual," March 11, 1949.

invitation, the ROC did not have to reactivate its membership to ensure the Communists' exclusion.[84] Interestingly, as I will explore in more detail in Chapter 7, the People's Republic of China (PRC) also resisted joining the WHO based on concerns about American dominance of the organization and the expectation that the PRC would have to contribute financially to the WHO. Though the WHO's founding members had stressed that the organization would be purely technical in nature, neither the ROC nor the PRC had ever seen their relations with the organization as a form of purely technical collaboration on health matters, but always considered them within the context of the Cold War. The ROC, which still officially represented China within the United Nations system, clearly saw the WHO in political terms during the 1940s and 1950s. The WHO courted the ROC as part of its efforts to gain more members and live up to its name as a "world" health organization. After negotiating with Liu Ruiheng (historically known as J. Heng Liu), a New York-based adviser to the ROC's NHA, the WHO agreed to give the ROC preferential treatment to encourage its re-entry. Under the agreement, the ROC government had to contribute only a symbolic membership fee of $10,000.[85] The ROC rejoined the WHO in 1953 and represented all of China until 1971.

Although he successfully negotiated the ROC's re-entry, Liu was unable to remedy the disconnect between the WHO and the ROC regarding the core role played by the organization. The ROC continued to consider the WHO in terms of Cold War rivalries, and therefore remained passive in response to the WHO's suggestion that it remedy the administrative failures of its vital and health statistics collection. As the WHO proposed only short-term training, fellowships, and expert consultancy to improve epidemic- and death-reporting systems, the ROC government's involvement was limited to accepting consultants and sending statisticians to undertake fellowships and participate in WHO training.

In the end, the ROC health organizations did not undertake any concrete reforms of its vital and health statistics collection. A report by Cai Fu (Tsai Fu), the chief of the Taiwan provincial health administration's statistical office, offers an account of how the WHO's statistical network was failing at the national level. Cai received a WHO fellowship in 1952 for statistical training at the Japanese Public Health Institute. In his 30-page fellowship report, he recorded in detail his training in a variety of Japanese statistical and health administrations. In the last section of

[84] Waijiao bu, "Guanyu woguo yingfou jiaru shijie weisheng zuzhi shi," July 11, 1950.
[85] Liu Ruiheng, "Neizhengbu weishengsi [To Department of Health, Ministry of the Interior]," October 21, 1954, 028000002240A, Academia Historica.

his report, entitled "Suggestions," he mentioned the importance of combining household registration and demographic statistics collection.[86] It is unlikely that Cai's suggestions were implemented, however. He would not have been able to organize his office as he wished, since the Taiwan provincial health administration had a very small budget, and the statistical office was a low priority for the government. Without financial and political commitment from the ROC government, the WHO's efforts to train statistical officers did not make much difference in the implementation of statistical methods, as the officers did not have the authority or resources to reorganize statistical collection within the ROC health administration.

The limited impact of Cai's fellowship on the ROC's vital and health statistical system was partly due to limited administrative capacity, the second driver of the WHO reporting system's failure in Taiwan. Three years after Cai returned from Japan, the United Nations sent out three sets of questionnaires – on population statistics, vital statistics, and cause-of-death statistics – to the Taiwan provincial government. This troubled the ROC administration. By that time, the ROC was collecting vital statistics using two parallel systems. The Taiwan provincial civil administration was in charge of compiling birth and death numbers, while causes of death were to be reported by caregivers to the provincial health administration. These two branches were not informed of each other's responsibilities regarding vital and health statistics. In order to fill out the forms sent by the United Nations, the ROC government had to convene a meeting to determine which branch was qualified to do so. Participants in the meeting proposed giving the responsibility for filling out United Nations forms to the civil administration, while the statistical office of the health administration would be in charge of re-examining the completed forms.[87] This is illustrative of the disorganized nature of vital and health statistics collection within the ROC. In the 1950s, the government lacked not only reliable vital and health statistics, but also coordination between its civil and health administrations. Although the ROC government was perfectly willing to fill out United Nations statistical forms, it did not actually attempt to improve the quality of its statistics.

---

[86] Cai Fu, "Fu Riben jinxiu weisheng tongji baogaoshu [Report on Health Statistics Training in Japan]," August 1952, 028000002830A, Academia Historica.

[87] Neizheng bu [Ministry of the Interior], "Tigong lianheguo renkou shengming ji siyin tongji ziliao zuotanhui jilu [Minutes of the Meeting on Providing the United Nations with Vital and Cause-of-Death Statistics]," May 31, 1955, 028000002832A, Academia Historica.

Similar difficulties were encountered when attempting to implement the ICD in the ROC, not only because of the government's administrative failures, but also because the ROC did not place any importance on the collection of vital and health statistics. In 1955, the ROC government sent Guo Songgen, then the director of the public health school at the National Taiwan University, to participate in the seventh revision of the ICD. On his return, Guo drew up a report on his experience and listed the conclusions of the conference.[88] Although considerable efforts had been made to ensure the ICD-7 was applied in member states, Guo – despite taking part in the conference – did not recommend that his government use the updated list. Four years later, when the United States aid agency in Taiwan launched a program to improve the vital statistical system, researchers found that many local administrations were still using the death certificate form from the 1929 version of the ICD.[89]

Despite facing setbacks within the ROC administration, the WHO's statistical initiatives were not completely useless. For one thing, they raised ROC officials' awareness about integrating statistical practices into health administrations. In 1955, the WHO proposed sending consultants to improve statistical collection in the ROC. The Executive Yuan, the executive branch of the ROC government, convened a meeting of all statistical officials to discuss this proposal. The debate was heated, with participants taking turns to complain about the difficulties they encountered when collecting statistics. For instance, due to a lack of training and awareness about the importance of statistics, collection on the ground had limited oversight; there were no trained staff to verify death certificates filled out by civilians; and a lack of doctors paralyzed the process of designating causes of death.[90] The director of the provincial statistical bureau concluded that "our statistics [for the whole ROC] were merely decorative."[91] As a result, participants unanimously agreed to accept a visit from WHO consultants, and suggested that the Ministry of the Interior set up a committee for vital statistics and survey design.

---

[88] Quo Songgen, "Fengpai daibiao woguo canjia lianheguo shijie weisheng zuzhi diqici guoji jibing mingcheng ji siwang yuanyin huiyi baogaoshu [Report on the 7th Revision of the International List of Diseases and Causes of Death]," February 1955, 028000002300A, Academia Historica.

[89] JCRR Rural Health Department, "Minutes of the Discussion Meeting on Vital Statistics," June 26, 1959, 286/150/38/08.09/06.07.01/8, National Archives and Records Administration, College Park.

[90] Neizheng bu [Ministry of the Interior], "Neizheng bu guanyu shengming tongji an huiyi jilu [Minutes of Meeting of the Ministry of the Interior on Matters of Vital Statistics]," August 19, 1955, 028000002832A, Academia Historica.

[91] Ibid.

Limited central health administration capacity gave rise to the third driver of the WHO reporting system's failure in Taiwan. As public health affairs remained marginal and underfunded within the ROC central government and the Taiwan provincial government, vital and health statisticians began to leave Taiwan for more promising careers with the WHO. Tellingly, although the ROC's own vital and health statistics were poorly organized, Guo, an ROC national, was the regional statistician for the WHO Western Pacific Regional Office from 1957 and traveled between countries to give suggestions on the use of statistics.[92] Guo was a Taiwanese physician who had worked in Manchuria during the Second Sino-Japanese War. He had also worked with the UNRRA to organize the return of Taiwanese people from Manchuria. In 1950, he received biostatistics training at the JHSPH through a fellowship paid for by the American Bureau for Medical Aid to China.[93] Upon his return to Taiwan, he served as the director of the NHA and a professor at the National Taiwan University School of Public Health, before joining the WHO as a regional statistician. Although there are no sources that directly indicate the precise reason why Guo left Taiwan, according to his former colleague at the National Taiwan University, Chen Jingsheng (Ch'en Ching-Sheng), Guo was sidelined within the school of public health after returning from his position at the NHA – a position that did not have much budget or power by that time[94] – and it was this slight that made him decide to work for the WHO.[95] Another example was that of Rong Qirong, a port health specialist who had acted as the director of the China Epidemic Prevention Bureau in the interwar years and then as an NHA statistician during the Second Sino-Japanese War. When the ROC government retreated to Taiwan in 1949, political instability probably drove Yung to leave and accept the WHO's invitation to work for the Eastern Bureau in Singapore.[96] Neither Guo nor Yung ever returned to work for the ROC, except when sent by the WHO as short-term consultants on

---

[92] Quo, "Activity Reports by the WPRO Regional Adviser on Health Statistics."

[93] ABMAC, "1950 US Fellows," 1955, 63/Fellowship 1946–1955 information, American Bureau for Medical Aid to China Records, Columbia University Libraries.

[94] From 1949 to 1971, the ROC's budget for public health was mostly limited to the Taiwan provincial government and two special municipalities: the cities of Taipei and Kaohsiung. The NHA performed only limited functions since it did not receive much funding from the central government.

[95] Chen Jinsheng, "Taiwan weisheng xingzheng he yixue jiaoyu yibainian shi [One Hundred Years of Public Health Administration and Medical Education in Taiwan]" (2006), 111, 410.3 7582, National Taiwan University Library.

[96] Winston Yung, "Report of the Singapore Epidemiological Intelligence Station for the Month of May, 1949," June 10, 1949, 452-6-13, World Health Organization Archives.

WHO salaries.[97] Notably, Yuan Yijin, the first Johns Hopkins-trained public health statistician in China (see Chapter 2), also worked on tuberculosis statistics at the WHO at times. Yuan, however, was affiliated with Academia Sinica, the ROC's highest research institution.

When we juxtapose the ROC's rustic statistical system with the career paths of its health statisticians, the limits of the WHO's network for transferring statistical standards becomes apparent. Although the WHO expected ROC statisticians to integrate statistical knowledge into the administration, the statisticians found themselves at an impasse, as the ROC government did not prioritize reform of its vital and health statistical systems. Due to lack of funding, and despite several statisticians receiving training at the WHO, health statistics collection and civil registration remained siloed within the ROC's administration, and the reliability of its vital and health statistics remained questionable.

*

This chapter has outlined how the international health statistics reporting system was revived and implemented from Geneva to Washington, DC, to China and Taiwan. Compared to the LNHO's patchwork authority, the UNRRA and the WHO's takeover of the system was much more straightforward. The WHO aspired to centralize all types of statistics collected in administration, research, and policy-making. WHO statisticians aimed to take local variation into account in their policy-making, while creating a regional tier of statisticians to mediate knowledge and practices between international, regional, and national statistical administrations. Despite these innovations, the WHO's statistical policies came up against a challenging geopolitical context and local administrative failures, the same faced by its predecessors, the UNRRA and the WHOIC. The epidemiological intelligence system during the UNRRA and WHOIC years consisted of two separate circuits of transfer: the UNRRA and the NHA shared epidemiological information with each other, whereas field staff based their day-to-day decisions on the number of patients admitted to local health services, which they communicated among themselves but never reported to the UNRRA. The WHO's limited success in implementing its reporting system in Taiwan highlights the decisive role of the Cold War rivalry as well as the considerable administrative constraints in place.

---

[97] Chen Jinsheng, "Taiwan weisheng xingzheng he yixue jiaoyu yibainian shi," 118.

Not all of the WHO's statistical initiatives failed. Statistics were integrated into WHO-sponsored disease control programs and were collected and analyzed in both Geneva and Taipei. In the next chapter, I will discuss the strategies used by public health experts to collect and report statistics related to such programs, and the extent to which those experts' statistical practices influenced global health policy-making.

# 6    The Art of Rhetoric
Statistical Standards at Work, from Fieldwork
to World Policy-Making

Public health, in my mind, is a practical science. Our aim is to get
the best benefit for our people's health with up-to-date knowledge and
available resources of personnel and facilities within a minimum of
time. Health workers should not satisfy themselves with a few training
centers or a few demonstration centers. The success of such trainings or
demonstrations lies [in] whether these would solve the existing health
problem and whether these are practical.[1]

By repeatedly stressing the term "practical," Tao Rongjin (T'ao Jung-
Chin), the leading expert at the tuberculosis control program supported
by the World Health Organization (WHO) in Taiwan, exemplified the
pragmatism shared by most of his colleagues in Taiwanese health organizations. Tao was part of a cohort of Taiwanese public health experts,
trained in the United States and employed by the health administration and research institutes of the Republic of China (ROC), which had
been based in Taiwan since 1949. Such experts acted as intermediaries
for international organizations and the ROC's health agencies, and they
strove to obtain financial and technical aid from foreign health organizations so as to implement public health measures in Taiwan. Statistics, as
the lingua franca of health programs within the framework of the WHO,
served as an essential tool for communicating with the organization's
headquarters in Geneva.

In this chapter, I explore these experts' practices and strategies with
regard to the statistical collection systems used in the WHO's epidemic control campaigns from 1948 to the 1960s: a period in which the
WHO initially expanded its budget for programs centered on a single
technology. It was also a period that Anne-Emanuelle Birn describes

[1] Jung-Chin T'ao, "To Elizabeth W. Bracket," October 2, 1957, RG469/ICA US
Operations Mission, Taiwan, Public Health Division: Subject Files, 1952–1961/box
12, National Archives and Records Administration, College Park.

as the "bureaucratization and professionalization" stage of international health, when international health collaboration was centralized under the auspices of the WHO thanks to its more extensive membership in comparison with its predecessors.[2] As presented in the previous chapter, the WHO aimed to centralize all statistics for administration, research, and policy-making. The organization's founding staff saw statistics as a medium for sharing information between health administrations, researchers, and policy-makers. The WHO health statistics division thus became the rule-setter for epidemic control programs. This chapter will examine how experts, including those based in Geneva and Taiwan, integrated statistical collection into WHO-led disease control fieldwork, and how numbers were mobilized in the WHO's policy-making process.

Existing historiographies have shed light on how statistics were omnipresent in programs such as epidemic control, family planning, nutrition, and psychiatry.[3] I take the further step of investigating how statistical practices were designed and implemented, and how statistical practices changed the course of public health programs. Drawing on WHO archives as well as the ROC government archives in Taiwan, I examine how WHO statisticians designed statistical practices for its malaria control program (which later became the Global Malaria Eradication Program [GMEP]) and tuberculosis control program, the two flagship efforts of the WHO's first decade. I also detail how the WHO's statistical system for planning and evaluating campaigns on the ground was taken up by Taiwanese experts. Historiographies that cover the Taiwanese government's interactions with foreign aid agencies (including United Nations agencies, the United States government aid agency, and other philanthropic foundations) often focus on a specific program, such as malaria control, tuberculosis control, or family planning.[4] This group

---

[2] Anne-Emanuelle Birn, "The Stages of International (Global) Health: Histories of Success or Successes of History?" *Global Public Health* 4, no. 1 (2009): 56; Birn, Pillay, and Holtz, *Textbook of Global Health*, 53–9.

[3] For example: Matthew Connelly, *Fatal Misconception: The Struggle to Control World Population* (Cambridge, MA: Harvard University Press, 2008); Nick Cullather, *The Hungry World: America's Cold War Battle against Poverty in Asia* (Cambridge, MA: Harvard University Press, 2010); Packard, *The Making of a Tropical Disease*; Harry Yi-Jui Wu, *Mad by the Millions: Mental Disorders and the Early Years of the World Health Organization* (Cambridge, MA: MIT Press, 2021).

[4] See, e.g.: Kuo Wen-Hua, "Yijiuwuling zhi qiling niandai Taiwan jiating jihua: Yiliao zhengce yu nuxing shi de tantao [Family Planning in Taiwan from 1950 to 1970: An Exploration of Medical Policy and Women's History]" (Hsinchu: Institute of History, National Tsing Hua University, 1997); Chang Shu-Ching, "Fanglao tixi yu jiankong jishu: Taiwan jiehebing shi yanjiu (1945–1970s) [The System of Tuberculosis Control and the Techniques of Surveillance: The History of Tuberculosis in Taiwan (1945–1970s)]" (Hsinchu: National Tsing-Hua University, 2004); Wu Meng-Hui,

of historiographies lays a solid foundation; however, it pays little attention to how statistical information collected in public health fieldwork was shared and used in policy-making between the ROC government and the WHO.

I will begin by offering an account of the core roles accorded to statistics by the WHO for connecting fieldwork administration, research, and policy-making within the malaria and tuberculosis control programs; the organization relied here on quantified standards and collected numbers to govern the programs from a distance. This statistical system – which connected WHO experts, Taiwanese officers, and field staff – had a serious potential for impact, as producing favorable numbers eventually became the main aim of fieldwork. Statistics became a pervasive part of policy advocacy as experts presented, cited, and discussed numbers as part of the policy-making process. Though the experts ceded some of their authority to numbers, they were still a salient part of the policy-making process thanks to their role in curating and making sense of those numbers.

## Fieldwork Administration, Research, and Policy-Making in Disease Control Programs

The WHO's founding statisticians were in charge of setting standards for statistical practices within the organization's public health programs. To ensure the reliability of statistics collected in the field, Satya Swaroop, a former associate professor at the All India Institute and chief of the

"Zhanhou Taiwan de feijiehebing fangzhi (1950–1966) [Prevention of Pulmonary Tuberculosis in Taiwan after the Second World War (1950–1966)]" (Nantou: National Chi-Nan University, 2004); Kuo Wen-Hua, "Meiyuan xia de weisheng zhengce: 1960 niandai Taiwan jiating jihua de tantao [Public Health Policy with US Aid: Discussions of Taiwan's Family Planning in the 1960s]," in *Diguo yu xiandai yixue [Empires and Modern Medicine]*, eds. Li Shang-jen (Taipei: Linking Publishing, 2008), 325–65; Chang Shu-Ching, "1950 & 60 niandai Taiwan de kajiemiao yufang jiezhong jihua [The BCG Vaccination Program in Taiwan in the 1950s and 1960s]," *Keji, yiliao yu shehui [Taiwanese Journal for Studies of Science, Technology and Medicine]*, no. 8 (2009): 121–72; Yi-Ping Lin and Shiyung Liu, "A Forgotten War: Malaria Eradication in Taiwan 1905–1965," in *Health and Hygiene in Chinese East Asia: Policies and Publics in the Long Twentieth Century* , eds. Angela Ki Che Leung and Charlotte Furth (Durham, NC: Duke University Press, 2010), 183–203; Michael Shiyung Liu, "From Japanese Colonial Medicine to American-Standard Medicine in Taiwan: A Case Study of the Transition in the Medical Profession and Practices in East Asia," in *Science, Public Health and the State in Modern Asia*, eds. Liping Bu, Darwin H. Stapleton, and Ka-Che Yip (London: Routledge, 2012), 161–76; Hsu Feng-Yuan, "Shijie weisheng zuzhi yu Taiwan nueji de fangzhi (1950–1972) [Taiwan–World Health Organization Malaria Control Measures (1950–1972)]" (Taipei: National Chengchi University, 2013).

statistical studies section of the WHO's health statistics division, organized expert committees to discuss discrepancies between methodology
and reality.[5] Participants in the committees discussed sampling methodologies for morbidity statistics in 1958, the conduct of health surveys
in 1960, and the uses of statistics in public health fieldwork studies in
1972.[6] During these discussions, a wide range of sampling and survey
approaches were listed, with the aim of integrating laboratory principles
into public health fieldwork by devising control groups and treatment
groups, then comparing the results.

The statisticians' focus on survey methodologies vividly demonstrates
the WHO's hopes of relying on quantification to govern from a distance.[7]
Through rigorously devised methods, the organization aimed to impose
a grammar on the language of statistics and paint a reliable picture of
the situation on the ground that experts – whether based in Geneva or
within local health authorities – could comprehend.[8] Following the same
rationale, WHO statisticians also devised a statistical apparatus within
the organization to oversee and manage the statistics collected from epidemic control initiatives. For each initiative, the health statistics division
published instructions for collecting and analyzing quantitative data.

A prime example was the GMEP, launched by the WHO in 1955. Having witnessed the early success of insecticide DDT (dichloro-diphenyl-
trichloroethane) spraying campaigns against malaria in Europe and Latin
America, the WHO used DDT spraying for its malaria control program
since the organization opened its door. In 1955, the organization further
decided that the GMEP could reduce its budget for malaria control by rapidly eradicating the disease once and for all through intense DDT spraying
that would kill mosquitoes and stop malaria transmission before mosquitoes became resistant and the chemical lost its effectiveness.[9] The original

[5] WHO, "Expert Committee on Health Statistics Sixth Report," 3, Geneva, WHO,
1957; "Expert Committee on Health Statistics Seventh Report," 11, Geneva:
WHO, 1961; "Expert Committee on Health Statistics Fifteenth Report," Geneva:
WHO, 1972.
[6] WHO, "Expert Committee on Health Statistics Sixth Report," 3; "Expert Committee
on Health Statistics Seventh Report," 11; "Expert Committee on Health Statistics
Fifteenth Report."
[7] The statistics' characteristic for governance from a distance is discussed in: e.g. James
C. Scott, *Seeing Like a State: How Certain Schemes to Improve the Human Condition
Have Failed* (New Haven, CT: Yale University Press, 1998); Espeland and Stevens,
"A Sociology of Quantification," 415; Wendy Nelson Espeland and Michael Sauder,
*Engines of Anxiety: Academic Rankings, Reputation, and Accountability* (New York:
Russell Sage Foundation, 2016).
[8] This insight comes from Espeland and Stevens, "A Sociology of Quantification," 405.
[9] Randall M. Packard, "Malaria Dreams: Postwar Visions of Health and Development
in the Third World," *Medical Anthropology* 17, no. 3 (1997): 279; WHO, "Expert
Committee on Malaria Sixth Report," Geneva: WHO, 1957.

malaria control programs had had the same budget every triennium, and the GMEP would cap that budget. Moreover, WHO experts contended that money spent on the GMEP was an investment with a foreseeable return: more available manpower.[10] The GMEP was the WHO's core project during the 1950s and 1960s. By the time it ended in 1969, a total of $1.4 billion had been spent on it.[11]

WHO staff believed that statistics collected from fieldwork would be the key to eradicating malaria quickly, allowing them to keep track of existing malaria cases and report to the administration for follow-up.[12] The Sixth Expert Committee on Malaria expressed the WHO's official vision: the GMEP was a "well-administrated attack based on epidemiological studies." WHO experts further explained, in a technical report, that "it [was] not only necessary to make plans sufficiently in advance, but to keep data and their analysis flowing at a speed that [would] allow profitable use of the information and the prompt correction of errors."[13] Committee members thus had faith that statistics would lead to rapid policy adjustments.

For similar reasons, the health statistics division published statistical manuals for malaria control fieldwork as early as 1956, one year after the launch of the GMEP. Swaroop first published *Statistical Notes for Malaria Workers* in 1956, and an amended version, *Statistical Methodology in Malaria Work*, in 1957. These manuals set forth methodologies for sampling and recording health statistics in the field and explained the principles behind statistical tests.[14] Swaroop subsequently published books on statistical practices that were even more tailored to the implementation of the GMEP: *Statistical Considerations and Methodology in Malaria Eradication* (1959) and the posthumous *Statistical Methods in Malaria Eradication* (1966), which set forth standardized collection procedures for the preparation, attack, consolidation, and maintenance phases of the GMEP.[15]

Every aspect of the GMEP was quantified in some way, whether in terms of standards or survey methods that aimed to quantify conditions on the spot. For instance, the Expert Committee specified the amount of

[10] WHO, "Expert Committee on Malaria Sixth Report," 9.
[11] Packard, *The Making of a Tropical Disease*, 159.
[12] WHO, "Expert Committee on Malaria Sixth Report," 9.
[13] Ibid., 19.
[14] Swaroop, Satya and WHO, *Statistical Notes for Malaria Workers* (Geneva: WHO, 1956), http://apps.who.int/iris/handle/10665/64526; Satya Swaroop and WHO, *Statistical Methodology in Malaria Work* (Geneva: WHO, 1957), https://apps.who.int/iris/handle/10665/64527.
[15] Satya Swaroop and WHO, "Statistical Considerations and Methodology in Malaria Eradication" (World Health Organization, 1959), https://apps.who.int/iris/handle/10665/64660; Satya Swaroop, Alan Brownlie Gilroy, Kazuo Uemura, and WHO, *Statistical Methods in Malaria Eradication* (Geneva: WHO, 1966), https://apps.who.int/iris/handle/10665/41775.

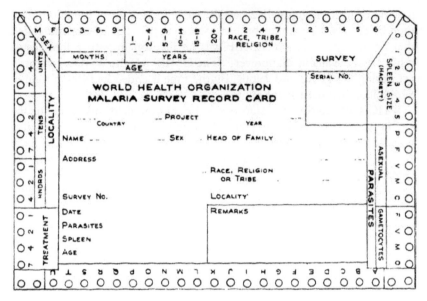

Figure 6.1 An example of a punch card used in the WHO's malaria survey.
Reproduced from "Statistical Considerations and Methodology in Malaria Eradication," Satya Swaroop and WHO, Designing Record Cards, p. 52, Copyright (1959).

DDT spray required to meet the normal criterion of efficacy, a dose of 2.0 g/m², stating that this was more likely to be effective on most types of surfaces.[16] And Swaroop's manuals contained statistical methods for evaluating the resistance of the *Anopheles* mosquitoes to DDT and the proper sampling methods for evaluating residual DDT on household surfaces.

The image above illustrates how the GMEP was administered from a distance using statistical practices. A punch-card system, designed by Swaroop, facilitated the calculation and monitoring of malaria cases around the world.[17] On the ground, health service providers recorded each malaria patient on a punch card that also contained their personal information and symptoms (see Figure 6.1). The cards were then sent to a national malaria research center, supported by the WHO, for further analysis. The research center then reported the raw data, along with its analysis, to the WHO.

[16] WHO, "Expert Committee on Malaria Fifth Report," 7, WHO Technical Report Series 80 (Geneva: WHO, 1954).

[17] Swaroop and WHO, "Statistical Considerations and Methodology in Malaria Eradication," 51.

Statistics were used to convey the local situation to Geneva (the center of policy-making), but experts made use of their own knowledge to decide how to present the quantified outcomes. In 1966, eleven years after the official launch of the GMEP, the Expert Committee on Malaria published a map that showed all fifty-two countries that had taken part in the GMEP, even though only ten of them had actually eradicated malaria.[18] The results were not as good as expected, but the committee did not acknowledge that in its discourse. Instead, it attributed the disappointing results to external causes and insisted on the GMEP's potential for success. The committee explained that they "acutely realize[d] the differences between different regions of the world," and that the GMEP's previous level of funding was insufficient because the value of local currencies was dropping,[19] all the while stressing the program's significance by enumerating how many people it covered.[20] The poor quantified results did not lead to the immediate discontinuation of the program. It was not until three years later that the World Health Assembly finally ended the GMEP, as the growing financial burden, resistance to DDT and antimalarial drugs, and a lack of flexibility in implementation had exhausted member states' enthusiasm for the program.[21]

The GMEP was not the only program to be managed through extensive quantification. During the same period, the WHO's tuberculosis control program also made use of an overarching statistical system, including standardized punch cards for recording cases and a random sampling methodology applied to prevalence surveys. To ensure the system was implemented, the WHO dispatched epidemiological experts either to supervise the use of statistical methods in the field or to implement such methods themselves. In 1957, for example, the WHO sent a consultant, Truls Zeiner-Henriksen, to Taiwan for six months to establish a central tuberculosis registry there.[22] And in 1960, F. A. Assad, an epidemiologist and statistician from the United Arab Republic, was sent to standardize the coding numbers of punch cards based on a recording system set forth in document WHO/CENTS/53/3, with

[18] WHO, "Expert Committee on Malaria Thirteenth Report," 6, WHO Technical Report Series 357 (Geneva: WHO, 1967).
[19] Ibid.
[20] Ibid., 3, 22.
[21] Packard, *The Making of a Tropical Disease*, 150–71.
[22] The Coordination Committee, "Minutes of the Meeting (182) of the Coordination Committee on Foreign Aid in Medicine and Health," March 9, 1957, 286/150/38/08.09/06.07.01/1, National Archives and Records Administration, College Park.

the United Nations Children's Fund (UNICEF) providing funding for machine tabulation.[23]

Just as with the GMEP, the WHO relied on quantification to provide preliminary answers and to govern its tuberculosis program from a distance. Unlike for malaria, WHO staff did not have an official stand on the best way to tackle tuberculosis across the world, although a resolution had been adopted at the First World Health Assembly in 1948 that made the Bacillus Calmette–Guérin (BCG) vaccine an integral part of the organization's tuberculosis control program.[24] Given the controversy surrounding the efficacy of the BCG vaccine, the WHO was unwilling to embrace a mass vaccination campaign right away. Instead, it established the Tuberculosis Research Office in Copenhagen, which placed strong emphasis on statistical methods. Citing the "operational research" method, in which mathematical models are used to determine the best solution in military situations,[25] the Office called for the use of standardized statistical methods to collect global tuberculosis statistics so as to determine the best way to respond to epidemics.[26] The Office was responsible for surveying tuberculosis prevalence rates before launching mass immunization campaigns, recording the results of tuberculin tests on schoolchildren, and examining changes in prevalence rates after the implementation of BCG vaccination campaigns. As part of an international tuberculosis control campaign supported by UNICEF and Scandinavian voluntary organizations – which hoped to implement BCG vaccination all over the world – the Tuberculosis Research Office dispatched Chinese expert Yuan Yijin, the first statistician trained at Peking Union Medical College (PUMC) (see Chapter 2), to countries such as Greece, Syria, Egypt, India, and Ecuador from 1948 to 1951 to compile statistical data on tuberculosis and the BCG vaccine.[27]

Contrary to expectations, the mass collection of statistical data did not provide a firm answer as to the efficacy of the BCG vaccine. For instance, although some BCG vaccination campaigns had satisfying results, United

---

[23] Alan Penington, "Final Report – June 1956–March 1960," May 24, 1960, 7–8, 286/150/38/08.09/06.07.01/15, National Archives and Records Administration, College Park; "United Nations Technical Assistance Personnel in China as of June 1961," June 23, 1961, 8–9, 286/150/38/08.09/06.07.01/10, National Archives and Records Administration, College Park.

[24] WHO, "Official Records of the WHO, Vol.13," n.d., 300, cited in: Brimnes, "BCG Vaccination and WHO's Global Strategy for Tuberculosis Control 1948–1983," 865.

[25] See, e.g.: Maurice W. Kirby, *Operational Research in War and Peace: The British Experience from the 1930s to 1970* (London: Imperial College Press, 2003).

[26] WHO, "Bureau de Recherches sur la Tuberculose (Copenhague)," 2–3.

[27] In total, Yuan worked in Czechoslovakia, Poland, Syria, Israel, Malta, Tunisia, Ecuador, Austria, Morocco (and Tangiers), Greece, and Yugoslavia (ibid., 36).

States Public Health Service trials in Puerto Rico and the American states of Georgia and Alabama showed protection rates of only 31 percent and 36 percent, respectively.[28] It was thus up to WHO experts to decide which strategy to adopt and how to justify it. As Christian McMillen has convincingly argued, the WHO's policy choices were not solely dependent on statistical results but in large part based on experts' understanding of public health work in different regions of the world. Halfdan Mahler, by that time a WHO tuberculosis adviser, favored BCG vaccination and argued that tuberculosis required a pragmatic solution. Mahler also contended that, as properly administrated in-home treatment was not feasible in poorer countries, the BCG vaccine was an ideal compromise owing to its low cost and lack of side effects.[29] McMillen presents a convincing case that numbers played a greater role in justifying policy choices than in actually making those choices, as Mahler turned to old data to bolster his argument. Because recent projects had failed to produce significant results, Mahler instead cited statistics from Joseph Aronson's 1938 trial, which showed 80 percent efficacy.[30] Notably, this 80 percent efficacy was not enough to convince WHO experts to fully embrace the BCG vaccine in the late 1940s, and yet this efficacy rate eventually became the best known statistic in the 1950s, and continued to be cited by Mahler, who went on to become chief of the tuberculosis unit in 1962.[31]

Mahler was not alone in cherry-picking statistics to support his policy choices. In published reports, other WHO experts also used their overall knowledge of the vaccine and the trial designs to challenge the quantified results produced by field trials, which had put the BCG vaccine's reputation in danger. As Niels Brimnes writes, WHO experts consistently used the inclusion of individuals of low-grade sensitivity and the existence of various BCG sub-strains as a "joker card" – to use Brimnes' wording – to explain why field trials did not show a sufficient degree of protection.[32]

---

[28] WHO, "Review of BCG Vaccination Programs," May 1959, 21–3, cited in: Brimnes, "BCG Vaccination and WHO's Global Strategy for Tuberculosis Control 1948–1983," 867.

[29] McMillen, *Discovering Tuberculosis – A Global History, 1900 to the Present*, 100–1.

[30] Aronson organized his trial in an Indian conservatory, with approximately 1,500 people in the test group and the same number in the control group. He stressed that his trial had controls for the age, sex, and living area of test subjects, and that only social conditions were not fully controlled. Although people from both groups died from tuberculosis, and despite the fact that overall tuberculosis prevalence was already declining in the area when the trial took place, Aronson concluded that his trial showed the BCG vaccine to be 80 percent effective (ibid., 83).

[31] Ibid., 112–13.

[32] Brimnes, "BCG Vaccination and WHO's Global Strategy for Tuberculosis Control 1948–1983," 864.

Specifically, WHO experts used such arguments to invalidate trials that showed a low degree of protection. In this way, they were able to claim that the BCG vaccine's degree of protection remained unknown. For example, experts participating in a WHO-sponsored seminar on tuberculosis in Nairobi in the 1960s again insisted on the value of the vaccine, despite a lack of direct proof as to its degree of protection.[33]

Similar methods of selectively presenting statistics were also employed in support of in-home therapy for tuberculosis patients. The WHO exhibited varying attitudes regarding field trials of in-home therapy organized by the Tuberculosis Chemotherapy Center in Madras, India. Established in 1956 in partnership with the Indian Council of Medical Research, the Madras state government, and the British Medical Research Council, the center's first trial was a controlled experiment on the effectiveness of in-home treatment of pulmonary tuberculosis using chemotherapy and isoniazid, as compared to treatment in a sanatorium.[34] In the experiment, the center dispatched public health nurses to follow up on tuberculosis patients' home care, including pill-taking and home quarantine. The experiment demonstrated that the group of patients who had received in-home treatment had the same rate of recovery as those treated in sanatoria. The results were published in the *Bulletin of the World Health Organization*, the foremost WHO publication on public health research.[35] However, when a subsequent trial in Madras suggested that drug resistance to isoniazid was pervasive, the Expert Committee on Tuberculosis showed great reluctance to take the new findings into account, fearing it would devalue isoniazid – and in so doing, in-home therapy. Eventually, without invalidating isoniazid, the technical report conservatively stated that "adequate information on the present prevalence of primary resistance is still not available," downplaying the large quantity of data pointing to isoniazid resistance that had been collected through trials in Hong Kong, Ghana, South Africa, and other places.[36] Just as they had when promoting the BCG vaccine, WHO experts replaced unfavorable results with vague statements, such as there being a lack of proof as to the efficacy of isoniazid.

The examples of the GMEP and the tuberculosis control programs shed light on how statistical practices were implemented in the WHO's epidemic control initiatives. Both examples show that WHO statisticians

[33] McMillen, *Discovering Tuberculosis – A Global History, 1900 to the Present*, 113.
[34] "Tuberculosis Chemotherapy Centre, Madras," *Tubercle* 49, no. 1 (1968): 114.
[35] S. Velu, R. H. Andrews, S. Devadatta, et al., "Progress in the Second Year of Patients with Quiescent Pulmonary Tuberculosis after a Year of Chemotherapy at Home or in Sanatorium, and Influence of Further Chemotherapy on the Relapse Rate," *Bulletin of the World Health Organization* 23, no. 4–5 (1960): 511–33.
[36] McMillen, *Discovering Tuberculosis – A Global History, 1900 to the Present*, 147.

devised a circular system that connected fieldwork administration, research, and policy-making: statistical practices were to guide fieldwork, which would provide data for research and eventually inform the WHO's policies. Under this system, however, WHO experts were still able to use their pre-existing knowledge on a given public health technology to select, invalidate, or interpret statistics collected from fieldwork. In both the GMEP and the tuberculosis control programs, WHO experts were able to decide which field statistics were reliable, and how to attribute the causes of unexpected quantified results. In this sense, WHO experts used statistics not only as a language to communicate the situation in the field, but also as a rhetorical instrument to reinforce their policy decisions. The way these experts selectively presented statistics (and commented on the lack of quantified proof for policies that were not supported by the numbers) also clearly demonstrates that statistics had an independent authority of their own, as experts were nonetheless obliged to cite – and make peace with – the numbers in their reports.

## The Chishan Experiment: Tailoring GMEP Methods to Taiwanese Conditions

Geneva-based experts were not the only ones to contribute and analyze statistics for the WHO's disease control programs. At the local level, ROC officials also played a role in the communication of field statistics to WHO headquarters.

The ROC's inclusion in WHO disease control programs can be traced back to 1950. Between 1950 and 1951, shortly after the ROC central government had retreated to Taiwan, the government signed agreements with the WHO and UNICEF on a wide array of programs, including malaria and tuberculosis control.[37] In these agreements, the WHO stipulated that beneficiary countries must share their data with

---

[37] The agreements required both sides to take on specific responsibilities: whereas UNICEF's budget often included a considerable amount of donated medical materials and vaccines, the WHO agreements focused on the transfer of public health knowledge by paying the salaries of foreign consultants and funding fellowships for ROC officials. The WHO and UNICEF coordinated their contributions to implement technology-centered programs (e.g. DDT spraying for malaria and the BCG vaccine for tuberculosis). As historians have observed, the strategy employed by United Nations public health programs during the 1950s and 1960s was to roll out what were presumed to be the most advanced technologies into member states. See, e.g.: Sunil Amrith, "In Search of a 'Magic Bullet' for Tuberculosis: South India and ʾond, 1955–1965," *Social History of Medicine* 17, no. 1 (2004): 113–30; Theodore ʾown, Marcos Cueto, and Elizabeth Fee, "The World Health Organization and ʾnsition from 'International' to 'Global' Public Health," *American Journal of ʾlth* 96, no. 1 (2006): 62–72.

the organization for publication.[38] Under the framework of the agreements, the WHO sent consultants to Taiwan from time to time to monitor fieldwork, and Taiwanese public health workers were trained to take up statistical practices not only for fieldwork administration but also to provide data for public health research.

Public health officials in Taiwan, trained either in the Japanese medical system (during the colonial period) or at American-funded public health schools in China and the United States (during the interwar period), were already familiar with public health administration and research. For instance, Tao Rongjin (T'ao Jung-Chin), the director of the Taipei Tuberculosis Control Center, was trained at PUMC from 1938 to 1942, then worked as a technical expert on tuberculosis at the Central Field Health Station from 1943 to 1946 before being sent on a fellowship to the Johns Hopkins School of Public Health (JHSPH) in 1947.[39] The head of the malaria control program in Taiwan, Liang Guangqi (Liang Kuang-Ch'i, K. C. Liang), graduated from Taipei Imperial University in 1945 and worked as the acting vice-director of the Rockefeller-funded Taiwan Malaria Research Institute (TMRI) from 1946 to 1949; when the Rockefeller Foundation left Taiwan, Liang studied at the JHSPH on a Rockefeller-funded fellowship. Upon his return, he was promoted to director of the TMRI and was put in charge of research activities for the WHO's malaria control programs in Taiwan.[40] In addition to Liang, sixty-four staff from the TMRI were trained by the Rockefeller Foundation from 1946 to 1949.[41] When the WHO began its epidemic control

[38] WHO, "Supplementary Agreement to the Basic Agreement Between the Government of the Republic of China and the World Health Organization for the Provision of Technical Advisory Assistance," n.d., 4, 286/150/38/08.09/06.07.01/16, National Archives and Records Administration, College Park.
[39] Tao had specialized in tuberculosis control since finishing his studies at PUMC. From 1943 to 1944, he was the physician in charge of the tuberculosis clinic in Chongqing, and in 1947 he was transferred to the Nanjing tuberculosis center (Jung-Chin T'ao, "Personal History Record and Application for Fellowship: T'ao Jung-Chin," March 25, 1947, rf/10.1/601E/ Fellowship Files, Rockefeller Archive Center).
[40] Liang K'uang-Ch'i, "Personal History Record and Application for Fellowship: Liang K'uang Ch'i," February 15, 1950, RF/10.1/601E/ Fellowship Files, Rockefeller Archive Center; Tsai Duu-Jian and Yu Yumei, eds., *Taiwan yiliao daode zhi yanbian – ruogan licheng ji gean tantao [The Evolution of Medical Ethics in Taiwan: Selected Histories and Case Studies]* (Taipei: National Health Research Institutes, 2003), 208; Liang Fei-Yi and Tsai Duu-Jian, "Liang Kuangqi koushu lishi [Oral History of Liang Kuangqi]," *Taiwan fengwu [The Taiwan Folkways]* 59 (2009): 9–39.
[41] Donald J. Pletsch, "Terminal Report: Covering the Period of Service from May 15, 1952 to September 1, 1955," September 12, 1955, 2, 286/150/38/08.09/06.07.01/1, National Archives and Records Administration, College Park. Since TMRI staff members had received training on malaria control while the Rockefeller Foundation was still present, they remained key actors even after the ROC central government arrived in Taiwan. From the 1940s to the 1950s, all TMRI staff were Taiwanese,

programs in collaboration with the ROC government, these local experts were trained in the WHO's latest policies and methods of operation. They would go on to become key actors within the international system of fieldwork statistics.

The TMRI was put in charge of preparing to implement the WHO's malaria control program. The first step was to establish the situation in the field. The TMRI staff first undertook malaria prevalence surveys and malariometric and entomological experiments to learn about malaria conditions on the island. In 1951, Liang prepared a blood smear census in collaboration with malaria control stations and health stations throughout the island.[42] On 17 December 1951, workers from malaria control stations visited elementary schools in their districts, sampling 100 schoolchildren between the ages of two and seven and collecting blood smears. All smears were sent to the TMRI to determine whether plasmodium was present. It was the ROC's first island-wide investigation into the health status of the population in Taiwan. The results showed an average of 8.63 percent plasmodium in the blood smears. Based on the results of each village, the TMRI drew a malaria map of Taiwan, which would serve as the basis for the WHO's design of its malaria control programs there.[43] From then on, every 17 December, all malaria control stations conducted a blood smear census to track changes in malaria prevalence rates.[44]

Once the facts were established, it was time to determine the most suitable way to scale-up DDT spraying in the local conditions. In May 1952, the WHO sent E. A. Demos (a Greek malariologist), Donald J. Pletsch (an American entomologist), and P. S. Echavez (a Filipino sanitary engineer) to tackle the task.[45] The three experts set up malariometric

which was rare for a public service at that time (Hsu Sheng-Kai, *Rizhi shiqi Taipei gaodeng xuexiao yu jingying yangcheng [Higher Education and Elite Formation in Taipei during the Japanese Rule Period]* (Taipei: Airiti Press, 2012), 263).

[42] A total of 155 malaria control stations were established during the Japanese colonial period. They were abandoned several years after the ROC took over Taiwan in 1945, and it was not until in 1952, when the WHO launched its malaria control program in Taiwan, that all 155 of the prewar stations were reopened (Michael Shiyung Liu, "The Theory and Practices of Malariology in Colonial Taiwan," in *Disease, Colonialism, and the State: Malaria in Modern East Asian History*, ed. Ka-Che Yip (Hong Kong: Hong Kong University Press, 2009), 49–60; Liu, "From Japanese Colonial Medicine to American-Standard Medicine in Taiwan: A Case Study of the Transition in the Medical Profession and Practices in East Asia").

[43] Department of Health, *Taiwan punue jishi [Malaria Eradication in Taiwan]*, 2nd ed. (Taipei: Centers for Disease Control, Department of Health, 2005), 113.

[44] Ibid., 111.

[45] "List of the UNICEF and WHO Personnel in Taiwan, China," 1954, 028000001990A, Academia Historica.

and entomological experiments in Chishan, a township in Kaohsiung municipality, where they expected to derive benchmarks for subsequent DDT spraying.[46]

Chishan thus became a laboratory for DDT spraying. Much like the Milbank health demonstration in New York (see Chapter 4), Chishan was selected based on statistical reasoning, given the presence of malaria there: the original candidate town, Chaojhou (where the TMRI was based), had too low a malaria prevalence rate to provide significant results.[47] The WHO and TMRI experts were more thorough than those from Milbank, however, in following controlled laboratory principles. They divided the township into three areas; these would undergo full, selective, and zero DDT spraying, respectively (see Figure 6.2).[48] In each area, TMRI technicians collected *Anopheles* mosquitoes every two weeks and conducted home visits to convince inhabitants to provide blood smears by informing them that parents who accepted the procedure being conducted on their babies under age one would receive milk powder donated by UNICEF.[49] All schoolchildren in Chishan were gathered every two weeks to undergo a spleen size check and blood smear sampling; those who were absent received visits from the TMRI staff.[50] Seven months later, the three WHO experts again went to Chishan to conduct a similar check. They discovered that spleen sizes were dropping in the selectively and fully sprayed areas; in fact, they had dropped the most in the area that had undergone selective spraying. However, despite proclaiming that the zero-DDT-spraying area served as the control group, the TMRI did not carry out a spleen size check or *Anopheles* sampling in that area. Moreover, because people living in the control area protested about being left out, in 1953 the TMRI implemented DDT spraying there as well. The Chishan experiment's control area hence existed only for a short period in 1952.[51]

As of 1952, the Chishan experiment was not statistically significant. All data collected were merely descriptive statistics without statistical hypothesis testing.[52] Although there was no clear explanation as to why the selective spraying area had experienced the largest drop in spleen size among schoolchildren, the experts nonetheless decided that the

[46] Pletsch, "Terminal Report: Covering the Period of Service from May 15, 1952 to September 1, 1955."
[47] Department of Health, *Taiwan punue jishi*, 56.
[48] Ibid., 57.
[49] Hsu, "Shijie weisheng zuzhi yu Taiwan nueji de fangzhi (1950–1972)," 92.
[50] Tsai and Yu, *Taiwan yiliao daode zhi yanbian*, 121.
[51] Department of Health, *Taiwan punue jishi*, 72.
[52] Hsu, "Shijie weisheng zuzhi yu Taiwan nueji de fangzhi (1950–1972)," 94–5.

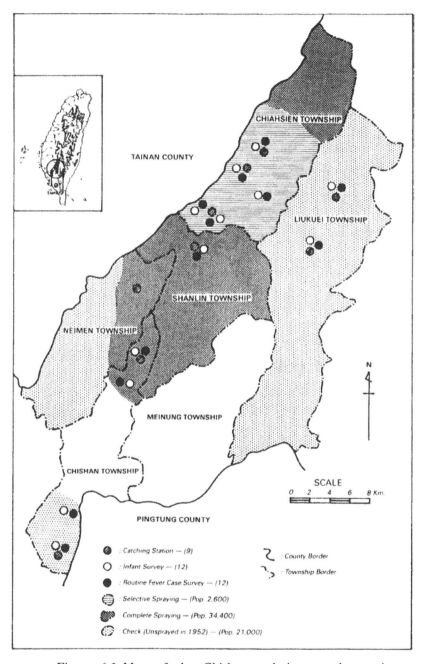

Figure 6.2 Map of the Chishan malaria control experiment. Department of Health, Malaria Eradication in Taiwan, 2nd ed. (Taipei: Centers for Disease Control, Department of Health, 2005), 75, www.cdc.gov.tw/InfectionReport/Info/etmdYAs54kXRRSHOiw 3C5A?infoId=mrl8S_96ADvSpl0j2kwX9A

reduction of malaria-bearing *Anopheles* mosquitoes and the drop in spleen size in the fully and selectively sprayed areas constituted strong enough evidence to validate DDT spraying in Taiwan. The WHO and TMRI staff approved DDT spraying as the main malaria control measure within the Taiwan program, and in 1954, due to the early success in investigated areas, the goal was modified from merely controlling malaria to totally eradicating it.[53]

An examination of the statistical practices used – and the decision to adopt DDT spraying – shows the distance that continued to separate statistics and policy-making, and the roles that experts played as intermediaries. Contrary to claims made at the beginning of the Chishan experiments, the results did not allow for a rigorous statistical test based on controlled laboratory principles. Possibly based on their general expertise and previous training, experts decided to approve DDT spraying in Taiwan despite the gaps in the quantified results. At the discursive level, quantification held considerable sway, and every report written by the WHO, the ROC government, and the United States aid agencies emphasized that the pre-operational survey in Chishan had played a salient role in determining the benchmark for the subsequent malaria control program.[54] In reality, the statistical practices used in the Chishan experiments resembled those used for the BCG vaccine: both reveal that experts had some leeway to select and interpret the numbers in such a way that they supported the WHO's ongoing policies.

## An Island-Wide Monitoring System, Based on Statistics

In addition to the Chishan experiments, Demos, Pletsch, and Echavez (the three WHO experts who had devised them) also collaborated with the TMRI to tailor the WHO's preferred policy – the use of DDT for malaria control – into a set of quantified standards so that implementation would be thorough and consistent. Based on a sample population of two villages (amounting to ninety-seven households or 704 total inhabitants), the experts concluded that the average spraying surface per person was $52.6 \text{ m}^2$,[55] that the ideal DDT concentration was $1.86 \text{ g/m}^2$,[56] and that spraying should be carried out every year, as the housing materials

---

[53] Pletsch, "Terminal Report: Covering the Period of Service from May 15, 1952 to September 1, 1955," 1.

[54] Ibid., 3.

[55] Department of Health, *Taiwan punue jishi*, 77.

[56] Tellingly, a concentration of DDT spray at $2 \text{g/m}^2$ (the WHO official standard) was used for DDT spraying operations across Taiwan, despite the Chishan experiment indicating that the ideal concentration was only $1.86 \text{ g/m}^2$ (ibid., 77).

did not absorb DDT.[57] A unit of seven workers could cover 356.71 m$^2$ per hour.[58] The cost per capita was 2.35 New Taiwan Dollars (about $0.23), of which 63.54 percent was spent on the DDT, 20.81 percent on worker salaries, and 15.65 percent on other expenses.[59] The experts noted that these costs would be adjusted annually.[60]

The TMRI established a roadmap for action in which it identified priority spraying areas through an island-wide spleen size survey, sampling 140,000 schoolchildren to determine the malaria prevalence in an area of 35,980 km$^2$, almost the entire island.[61] The institute also organized short-term training programs for DDT sprayers to distribute the quantified standards. During training, the workers (mostly twenty- to thirty-year-old men recruited on a temporary basis), learned and practiced standardized techniques for DDT spraying, including how to install the sprayer, prepare the liquid, and hold the nozzle at the proper angle to the wall during spraying.[62] One worker still clearly recalled the standardized method more than forty years later:

The optimal concentration of DDT was 75 percent and every m$^2$ had to be sprayed with 2 gm pure DDT. Based on this rule, we had to calculate how much DDT liquid should be prepared every minute, how much liquid should be sprayed every minute, and what the strength of the spray was, so that the DDT would not drip down on the wall. ... With the DDT sprayers that we used, the sprinkler had to be kept at 80 degrees to the wall, at a distance of 45 cm from the wall.[63]

The TMRI devised an island-wide network for malaria control that would be monitored using statistics. This monitoring system relied on more than 300 health centers dispersed throughout Taiwan.[64] Medical

---

[57] Hsu, "Shijie weisheng zuzhi yu Taiwan nueji de fangzhi (1950–1972)," 101.

[58] Department of Health, *Taiwan punue jishi*, 66.

[59] Ibid., 78.

[60] Pletsch, "Terminal Report: Covering the Period of Service from May 15, 1952 to September 1, 1955"; Department of Health, *Taiwan punue jishi*, 110.

[61] Pletsch, "Terminal Report: Covering the Period of Service from May 15, 1952 to September 1, 1955," 3.

[62] Department of Health, *Taiwan punue jishi*, 89.

[63] Translated from: Tsai and Yu, *Taiwan yiliao daode zhi yanbian*, 122.

[64] In 1949, prior to the agreements between the WHO/UNICEF and the ROC government, the Sino-American Joint Commission on Rural Reconstruction (JCRR), a United States aid agency in Taiwan, launched construction projects aimed at establishing a health center in every village in Taiwan. The JCRR planned for each health center to serve 20,000 to 30,000 local inhabitants and employ one or two doctors, two to five nurses, and one to four other health workers, including sanitary workers, to take on work that included clinical services, obstetric examinations, and immunizations. In less than two years, the number of health centers grew rapidly, from 101 to 343; in 1957, there were a total of 372 health centers across Taiwan. Since the WHO/UNICEF programs began in Taiwan in 1951, these health centers acted as the basic

officers at the health centers were involved in collecting statistics in the field to be communicated to higher-level health authorities.[65] Health center workers and malaria detection teams toured rural areas conducting daily door-to-door surveys on fever cases and taking blood smears. Meanwhile, TMRI technicians collected mosquitoes to examine the overall malaria levels of the area.[66] Malaria prevalence studies and fieldwork were followed by laboratory examinations at the TMRI. Through blood smear exams and wall sample checks, the status of malaria in Taiwan was constantly under the microscope. The TMRI staff took samples from sprayed households (by cutting a 10 cm$^2$ piece out of the wall) and sent them to the TMRI laboratory so it could determine if DDT spraying was in line with the benchmark.[67] The DDT spraying teams worked in a different part of the island and were required to submit a diary that included work hours, travel hours, working staff, number of villages, and beneficiary population numbers.[68]

The circuit of information described above was maintained by individuals whose work was tightly controlled through a system of punishments and rewards. Private medical practitioners were encouraged to take blood smears from their patients, and for every blood smear that contained plasmodium, the practitioner received a bonus from the TMRI.[69] The TMRI laboratory workforce was also monitored using statistics. Every staff member was required to examine seventy blood smears per day, and to ensure the quality of the examinations, each smear was double-checked by a different staff member. For every smear incorrectly labeled as clean, the lab worker lost a third of his or her salary. Three mistakes would cost the worker a whole month's pay.[70]

This statistics-based system of punishments and rewards, though somewhat draconian, was presented by Taiwanese health experts in their reports to the WHO as an indicator of self-sufficiency and local participation: a sign of full collaboration with WHO policy. Pletsch,

administrative units for related fieldwork (The ROC Ministry of the Interior, "Health Situation of Republic of China," August 1957, 028000002350a, Academia Historica; JCRR, "Shijie weisheng zuzhi shizhounian tekan [World Health Organization 10th Anniversary Special Issue]," 1959, 11-11-09-08-134, Archives of Ministry of Foreign Affairs of the Republic of China, Academia Sinica).

[65] Pletsch, "Terminal Report: Covering the Period of Service from May 15, 1952 to September 1, 1955."
[66] Ibid.
[67] Tsai and Yu, Taiwan yiliao daode zhi yanbian, 124.
[68] Department of Health, Taiwan punue jishi, 106–7; Hsu Feng-Yuan, "Shijie weisheng zuzhi yu Taiwan nueji de fangzhi (1950–1972)," 108.
[69] Tsai and Yu, Taiwan yiliao daode zhi yanbian, 126.
[70] Ibid., 127.

the leader of the WHO malaria and insect control team in Taiwan, was critical of statistics' capacity to properly represent the passion and self-sufficiency of Taiwanese public health workers. As he wrote in a report to the WHO: "The co-operation, enthusiasm and diligence of the Malaria Institute and local health personnel have made possible extensive training and spraying operations which are expressed very inadequately by cold statistics."[71] In fact, underlying the positive image evoked by Pletsch was the autocratic nature of the local regime. The period from 1947 to 1987 is known in Taiwan as the White Terror, a period in which the ROC government applied martial law and strict censorship. The public health surveillance system functioned similarly to the police in Taiwan at the time,[72] with public health nurses acting much like police officers, knocking on doors, following patients, and reporting them to research institutes. It is possible that this authoritarian atmosphere facilitated the implementation of the WHO's programs, making Taiwan one of the rare places to successfully eradicate malaria through the GMEP.

Malaria control was not the only public health program that used a statistical system to administer fieldwork. The tuberculosis control program in Taiwan included a similar system to connect public health services at different levels. The Taipei Tuberculosis Control Center acted as the central organization of the WHO's tuberculosis control program in Taiwan, the equivalent of the TMRI in the malaria control program. From this center, the statistical system was propagated to Taiwanese villages. As in the malaria control program, statistics were used to supervise progress on the ground and monitor the epidemiological situation. Specifically, the system comprised a large variety of tuberculosis detection organizations at different administrative levels, ranging from a specialized research and training institute (the Taipei Tuberculosis Control Center) to district chest clinics, health centers, health stations, and field units (such as mobile X-ray units).[73] In the field, statistics were collected

---

[71] Pletsch, "Terminal Report: Covering the Period of Service from May 15, 1952 to September 1, 1955," 3.

[72] Though they do not go into detail, some historians mention the resemblance of the epidemic surveillance system to the ROC government's mind-control techniques employed during the Cold War. See, e.g.: Chang, "Fanglao tixi yu jiankong jishu: Taiwan jiehebing shi yanjiu (1945–1970s)"; Kuo Wen-Hua, "Ruhe kandai Meiyuan xia de weisheng? Yi ge lishi shuxie de fanxing yu zhanwang [How to Write a History of Public Health under US Aid in Taiwan: A Critical Review]," *Taiwan shi yanjiu [Taiwan Historical Research]* 17, no. 1 (2010): 191.

[73] WHO, "Tuberculosis Control in Taiwan Province: Plan for Future Development by Means of a Fully Integrated Program," March 1955, 10, 22–23, 11-11-09-08-046, Archives of Ministry of Foreign Affairs of the Republic of China, Academia Sinica.

directly by health service providers. Nurses in health centers were responsible for supervising medication, carrying out sputum and tuberculin testing, arranging X-ray exams, publicizing tuberculosis control methods, administering the BCG vaccine, and reporting the quantity of services provided to their district supervisors.[74] Every mobile X-ray unit had two clerks to record and report the number of X-ray tests and sputum checks to the Taipei Tuberculosis Control Center; any tuberculosis cases identified were to be reported for follow-up.[75] The Center had a statistical unit with one statistician, five clerks, and IBM machines for analyzing the numbers sent in by the nurses and X-ray units. The Center also organized training for five to seven statisticians each year to ensure statistical practices conducted in local organizations conformed to WHO standards.[76]

In 1956, the ROC signed a supplementary agreement with the WHO. Stressing the importance of early detection and promoting in-home chemotherapy for tuberculosis patients, this agreement expanded the statistical system by increasing the number of local workers for detecting tuberculosis cases.[77] Tao Rongjin, the director of the Taipei Tuberculosis Control Center, also sought financial support from American aid agencies to hire non-professionals for tuberculosis control. Ambitiously, Tao contended that the Center was "going to examine half a million of people a year and more than 10,000 cases would be discovered."[78] Taiwan's tuberculosis control program gradually became a social program supervised by statistical data. The program's workers had minimal medical training: all were unmarried women with a middle-school education. They were trained in social work and interviewing skills and put in charge of conducting "social control": knocking on doors and persuading people to accept X-ray screening, handing over drugs to patients, calling patients for follow-up examinations, and collecting specimens for

<hr>

[74] Chang, "Fanglao tixi yu jiankong jishu: Taiwan jiehebing shi yanjiu (1945–1970s)," 95.
[75] WHO, "Zhonghua Minguo zhengfu yu Lianheguo shijie weisheng zuzhi ji Lianheguo ertong jijinhui youguan jishu jiben xieding zhi butong xieding dingan [Supplementary Agreement to the Basic Agreement Between the Government of the Republic of China and the WHO and UNICEF for the Provision of Technical Advisory Assistance]," 1959, 6,14, 11-11-09-08-138, Archives of Ministry of Foreign Affairs of the Republic of China, Academia Sinica.
[76] WHO, "Tuberculosis Control in Taiwan Province: Plan for Future Development by Means of a Fully Integrated Program," 20–1.
[77] The ROC Ministry of Health, "The ROC's Request to the WHO for Tuberculosis Control for 1960," n.d., 11-11-09-08-119, Archives of Ministry of Foreign Affairs of the Republic of China, Academia Sinica.
[78] T'ao, "To Elizabeth W. Bracket," October 2, 1957, 3.

sputm tests.[79] Because all those conducting home visits were required to report on their daily services and meet their assigned benchmarks, numbers became the main focus of the tuberculosis reports.[80] The statistics collected were descriptive but very detailed in their depiction of the achievements of the program. In every report submitted to sponsors – including the WHO, UNICEF, and American aid agencies – numbers on tuberculin tests, X-rays, and BCG vaccinations were presented again and again.[81]

This single-minded focus on statistical data was not without repercussions. As Wendy Espeland and Michael Sauder's research on quantification has shown, a focus solely on the numbers created a "selective accountability" in that dimensions that were quantified and recorded were taken into account, while other aspects tended to be overlooked.[82] The final mission report of Alan Penington, the WHO's senior adviser on tuberculosis, provides a lucid account of this phenomenon: "The performance of a large number of X-ray examinations may appear impressive, but has little significance unless all suspect cases found are adequately followed and brought under study."[83] He concluded: "There is a very real danger of seeking the accumulation of figures which are not genuinely significant."[84] In expressing his concerns about the limits of statistics, Penington underscored the importance of following up on patients' conditions after massive case-finding. However, his reflections had no influence on later projects and reports, in which statistical data remained central. For example, in its five-year plan for the tuberculosis control program, the Taiwan provincial health administration again

---

[79] Ibid. Gender stereotypes played a major role in how non-professionals were recruited to conduct home visits. Tao explicitly called for young women to be hired, as they were considered to be "prone to gain the population's trust" (Chang Shu-Ching, "Zhanhou Taiwan de fanglao baojianyuan [Lay Home Visitors in Tuberculosis Control after World War II in Taiwan]," *Jindai zhongguo funushi yanjiu [Research on Women in Modern Chinese History]* 14 (2006): 89–123).

[80] Chang, "Zhanhou Taiwan de fanglao baojianyuan [Lay Home Visitors in Tuberculosis Control after World War II in Taiwan]."

[81] WHO, "Zhonghua Minguo zhengfu yu Lianheguo shijie weisheng zuzhi ji Lianheguo ertong jijinhui youguan jishu jiben xieding zhi butong xieding dingan [Supplementary Agreement to the Basic Agreement Between the Government of the Republic of China and the WHO and UNICEF for the Provision of Technical Advisory Assistance]"; Alan Penington, "Final Report – June 1956–March 1960"; Taiwan Provincial Health Administration, "Taiwansheng Fanglao Wunian Jihua Gangyao [Five-Year Plan for Tuberculosis Control in Taiwan," 1963, 286/150/38/08.09/06.07.01/15, National Archives and Records Administration, College Park.

[82] Espeland and Sauder, *Engines of Anxiety*, 7.

[83] Penington, "Final Report – June 1956–March 1960," 18.

[84] Ibid., 18.

contented itself with listing numbers that showed the efforts they had made in hunting down tuberculosis cases in every corner of the island.[85]

In its efforts to fight both malaria and tuberculosis in Taiwan, the WHO worked with local health organizations to construct statistical surveillance systems aimed at ensuring that the standards used to control the diseases were correctly implemented throughout the island. Actors at different levels were connected by statistical systems. From quantified DDT spraying efforts to benchmarks for fieldworkers, numbers allowed experts to govern from a distance, even though those experts were aware of the negative impact of this reliance on numbers.

### Present, Convince, Support: From Local Statistics to Global Knowledge

The administration of local fieldwork was not the only reason statistical practices were integrated into public health programs. In fact, at the outset of every field research project, public health experts such as Liang and Tao envisaged their fieldwork as contributing to the overall scientific understanding of a given public health measure. Liang's opening address at a training session for DDT sprayers, for instance, shows that he equated fieldwork with experimentation; this was reminiscent of his interwar predecessors, who considered health demonstrations to be laboratories of a sort (see Chapter 4). Encouraging field workers to report statistics honestly, Liang stated:

The experiment cannot be faked; fake numbers cannot produce good experiment results. We should always be honest. ... Medical science cannot be faked, once you have faked, everything will become fake.[86]

After compiling statistics from fieldwork, ROC experts working at each program's headquarters (the TMRI and the Taipei Tuberculosis Control Center, respectively) published their statistical "findings" (sometimes a mere compilation of field reports) in scientific journals. Liang himself also presented data collected in the field to the WHO Expert Committee on Malaria.[87] Through such efforts, public health programs in Taiwan became scientific experiments that served as models, or references, for similar programs across the world.

By showcasing the programs in Taiwan, public health experts promoted their know-how, which also made them fitting candidates for

[85] Translated from: Taiwan Provincial Health Administration, "Taiwansheng fanglao wunian jihua gangyao."
[86] Translated from: Tsai and Yu, *Taiwan yiliao daode zhi yanbian*, 119.
[87] WHO, "Expert Committee on Malaria Sixth Report."

implementing analogous programs. It is significant that, once the Taiwan programs were fully established, the experts who devised them were
recruited by the WHO to design similar programs in other countries.[88]
Liang and Tao, for example, who had published their results in academic
journals and/or participated in WHO expert committee meetings, were
both recruited in this manner. Tao became the tuberculosis expert at the
WHO's Western Pacific Regional Office in 1959 and was sent by the organization to mainland China in the 1980s. Liang, on the other hand, was
recruited by the Pan American Health Organization in 1957 and worked
there until his retirement in 1981. TMRI expert Chen Wanyi (Ch'en
Wan-I) also ended up working for the Pan American Health Organization for twelve years; Chen Xixuan (Ch'en Hsi-Hsuan) worked for the
WHO for twenty, traveling from Vietnam to the Solomon Islands devising malaria control programs.[89] A total of twenty-nine other Taiwanese
nationals were also recruited by the WHO between 1949 and 1971. All
except Fang Yiji (I. C. Fang) – who became the director of the Western
Pacific Regional Office – were recruited as experts in a specialized field,
such as malaria, tuberculosis control, and public health administration.[90]

   To shed light on these experts' publication of statistics collected in the
field, I conducted research on PubMed, a leading database comprising
more than 26 million citations for biomedical literature, and searched
for articles authored by Liang and Tao, the two key experts who worked
on malaria and tuberculosis, respectively.[91] There are eight articles by
Liang (the director of the TMRI until 1957) in the database.[92] They can

[88] Chu Chen-Yi, "Nueji yanjiusuo ji zaoqi fuwu de qianbei – shang [The Taiwan
    Malaria Research Institute and its Staff during its Founding Years. Part I]," *Taiwan
    Yijie [Taiwan Medical Journal]* 52, no. 3 (2009): 58–61; Chu Chen-Yi, "Nueji yanji-
    usuo ji zaoqi fuwu de qianbei – xia [The Taiwan Malaria Research Institute and its
    Staff during its Founding Years. Part II]," *Taiwan Yijie [Taiwan Medical Journal]* 52,
    no. 5 (2009): 53–6.
[89] Chu, "Nueji yanjiusuo ji zaoqi fuwu de qianbei – xia," 54.
[90] Weisheng bu [Ministry of Health], *Taiwan diqu gonggong weisheng fazhan shi (er) [The
    History of Public Health Development in Taiwan Vol. II]* (Taipei: Weisheng bu [Ministry
    of Health], 1995), 963–4.
[91] Pubmed Development Team, "Home – PubMed – NCBI," accessed October 4, 2016,
    www.ncbi.nlm.nih.gov/pubmed.
[92] I collected the following list of articles from *PubMed*: R. B. Watson and K. C. Liang,
    "Seasonal Prevalence of Malaria in Southern Formosa," *Indian Journal of Malariology*
    4, no. 4 (1950): 471–86; J. H. Paul, R. B. Watson, and K. C. Liang, "A Further
    Report on the Use of Chloroguanide (Paludrine) to Suppress Malaria Prevalence
    in Southern Formosan Villages," *Journal National Malaria Society (US)* 9, no. 4
    (1950): 356–65; C. Y. Chow, K. C. Liang, and Donald J. Pletsch, "Observations
    on Anopheline Populations in Human Dwellings in Southern Taiwan (Formosa),"
    *Indian Journal of Malariology* 5, no. 4 (1951): 569–77; H. C. Hsieh and K. C. Liang,

be broadly categorized into two groups: those that focus on demonstrating the behavioral patterns of *Anopheles* mosquitoes in Taiwan, which were published in the *Journal of Indian Malariology*, in collaboration with Robert Watson of the Rockefeller Foundation and Pletsch of the WHO; and those that recount the malaria control program in Taiwan, which were published in WHO's *Bulletin* and *Chronicle*. Tao, for his part, is the author of nine articles in the database. The earliest set of articles presents facts collected during Taiwanese tuberculosis control fieldwork, including vital statistics, prevalence rates, and death rates among tuberculosis patients;[93] a later set, published in the 1970s, frame Taiwan's tuberculosis control program as a success owing to its low costs.[94] Though there is some divergence in Liang and Tao's publications, partially due to the different epidemiological patterns of malaria and tuberculosis, both used statistics to present their programs to the scientific community. Both had been trained at the JHSPH,[95] and thus it was highly possible that they

---

"Residual Foci of Malarial Infection in the DDT-Sprayed Area of Taiwan," *Bulletin of the World Health Organization* 15, no. 3–5 (1956): 810–13; C. T. Ch'en and K. C. Liang, "Malaria Surveillance Programme in Taiwan," *Bulletin of the World Health Organization* 15, no. 3–5 (1956): 805–10; K. C. Liang, "The Priority of Malaria Eradication Programs," *Bulletin of the Pan American Health Organization* 9, no. 4 (1975a): 295–9; K. C. Liang, "Priorities of the malaria eradication program," *Boletin de la Oficina Sanitaria Panamericana. Pan American Sanitary Bureau* 79, no. 6 (1975b): 508–13; K. C. Liang, "Historical Review of Malaria Control Program in Taiwan," *The Kaohsiung Journal of Medical Sciences* 7, no. 5 (1991): 271–7.

[93]    Jung-Chin Tao, "Tuberculosis in Taiwan (Formosa)," *American Review of Respiratory Disease* 80, no. 3 (1959b), 359–70.

[94]    I collected the following list of articles from PubMed: J. C. Tao, "Pulmonary Tuberculosis in Chinese Students," *American Review of Tuberculosis* 56, no. 1 (1947): 22–6; Tao, "Tuberculosis in Taiwan (Formosa)"; J. C. Tao, "Community Approach to Tuberculosis," *Journal of the American Medical Women's Association* 14, no. 12 (1959): 1077–83; J. C. Tao, "Organizing a Simplified Case-Finding Service for Developing Countries. People with Little Formal Education Can Be Trained to Examine the Sputum," *Bulletin – National Tuberculosis and Respiratory Disease Association* 56, no. 2 (1970a): 9–11; J. C. Tao, "Tuberculosis. Training, Supervision and Motivation of Personnel," *Bulletin of the International Union Against Tuberculosis* 43, no. 6 (1970b): 87–92; J. C. Tao, "The Fight against Tuberculosis. A Cheap and Efficient Case-Finding Method," *Journal of the West Australian Nurses* 37, no. 1 (1971): 20–2; J. C. Tao, "Tuberculosis Control in the Western Pacific Region of WHO 1951–1970," *WHO Chronicle* 27, no. 12 (1973): 507–15; J. C. Tao, "BCG Vaccination in the Control of Tuberculosis and the Organisation of a National BCG Vaccination Programme," *Bulletin of the International Union Against Tuberculosis* 49, suppl. 1 (1974a): 154–60; J. C. Tao, "Tuberculosis in the Western Pacific Region," *Bulletin of the International Union Against Tuberculosis* 49, suppl. 1 (1974b): 18–23.

[95]    Tao was trained at the PUMC and later worked at the Central Field Health Station, an organization designed by the LNHO (see Chapter 4). He was therefore a product of the American public health tradition. Liang, on the other hand, was trained in the Japanese tradition at Taipei Imperial University. He later became acquainted with the American tradition while working at the TMRI, which was funded by the

had a positive view of public health technologies and statistical practices that they shared with their counterparts in Geneva. Liang and Tao did not only use statistics to increase the visibility of their programs: through analysis, they also presented their fieldwork as meaningful case studies of the WHO's disease control policies. By imposing the grammar of statistics, they made public health fieldwork in Taiwan legible to other public health researchers.

Beneath the general picture presented by their publications, what strategies did Taiwanese public health experts employ when using field statistics to feed into foreign organizations' policy-making process? I identified three types of argumentation used by Taiwanese experts: i) presenting quantified facts and making policy suggestions to the scientific community; ii) presenting Taiwan as a potential case study for new measures; and iii) providing facts relevant to the WHO's concerns under the framework of its ongoing policies.

The first category involved using statistics simply to present quantified facts and make policy suggestions. Most of the publications reviewed above fall into this category. Tao's article in *American Review of Respiratory Disease* provides an evocative example. In the twelve-page article, Tao used a total of fifteen graphs and tables to portray the decreasing trend in tuberculosis cases in Taiwan.[96] He did not make any argument based on the graphs, as the statistics were purely descriptive – there was no statistical hypothesis testing. In the final section, entitled "Discussion," Tao merely suggested that the main contribution of the tuberculosis control program in Taiwan was to give rise to "cultural change." He argued that, thanks to the program, Taiwanese people no longer considered tuberculosis an incurable disease affecting only the rich. Tellingly, Tao's argument was completely dissociated from the statistical facts to which he had devoted several pages. Despite the lack of a real argument, Tao's article nonetheless established solid facts regarding the program in Taiwan, and because it was published in a renowned scientific journal, it was considered as an important point of reference on tuberculosis control there.

The second type of argumentation adopted by the Taiwanese experts was to use quantified survey methods to present the island as a case study for new measures supported by foreign organizations. In doing

Rockefeller Foundation. Liang and Tao were both associated with public health programs funded by international health organizations when they were selected for the Rockefeller Foundation's international fellowship (T'ao, "Personal History Record and Application for Fellowship: T'ao Jung-Chin"; Liang K'uang-Ch'i, "Personal History Record and Application for Fellowship: Liang K'uang Ch'i").
[96] J. C. T'ao "Tuberculosis in Taiwan (Formosa)."

so, the experts influenced policy-making by introducing the latest and most advanced public health measures to the island, a possibility they relished. This finding contradicts historians' typical discourse on the implementation of public health programs in Taiwan. While most historians note that Taiwan rolled out in-home therapy only a year after the Madras domiciliary therapy experiment, despite no statistical proof that it was effective, this is generally considered an indicator of WHO experts' careless attitude toward their programs' benefit to countries.[97] The archival records show otherwise, however. In fact, it was Tao who sought to implement in-home therapy in Taiwan and brokered the arrangement with the foreign organizations involved. To potential sponsors, he presented Taiwan's tuberculosis prevalence rate as a reason the island would make an ideal case study for testing the effectiveness of in-home therapy. In 1956, during a stay in the United States, Tao gave a presentation on tuberculosis prevalence in Taiwan to Carroll Palmer, the tuberculosis expert at the United States Public Health Service and a consultant to the WHO on tuberculosis control. In his presentation, Tao argued that the high prevalence rate in Taiwan would make it a strong example for validating the effect of isoniazid in outpatient treatment regimens.[98] With Palmer's support, Tao developed a sampling plan for evaluating the prophylactic use of isoniazid for outpatient treatment, using high-school students in Taiwan as test subjects.[99] Guo Songgen (Quo Sung-Ken), by that time a statistician at the WHO's Western Pacific Regional Office, also visited Taiwan to review the sampling procedure and establish a tuberculosis registry center within the Taipei Tuberculosis Control Center.[100] Tao's strategy – presenting Taiwan as an ideal case study for testing isoniazid – successfully attracted additional financial support from the WHO and the United States government.

The third category of argumentation used in published articles involved providing facts that supported the WHO's ongoing policies. One significant instance was a research document entitled "Economic and Social Effects of Malaria Control with Some Specific Instances From

[97] Chang, "Fanglao tixi yu jiankong jishu: Taiwan jiehebing shi yanjiu (1945–1970s)," 89.
[98] Carroll Palmer, "To James Ward," February 29, 1956, 286/150/38/08.09/06.07.01/15, National Archives and Records Administration, College Park.
[99] Carroll Palmer, "To Dr. S. C. Hsu," February 4, 1956, 286/150/38/08.09/06.07.01/15, National Archives and Records Administration, College Park.
[100] The Coordination Committee, "Minutes of the Meeting (179) of the Coordination Committee on Foreign Aid in Medicine and Health," January 26, 1957, 179, 286/150/38/08.09/06.07.01/1, National Archives and Records Administration, College Park.

Taiwan," submitted by Pletsch and Chen Zhengde (Ch'en Cheng Te, commonly known as C. T. Ch'en) to the WHO Expert Committee on Malaria in 1956.[101] At the time, the WHO had just endorsed the GMEP based on the idea that eradicating malaria would help to conserve the workforce in tropical countries.[102] Aiming to test the validity of this notion, Pletsch and Chen Zhengde presented statistics on the loss of working days and calculated the total loss of salary during a malaria epidemic in Kaoshu, a town in southern Taiwan. In the conclusion, they nonetheless reported that the malaria epidemic had actually created jobs for people living in neighboring villages, meaning that the epidemic was partially beneficial to the local economy. Faced with two conflicting results, the duo chose to stand with the WHO by stating that Taiwan was, after all, "overpopulated".[103] This case provides a revealing example of how experts used statistics within the framework of WHO policy: Pletsch and Chen conducted a statistical survey based on WHO policy statements, and despite the fact that their data contradicted the WHO's official position (that malaria epidemics undermined the economy), they nonetheless expressed support for the existing policy in their core argument, even discarding some important findings from their survey. During the 1950s, Pletsch and Chen's investigation was never included in mainstream discourse. A progress report submitted to United States aid agencies again repeated the prevailing discourse about malaria causing a loss of manpower and working hours, writing that:

Until recent years, one of the most serious obstacles to economic progress in Taiwan was the loss of time caused by malaria. ... The avoidance of lost time due to illness on farms and in factories by the reduction of upwards of ninety nine percent in cases represents both a vast increase in productivity and a stupendous reduction in human suffering and poverty.[104]

It was not until the 1960s, when economic development policy peaked within the United Nations, that experts openly argued that malaria

---

[101] Donald J. Pletsch and C. T. Ch'en, "Economic and Social Effects on Malaria Control with Some Specific Instances from Taiwan," August 31, 1954, WHO Library, http://apps.who.int/iris/bitstream/10665/64287/1/WHO_Mal_108.pdf."

[102] Randall M. Packard, "Malaria Dreams: Postwar Visions of Health and Development in the Third World," *Medical Anthropology* 17, no. 3 (1997): 279–96; Packard, *The Making of a Tropical Disease.*

[103] Pletsch and Ch'en, "Economic and Social Effects on Malaria Control with Some Specific Instances from Taiwan,".

[104] ICA [International Cooperation Administration], "Public Health Division: Malaria Eradication- 484-51-125," 1960, 286/150/38/08.09/06.07.01/9, National Archives and Records Administration, College Park.

control programs had had only a limited impact on developing countries' economies.[105]

Although experts in Taiwan packaged their field numbers for the global stage, the above three types of argumentation showcase how experts and the statistics they collected had a limited impact on mainstream global health policy. Taiwanese experts' curation of numbers influenced policy only when they made Taiwanese fieldwork appear to uphold existing policies, which they then introduced to the island.

*

When we juxtapose the WHO's statistical system for disease control with that of its interwar predecessors, it is clear that numbers became more pervasive in public health experts' arguments and policy-making practices. In both Geneva and Taiwan, experts could not do as their interwar counterparts had done and simply denounce the unreliability of the existing statistics. Nor were they completely free to decide whether to cite statistics in their policy advocacy or the extent to which statistics from the field could be translated into policies (see Chapter 4). If the results of vaccine trials and pilot programs did not validate programs designed at the WHO's headquarters, experts instead used their public health knowledge to criticize the representativeness of the results.

In both Geneva and Taiwan, officers' statistical practices tended to support the WHO's ongoing policies despite failing to obtain positive quantified results from fieldwork. Still, their aims were conspicuously different, as the two groups were situated at different levels of the global health policy-making hierarchy: WHO experts aimed to produce evidence that supported the organization's ongoing general policy, whereas Taiwanese experts' priority was to secure resources from Geneva by presenting Taiwan as an eligible testing ground for WHO policies. Taiwanese experts therefore based the type of field observations they made – and the type of numbers they reported – on the WHO's policy advocacy statements. At the policy-making level, however, on-the-ground observations that went against WHO policy had little power to alter the policy in question. In this sense, the contention that public health technologies were validated by field experiments before being massively implemented in Taiwan and the rest of the world should not be taken entirely at face value. Although Taiwanese experts were clearly limited in their power to

---

[105] Randall M. Packard, "'Roll Back Malaria, Roll in Development'? Reassessing the Economic Burden of Malaria," *Population and Development Review* 35, no. 1 (2009): 61–70.

influence international health policy, they still became authorities thanks to their experiences in Taiwan, and many were recruited by the WHO to contribute to similar programs in other regions. Some went on to work for the WHO until their retirement.

Although statistics drew a sometimes unflattering picture of the WHO's technology-centered programs, it was not until the Alma-Ata Declaration of 1978 – in which the WHO's member states urged the organization to adopt a strategy on primary health care – that belief in technology-centered solutions began to wane, before being reignited by the eradication of smallpox in the 1980s.[106]

It should also be noted that the WHO's statistical system was not omni-present throughout the world. The next chapter will focus on another group of statisticians, working in the People's Republic of China, who were disassociated from the WHO's epidemiological reporting system and instead based their statistical methods on the socialist model.

---

[106] Marcos Cueto, "The ORIGINS of Primary Health Care and SELECTIVE Primary Health Care," *American Journal of Public Health* 94, no. 11 (2004): 1864–74; Packard, *A History of Global Health*, 177.

# 7    Another Way of Speaking?
## Public Health Statistics in the People's Republic of China

On 1 October 1949, Mao Zedong stood atop the Tiananmen Gate and proclaimed the People's Republic of China (PRC) to be the only legal government representing the Chinese people. From its inauguration, the PRC government adopted a "One China" policy and endeavored to disqualify the Republic of China (ROC) from representing China on the international stage. Considering the United Nations to be a proxy for the American-led capitalist camp, the PRC cut off relations with the United Nations system, including with the World Health Organization (WHO), thus ending its epidemic reporting to the organization. Despite its disassociation from the WHO, health statisticians in the PRC who had been trained at the Peking Union Medical College (PUMC) and/or the Johns Hopkins School of Public Health (JHSPH) before 1949 did not stop using statistics in their teaching and field research. Nevertheless, the ways in which they used statistics evolved in line with the central government's policies regarding numbers collection, which, in the 1950s, was largely influenced by statistical thinking from the Soviet Union.

By following the work of health statisticians in the PRC between 1949 and 1971, before it joined the WHO, this chapter explores another way in which the language of statistics was spoken. It serves to complement previous chapters by recounting the story of health statistics on the other side of the Iron Curtain, detailing the continuities and transformations in health statistics once the global health network led by the WHO lost its influence over mainland China. One of the major proofs that continuities existed nonetheless is that, when the PRC joined the WHO, Chinese health experts such as Chen Zhiqian (also known as C. C. Ch'en), who was educated at the PUMC and directly associated with the public health enterprises of the Milbank Memorial Fund and Rockefeller Foundation in interwar China, were presented as gurus within the Chinese health system and mediated between the WHO and the Chinese government. The PRC government promoted its community health system, designed by Chen, that relied on non-professionals with minimal training (commonly known as "barefoot doctors" during the Cultural Revolution) to the WHO. The WHO would take inspiration from this system in the Alma-Ata Declaration of the late 1970s.[1]

Important questions remain, however. What happened to public health experts when the newly established PRC cut off connections with the West in 1949? Did they manage to integrate their know-how into the Soviet model of health statistics adopted by the PRC? How were they influenced by the thought-reform initiatives that peaked during the Cultural Revolution (1966–1976) and targeted Western-educated Chinese? By mobilizing archival materials and works published during the period under study, this chapter follows the trajectories of health statisticians trained in the United States before 1949 during a period of significant political change. In particular, this chapter complements Arunabh Ghosh's research focused on the endeavors of the PRC State Statistics Bureau.[2] I will show that public health experts had a certain level of independence when it came to using the national statistical system that Ghosh describes. These experts used statistics to tackle public health work during the early years of the PRC; this chapter therefore also complements emerging literature on the history of public health in the PRC.[3] The literature unequivocally shows that reporting numbers was part of the PRC's public health policies, and that health workers in the field were required to meet quotas set by their superiors.[4] This chapter completes that picture by exploring the work of elite public health experts who used statistics, and the extent to which their statistical practices – and the central government's statistical

[1] The historian Zhou Xun has provided one of the most complete discussions on the influence of the PRC's "barefoot doctor" model within the WHO in the 1970s (Zhou, "From China's 'Barefoot Doctor' to Alma Ata: The Primary Health Care Movement in the Long 1970s"; Zhou, *The People's Health*).

[2] Based on archival materials from the State Statistics Bureau, as well as other publications from the time, Ghosh's work chronicles changes in the PRC's statistical policies during its early decades, work from which this chapter greatly benefited (Ghosh, *Making It Count*).

[3] See, e.g.: Gross, *Farewell to the God of Plague*; Xiaoping Fang, "Diseases, Peasants, and Nation-Building in Rural China. Social Conformity, Institutional Strengthening, and Political Indoctrination," in *Public Health and National Reconstruction in Post-War Asia: International Influences, Local Transformations*, eds. Liping Bu and Ka-Che Yip, 52–71; Mary Augusta Brazelton, "Western Medical Education on Trial: The Endurance of Peking Union Medical College, 1949–1985," *Twentieth-Century China* 40, no. 2 (2015): 126–45; Bu, *Public Health and the Modernization of China, 1865–2015*; Brazelton, *Mass Vaccination*; Zhou, *The People's Health*; Xiaoping Fang, *China and the Cholera Pandemic: Restructuring Society under Mao* (Pittsburgh, PA: University of Pittsburgh Press, 2021)

[4] See, e.g.: Brazelton, *Mass Vaccination*, 60–2; Zhou, *The People's Health*, 61–2, 89.

reporting system for health campaigns – ebbed and flowed during the early years of the PRC. In general, although the young government's central policies undermined the authority of the WHO – as well as that of the public health experts studied here – it continued to rely on numbers for its public health campaigns and put effort into organizing and reorganizing its reporting systems.[5] As this chapter will show, reliance on statistics grew during times of intense mass mobilization when experts lost their authority within the regime, thus illustrating the role of statistics as a substitute for expert authority, as observed by Porter.[6]

### Participation in Non-WHO International Health Collaboration

Despite the Cold War political climate and its policy of only accepting United Nations members, the WHO nonetheless sought to contact the PRC with the aim of fulfilling – at least partially – its promise of being a worldwide organization.[7] Nevertheless, just like the ROC, the PRC government considered its policy vis-à-vis the WHO within the Cold War context and was skeptical as to the benefits it would receive in exchange for the high membership fee. A document prepared by the PRC Ministry of Foreign Affairs spells out these considerations, listing the reasons why the PRC should not establish a relationship with the WHO:

1. All of the WHO's core staff were from countries in the United States–United Kingdom bloc. In addition, the organization collaborated closely with the United Nations Headquarters and the Pan American Health Organization. If China were to participate, the United States (an imperial power) would use the organization to collect intelligence about China and deceive backward-thinking people.
2. Only 50 percent of the WHO's 1948 budget was allocated to on-the-ground services. Its programs in China were superficial. The Russian, White Russian, and Ukrainian Soviet Socialist Republics had all left the organization in 1949 under the pretext that its work was unsatisfying and its budget too large. The PRC could refer to their reasons.

---

[5] I would like to thank an anonymous reader for this insight.
[6] Porter, *Trust in Numbers*.
[7] Waijiao bu [Minister of Foreign Affairs], "Guanyu woguo yingfou jiaru shijie weisheng zuzhi shi," July 11, 1950.

3. The PRC might have to pay a steep membership fee to the organization. Given the meager results expected, the PRC might as well use the money to improve its own medical and public health work.[8]

The first point reveals the PRC government's distrust of the WHO when it came to public health intelligence. The government was convinced that such information would be used against it, as the WHO was run by nationals of countries from the Western bloc. The PRC Ministry of Foreign Affairs explicitly prohibited the Ministry of Health from directly reporting epidemic statistics to the WHO's Singapore-based epidemiological intelligence service.[9] Instead, the government sought to partner with socialist countries to exchange epidemic information, and, as early as 1949, the PRC government had hosted visits from four Soviet epidemic control experts.[10]

The PRC's attitude toward the United Nations agencies was even colder than that of other socialist countries due to the United Nation's recognition of the ROC, now settled on the island of Taiwan, as the only legitimate representative of China. When the Soviet Union delegation in Geneva called on its allies to provide their own data to promote socialism within the United Nations, the PRC representative requested other members of the socialist bloc not to leak any Chinese information to United Nations agencies in the fear that agencies such as the WHO and the International Labour Office might use it to justify meddling in "Chinese domestic affairs."[11]

[8] Translated from: Waijiao bu [Minister of Foreign Affairs], "Guanyu Zhongguo yingfou canjia guoji laogong zuzhi, shijie baojian zuzhi de baogao [Report on Whether China Should Participate in the International Labour Organization and the World Health Organization]," December 23, 1949, 113-00044-02, Archives of Ministry of Foreign Affairs of China.

[9] Waijiao bu [Minister of Foreign Affairs], "Guanyu tingzhi xiang shijie weisheng zuzhi Xinjiapo yiqingzhan tigong woguo yiqing de wenjian [On Ending Epidemic Reporting to the WHO's Singapore Epidemiological Station]," 1950, 113-00044-04, Archives of Ministry of Foreign Affairs of China.

[10] Ibid.; Waijiao bu [Minister of Foreign Affairs], "Sulian fangyi zhuanjia jiedai baogao [Soviet Union Epidemic Control Experts Reception Report]," November 3, 1949, 117-00031-01, Archives of Ministry of Foreign Affairs of China.

[11] Translated from: Zhu Rineiwa Zong Lingshiguan [Consulate General in Geneva], "Xiongdi guojia changzhu Rineiwa guoji zuzhi daibiaotuan jihui qingkuang [Meeting of the Permanent Delegation of Brother Countries to the International Organizations in Geneva]," October 16, 1951, 113-00368-01, Archives of Ministry of Foreign Affairs of China; Waijiao bu [Minister of Foreign Affairs], "Waijiao bu quhan zhu Ruishi shiguan bing Zhu Rineiwa Zong Lingshiguan [The Ministry of Foreign Affairs Wrote to the Embassy in Switzerland and the Consulate General in Geneva]," October 27, 1951, 113-00368-01, Archives of Ministry of Foreign Affairs of China.

206 Another Way of Speaking?

Though it had cut off contact with the WHO, the PRC was an active participant in an international health event led by the Soviet Union during the 1950s. In the archives of the PRC Ministry of Foreign Affairs, a document about the PRC's delegate to the *Congrès mondial des médecins pour l'étude des conditions actuelles de vie* (World Congress of Doctors for the Study of Current Life Conditions) reveals that the PRC was active in Soviet Union-led international health events in the first half of the 1950s. In 1953, the World Congress of Doctors took place in Vienna. Led by the Soviet Union and with representatives from eleven countries from both sides of the Cold War rivalry,[12] the goal was to create a platform for information exchange among medical practitioners.[13] The use of the term "current life conditions" in the title is suggestive, in that it placed prime emphasis on social medicine, drawing a telling contrast with coeval WHO activities focused on epidemic control through mass distribution of vaccines and insecticide spray. The PRC was an active member of the Congress: it contributed to the publication of its papers, worked to recruit more Asian countries as participants, and introduced a session during the annual conference of the China Medical Association to discuss life conditions in China, a topic deemed important by the Congress.[14]

The archives of the PRC's Ministry of Foreign Affairs also contain clues as to the PRC's policy on international health collaboration in terms of accepting foreign patients for treatment in China. The PRC became an exporter of medical services by accepting foreign patients, who came to receive Chinese traditional treatments.[15] From 1957 to 1960, there were 186 requests for treatment in China, 90 percent of which came from the Soviet Union, Mongolia, Vietnam, and North Korea. Only eighty-three were accepted, as the PRC assessed in advance whether the treatment was likely to be effective, depending on the individual's condition.[16]

---

[12] Participating countries included Australia, the Soviet Union, China, France, the United Kingdom, the German Democratic Republic, Italy, Czechoslovakia, Denmark, India, and Chile.

[13] "Shijie yixue huiyi mishuchu huiyi qingkuang huibao [Summary of the World Congress of Doctors' Secretariat Meeting]," 1953, 113-00187-01, Archives of Ministry of Foreign Affairs of China.

[14] Bai Xiqing, "Women jihua jinhou jinxing de gongzuo [The Work We Plan to Do in the Future]," December 15, 1953, 113-00187-01, Archives of Ministry of Foreign Affairs of China.

[15] For the PRC's efforts in Traditional Chinese Medicine, see, e.g.: Kim Taylor, *Chinese Medicine in Early Communist China, 1945–63: A Medicine of Revolution* (London: Routledge, 2004).

[16] Waijiao bu [Minister of Foreign Affairs], "Guanyu guoji youren lai woguo zhibing wenti [On International Friends Coming to Our Country for Medical Treatment]," May 22, 1961, 113-00368-01, Archives of Ministry of Foreign Affairs of China.

Research institutions also received foreign medical experts, and not only from socialist countries. The Shanghai Medical College's chronicle shows visits by medical experts from Japan, Denmark, Sweden, and Italy in 1955 alone.[17] Most went first to Shanghai Medical College, then Shanghai First Medical School, to exchange surgical knowledge, and one visitor from Japan came to participate in snail fever control campaigns.[18]

These anecdotes show that the PRC did not lose all contact with other countries in terms of health affairs, despite cutting off its connection with the United Nations. Rather, it participated in a different, socialist-led global health network. It also exported Chinese traditional medicine to other regions of the world. Moreover, the government did not shy away from exchange with individual experts from the other side of the Iron Curtain when it came to acquiring medical and public health expertise.

### Economic Recovery Period (1949–1952): An Extension of the ROC's Statistical Practices

The PRC's domestic public health work during its early years resembled its work in border regions during the Second Sino-Japanese War. In 1950, Chen Zhiqian, the former Ding Xian health expert and an alumnus of the PUMC and the Harvard School of Public Health (see Chapter 4), led the PRC's First National Health Conference, which promulgated three principles of medical and public health work: i) prevention as the priority; ii) solidarity among workers, peasants, and soldiers; and iii) unification of traditional Chinese and Western medicine.[19] In line with these principles, the PRC's public health work differed from that of the ROC. Whereas the postwar ROC regime – which received support from United States aid agencies and the WHO – was focused on mass epidemic control campaigns based on "panaceas" such as vaccines or insecticide spray, the PRC devised its public health actions also with a focus on social hygiene, emphasizing the link between public health and living conditions, and therefore concentrated on sanitation in living environments and personal hygiene.

---

[17] Shanghai yike daxue jishi bianzuan weiyuan hui [Shanghai Medical College Chronicle Editorial Board], *Shanghai yike daxue jishi [Shanghai Medical College Chronicle (1927–2000)]* (Shanghai: Fudan University Press, 2000), 130–1.

[18] It is likely that the visit of the Japanese expert was arranged by the Chinese premier, Zhou Enlai, who had approached Japan for help with schistosomiasis control campaigns. For details on Japan's suggestions regarding the campaigns, see: Zhou, *The People's Health*, 92–4.

[19] Bu, *Public Health and the Modernization of China, 1865–2015*, 224.

Statistical collection, with its capacity for obtaining actual knowledge of the health and living conditions of the masses, continued to be a part of the PRC's public health work. From 1949 to 1952, before the Patriotic Health Campaign took place in November 1952,[20] statisticians who were trained and/or active during the interwar years adopted the same statistical practices, regardless of whether they were organizing health administrations or conducting research in universities. Xu Shijin (Hsu Shih-Chin), a PUMC- and JHSPH-trained statistician and a former staffer at the ROC Ministry of Health, took on a professorship at Shanghai First Medical School in 1949. Based in Shanghai, Xu expanded the vital and health statistics collection demonstration he had conducted in the prewar capital, Nanjing, to seventy-two localities across the Chinese mainland. In line with Xu's program, the Shanghai Municipal Health Bureau began organizing statistical training in 1950 to increase the quality of vital statistics and improve collaboration in epidemic control programs.[21] The training covered the use of various forms and reporting methods. Once investigators had completed the training, they were dispatched to health centers in greater Shanghai.[22]

Another example of a prewar statistician who went on to serve the PRC regime was Guo Zuchao. Guo was a public health statistics lecturer at the Central University in Nanjing who was sent on a WHO-sponsored fellowship in 1947 to receive training at the JHSPH. Upon his return, he continued to work at the Central University, specializing in vital and health statistics, before being hired by the Fifth Military Medical University, where he oversaw the use of statistical forms for public health matters within the People's Liberation Army. Guo's *Medical Science and Biostatistical Methods*, first published in 1948, would become a reference for later generations of PRC medical and public health statisticians. The 1948 edition contains text that is very similar to the training handouts on statistical analysis used in American public health schools. In it, Guo enumerates ways of analyzing statistics and presents basic concepts such as sampling, means, regression, and analysis of variance.[23]

---

[20] Claiming that the use of germ warfare by the United States in the Korean War was the source of China's ongoing epidemics, the PRC central government launched the Patriotic Health Campaign in 1952. This established a series of public health measures, such as mass vaccination campaigns and the elimination of several disease-carrying animals. I will elaborate on it in the following pages.

[21] Shanghai Municipal Health Bureau, "Shanghai shi shengming tongji gongzuo diyinian zongjie baogao [Shanghai City's Vital Statistics Activities, First Year Summary Report, 1950.07-1951.06]," 1951, B242-1-255, Shanghai Municipal Archives.

[22] There were thirty-one trainees at the 1950 session and eighteen at the 1951 session (ibid.).

[23] Guo Zuchao, *Yixue yu shengwu tongji fangfa [Medical Science and Biological Statistical Methods]* (Shanghai: Zhengzhong shuju [Cheng Chung Book Company], 1948).

Notably, he cited not only renowned scholarly publications on biostatistical methods from the United States and the United Kingdom, but also integrated Chinese research to serve as examples in exercises at the end of each chapter.[24] Four years later, Guo co-authored another manual, *Public Health*, which included a chapter on vital and health statistics. Focusing on administrative collection methods, the chapter introduced basic guidelines about vital and health statistics, including the data to be collected in vital registration, the international list of causes of death, and the methods for collecting and tabulating them. Citing John Snow's research during the London cholera epidemic, the authors emphasized the importance of observing changes in epidemic statistics to infer the causes of an epidemic.[25] Once again, their description of vital and health statistics was in accordance with the training he had received at JHSPH.

Neither Xu's nor Guo's work between 1949 and 1952 differed from their earlier work, when the ROC regime was still in power on the mainland. Publications by both would receive corrections in the following years, when the PRC regime started adhering to socialist statistics as introduced by the Soviet Union. The influence of socialist statistics was further reinforced during the period covered by the PRC's first five-year economic plan (1953–1957), when the Soviet Union increased its financial aid and sent experts of all sorts to the PRC in the hopes of demonstrating the effectiveness of the Soviet Union's socialist system in developing countries. Swayed by the Soviet model, the PRC closely followed the Soviet Union's administrative and economic consultancy during the first five-year economic plan, which also left its mark on vital and health statistics collection.

### The Implantation of Socialist Statistics and Their Limits in Public Health

The year 1952 is crucial to understanding the PRC's use of public health statistics over the following decades. This was the year when the Chinese Communist Party blueprinted two important programs: the first five-year plan; and the Patriotic Health Campaign. The two programs promoted distinctly different ways of using vital and health statistics. Whereas the first five-year plan was based on the principle of the uniform collection of all sorts of statistics using methods in line with socialist

---

[24] Ibid.
[25] Bi Rugang and Guo Zuchao, eds., *Gonggong weisheng [Public Health]* (Shanghai: Shangwu yinshuguan [The Commercial Press], 1953), 39.

ideology, the Patriotic Health Campaign – and its local implementation – was somewhat resistant to the dominance of socialist statistics.

The first five-year plan intensified programs based on socialist statistics. It represented the peak of the Soviet Union's influence in China, as it launched the Party's all-encompassing imitation of the Soviet nation-building efforts, with a Soviet Union loan supporting one-third of related programs. Soviet experts flocked to China to advise on nation-building matters ranging from transport infrastructure to the education system.[26] Among them were six statisticians, who successively served at the State Statistics Bureau, where they designed statistical collection systems, inspected local statistical work, assisted with the publication of Soviet Union textbooks, and trained Chinese statistical staff through lectures and discussions.[27] Following the lead of these Soviet Union statisticians, the PRC designed its statistical practices in the tradition of socialist statistics.

Specifically, socialist statistics stressed the political nature of statistical practices.[28] Under Marxism–Leninism, statistics were considered a social science, as they aimed to reveal existing social inequality. Socialist statisticians rejected the idea of statistics as a common discipline in which identical methods could be applied to anything from biology to physics to the social sciences.[29] For them, using statistics in such a way was dangerous, as it presumed that social inequality was biological and natural, and therefore could not be reversed. In that sense, a census including all social classes was crucial and could not be replaced by mathematical statistics that inferred an entire population's situation based on random samples. The mathematical statistics of Karl Pearson and his followers were condemned as a bourgeois scheme to conceal class inequality.[30]

[26] The PRC had in fact been hosting Soviet experts since 1949. The number of such experts in China increased in 1950, after the Communist Party signed the Sino-Soviet Treaty of Friendship, Alliance and Mutual Aid. For a complete history of China's learning from the soviet model, see, e.g.: Thomas P. Bernstein and Hua-Yu Li, eds., *China Learns from the Soviet Union, 1949–Present*, The Harvard Cold War Studies Book Series (Lanham, MD: Lexington Books, 2010).

[27] Ghosh, *Making It Count*, 77–88.

[28] Arunabh Ghosh provides a much-needed general account of socialist statistics (ibid., 62–74).

[29] Zhongguo kexueyuan hebeisheng fenyuan jingji yanjiusuo zichanjieji tongjixue pipan xiaozu [China Science Council's Critic Group Against Bourgeois Statistical Research] and Nankai daxue jingjixi zichanjieji tongjixue pipan xiaozu [Nankai University's Critic Group against Bourgeois Statistical Research], *Suqing zichan jieji tongji xueshu sixiang de liudu [Cleaning the Remaining Poison of Bourgeois Statistical Research]* (Shanghai: Shanghai renmin chubanshe [Shanghai People's Publishing House], 1958), 6, 11.

[30] Ibid., 6.

When it came to vital and health statistics, socialist statisticians advocated for the two categories to be kept completely separate. Vital statistics were to be confined to population statistics – births, deaths, and changes in the composition of the population – whereas health statistics were to focus on the quantity of public health services provided, disease case numbers, and height and weight statistics. The purpose of this separation of vital statistics from health statistics was to avoid attributing cases of unnecessary death and disease to individuals' poor hygiene, as socialist teaching held that any death or disease was closely related to social inequality. Gu Weilin, the translator of *The USSR's Public Health, Educational, and Cultural Statistical Organizations* (and possibly a statistical staff member within the PRC administration),[31] clearly articulates the socialist view of vital statistics in an article in the State Statistics Bureau's *Statistical Work Bulletin*:

The formulation of vital statistics allows the bourgeoisie to explain births, deaths, marriages and diseases from a biological perspective. Bourgeois statisticians must employ a biological perspective when conducting statistical studies on births, deaths, marriages and diseases in order to present demographic change and disease outbreaks as natural phenomena, disassociated from class relations. They chose to make the term "vital statistics" include birth, death, marriage and disease statistics precisely because the term "vital" is suggestive of biology, which allows them to present vital statistics as a branch of biology. ... Combining population statistics with public health statistics enables the bourgeoisie to obscure the goal of the people's struggle. The bourgeoisie often claims that the high mortality rate is due to problematic personal hygiene, and that any decrease in mortality rate is because of improved public health and medicine. They hope to use this theory to shift the focus of working people and oppressed groups [away from class inequality].[32]

Socialism-inspired statistical thinking left its mark on health statisticians' work. In 1954, Xu Shijin's vital registration demonstrations in seventy-two localities were all canceled. This was in line with the socialist principle that the collection of vital statistics tended to make ill health a matter of personal responsibility.[33] Instead, three years later, Xu and his students launched statistical surveys on community health and

---

[31] Shalobaofu [transliterated name], *Sulian baojian, jiaoyu he wenhua tongji zuzhi [The USSR's Public Health, Educational, and Cultural Statistical Organizations]*, trans. Gu Weilin (Beijing: Caizheng jingji chubanshe [Financial and Economic Publishing House], 1955).

[32] Translated from: Gu Weilin, "Wodui tingban shengming tongji shiban gongzuo de renshi [My Knowledge of the End of Vital Statistics Demonstrations]," *Tongji gongzuo tongxun [Statistical Work Bulletin]* , no.1 (1955): 38–9.

[33] Ibid.

researched hygiene levels in village coal mines near Shanghai.[34] More-over, in line with socialist statistical teaching, Xu's 1957 textbook *Common Public Health Statistical Knowledge in Factories* enumerated aspects that should be recorded regarding workers' health and the loss of man-power due to disease in factories, with no mention of mathematical statistics.[35] Although there is no archival evidence that proves a direct relationship between the changes in Xu's statistical practices and the PRC's national policy, it is informative to note that the PRC took a strong lead in standardizing the country's statistical collection follow-ing the Soviet Union model, including standardizing textbooks at the national level. Around the same time, the Party also implemented waves of thought-reform campaigns, with some directly aimed at intellectuals, particularly those educated in the West.[36] It is therefore reasonable to deduce that Xu had a strong incentive to follow state policy regarding vital and health statistics.

Notably, socialist statistics were not strictly applied to all public health programs. The concept of sampling, for example – inherent in the selection of a "demonstration" area prior to more extensive imple-mentation – did not disappear from public health work, despite being prohibited under socialist doctrine. A document from the Shanghai Municipal Archives, published only two years after the cancellation of Xu's vital registration demonstration, shows that the Shanghai Munici-pal Health Bureau nonetheless maintained three testing sites for such a system.[37] Faculty members at the Shanghai First Medical School also continued to implement random sampling in their health surveys. In 1956, Yang Guoliang, an American-trained dermatologist, led a group of students to survey yaws prevalence north of the Yangtze River in

---

[34] Wo Hongmei, "Zhongguo yixue tongjixue fazhan jianshi [Brief History of China's Medical Statistics, 1949–2012]" (Master's dissertation, Nanjing, Nanjing Medical College, 2013), 61.

[35] Xu Shijin, *Gongchang changyong weisheng tongji zhishi [Common Public Health Statistical Knowledge in Factories]* (Shanghai: Shanghai Public Health Publishing House, 1957).

[36] Fu Zhengyuan, *Autocratic Tradition and Chinese Politics* (Cambridge: Cambridge University Press, 1993), 256–87. For general accounts of the relationship between the PRC and its scientists/intellectuals, see, e.g.: Cong Cao, *China's Scientific Elite* (London: Routledge, 2004); Joel Andreas, *Rise of the Red Engineers: The Cultural Revolution and the Origins of China's New Class* (Stanford, CA: Stanford University Press, 2009); Timothy Cheek, *The Intellectual in Modern Chinese History* (Cambridge: Cambridge University Press, 2015).

[37] Shanghai Municipal Health Bureau, "Shanghaishi 1955 nian weishengfangyi gong-zuo jihua [Shanghai City's public health and epidemic control work plan for 1955]," 1955, 6, B242-1-793, Shanghai Municipal Archives.

Jiangsu Province.[38] Yang's survey method was to sample four counties and one city, where 14,000 inhabitants were examined. After finishing his survey, Yang published an article praising the superiority of both collective work and social institutions when seeking to develop statistics and a reporting system, asking: "[H]ow can a commander with no idea as to his enemies' situation devise an overall war plan?"[39] Yang's vision of statistics and their role in representing field conditions to aid policy-making was identical to that of his Western colleagues and pre-1949 Chinese public health experts.[40]

These fieldwork activities reveal some of the limits that socialist methods encountered during implementation. In 1952, the Patriotic Health Campaign also shaped the uses of statistics in public health domains. The Communist Party launched the Campaign in March in response to an alleged American bacteriological attack in North Korea and China during the Korean War (1950–1953). Fang Xiaoping posits that the germ-welfare allegation was of crucial importance for the PRC's early nation-building efforts, as public health programs were a good way of converting rural inhabitants to the Party's political ideology.[41] The main action taken under the Patriotic Health Campaign was the mobilization of administrations at all levels, along with the general population, to eliminate mice, flies, mosquitoes, fleas, snails, and other disease-carrying vermin. Though it remains a subject of debate among historians as to whether the alleged bacteriological attack even took place,[42] those specializing in public health generally agree that the PRC government

[38] Yang Guoliang, "Qu Subei diaocha yasi gongzuo de jingguo qingkuang he yixie tihui [My Field Survey on Yaws Work in Subei]," *The Magazine of the Shanghai First Medical School*, October 16, 1956.
[39] Translated from: Ibid.
[40] Ghosh also observes that the PRC attempted to use sampling methods to conduct economic surveys. See: Ghosh, "Accepting Difference, Seeking Common Ground."
[41] Fang, "Diseases, Peasants, and Nation-Building in Rural China," 63.
[42] For a long time, historians held different theories about the veracity of alleged American bacteriological attacks on China and North Korea during the Korean War. Though many well-respected historians, including John King Fairbank, Kathryn Weathersby, and Milton Leitenberg, all rebut the existence of the bacteriological attack, others consider that it did actually take place. In 2016, Leitenberg published the first article using Chinese sources to argue that the claims of bacteriological warfare were a well-articulated, but ultimately false, allegation. See: John K. Fairbank and Mary C. Wright, "Introduction," *The Journal of Asian Studies* 17, no. 1 (1957): 55–60; Kathryn Weathersby, "New Evidence on the Korean War," *Cold War International History Project Bulletin* 11 (1998): 176–99; Milton Leitenberg, "A Chinese Admission of False Korean War Allegations of Biological Weapon Use by the United States," *Asian Perspective* 40, no. 1 (2016): 131–46. For historians who consider the attacks to have actually taken place, see, e.g.: Stephen Lyon Endicott and Edward Hagerman, *The United States and Biological Warfare: Secrets from the Early Cold War and Korea* (Bloomington, IN: Indiana University Press, 1998).

used the allegation to stoke the population's patriotism and implement comprehensive public health programs, establishing the model for such programs over the following decades.[43]

During the Patriotic Health Campaign, the PRC central government relied on trained statisticians to estimate its public health capacities on the ground. For instance, the government mobilized statisticians to compile data on military health achievements during the Korean War. The statisticians Guo Zuchao and his colleague Xue Zhongsan, both alumni of JHSPH, were put in charge of completing the public health work begun during the Korean War.[44] At the domestic level, the Ministry of Health conducted a national survey on bed numbers in all public health facilities, including hospitals and county health centers. In 1953, officials surveyed 172 health units throughout China and concluded that the statistics were mostly false, either due to the staff members' absent-mindedness or attempts to exaggerate their achievements. The ministry then published the results in the State Statistics Bureau's *Statistical Work Bulletin*, listing the errors and calling for accurate statistical reporting. At the end of the article, the author quoted Zhu De, the PRC's vice-chairman: "[F]aking statistics is a crime against the country and the people."[45] These words are an evocative testament to the PRC leaders' frustrations regarding chaotic reporting in the field and their calls for improvement. Socialist statistics may have changed the way statistics were practiced, but the PRC officers did not abandon the use of numbers for governance.

In the same vein, statistics were the linchpin of the Patriotic Health Campaign itself. The Campaign's leaders published aggregated numbers on vectors eliminated, rubbish removed, and drainage systems and wells built; this showcased the broad impact of mass mobilization and created a sense of community among citizens. The Communist Party ordered public health experts to teach local cadres how to collect statistics on the ground and used statistics to plan public health campaigns. Although the existing historiographies do not indicate the names of the health experts who carried out the training, Xu was probably among them, as he was based in Shanghai and in charge of organizing statistical training for health officials, which matches Miriam Gross' account.[46]

[43] Gross, *Farewell to the God of Plague*, 23; Bu, *Public Health and the Modernization of China, 1865–2015*, 224, 233.
[44] Wo Hongmei, "Zhongguo yixue tongjixue fazhan jianshi [Brief History of China's Medical Statistics, 1949–2012]," 71.
[45] Translated from: Weisheng bu [Ministry of Health], "Guanyu jiancha tongji gongzuo de jianyao baogao [Brief Report on the Examination of Statistical Work]," *Tongji gongzuo tongxun [Statistical Work Bulletin]*, 11 (July 3, 1953).
[46] Gross, *Farewell to the God of Plague*, 224–5.

Gross argues that statistical practices were an important element in the Patriotic Health Campaign, allowing local Party cadres to obtain a basic understanding of science, even during the various thought-reform initiatives, when scientists were undermined and forced to leave their positions. Despite problematic reporting on the ground, the use of statistics in health campaigns helped to educate a group of Party officials, who were then able to grasp basic scientific research techniques and apply them to policy-making. Along with map-making techniques, the use of statistics ensured the spread of scientific thinking, even during the Cultural Revolution, when most scientists were persecuted by the regime.[47]

Also during the period under study, the Chinese statisticians educated at the JHSPH began very different career paths. Xu remained at Shanghai First Medical School, but Guo Zuchao and Xue Zhongsan were recruited by the People's Liberation Army to compile and publish information on the PRC's military health achievements during the Korean War. They both went on to become army health statisticians. Guo left Central University in 1951 and became a professor of public health statistics at the Fifth Military Medical University, where he oversaw statistical forms on public health matters within the army. He became a Party member in 1956. A year later, Guo published *Teaching Guidelines on the Public Health Statistical Practices of the People's Liberation Army*, which served as the reference for health-related statistical work in the army.[48] Xue left the Shanghai University of Finance and Economics to also become a professor at the army health laboratory at Shanghai's Secondary Military Medical University. He remained a member of the People's Liberation Army until his death in 1988.

## The Great Leap Forward: Anchored by Statistics

The period covered by the first five-year plan was marked by the Communist Party's efforts to consolidate its governance through nation-building and collectivized agriculture, which integrated the entire country into a national movement. The period immediately afterward was marked by the Great Leap Forward, during which efforts were focused on accelerating production by means of omnipresent control over the governance structure established under the plan. By the end of the first five-year plan,

[47] Ibid., 228, 235–6.
[48] Zhongguo renmin jiefangjun weisheng tongji gongzuo jiaofan. I was unable to acquire a copy of these guidelines. Guo's statistical work for the PRC military is described in: Wo Hongmei, "Zhongguo yixue tongjixue fazhan jianshi," 16.

China's economy was growing steadily following the Soviet Union's economic model. Mao's ambition, however, was to increase China's productivity and outstrip developed countries such as the United States and United Kingdom through mass mobilization. Mao began to implement his mass mobilization method as the first five-year plan was drawing to a close.[49] At that time, in 1957, agricultural collectivization – a system under which farmworkers were paid salaries, regardless of their output – had spread rapidly and extensively across China.[50] Mao discarded the draft for a second five-year plan, however, and instead launched the Great Leap Forward, with the official aim of accelerating economic production to exceed that of the United Kingdom and the United States in ten years. People's communes were established across the country, regrouping tens of thousands of households into farm collectives. The people's communes were put under pressure to accelerate production in both agriculture and steel, as production of the latter was considered the first step toward industrialization. Mao's ideas and methods diverged from those of Soviet Union experts, whose influence had waned significantly, especially following the Sino-Soviet split. In 1960, the Soviet Union recalled most of its experts from China.[51]

The PRC government simplified the many forms that statisticians, in consultancy with Soviet Union experts, had devised to document every aspect of the country's public administration.[52] And yet numbers remained central, at least as rhetorical tools, given that the Great Leap Forward was based on mass mobilization and officers used statistics as a way of gauging the progress achieved. Mao set quantitative goals on production, and statistical data were the core metric for assessing accomplishments. This was made explicit in an editorial that appeared in *Statistical Work*:

Now, people across the world are eagerly awaiting the output of our Great Leap Forward. In order to summarize and inform the world quickly of our accomplishments, we should strive for the Great Leap Forward of producing yearly

---

[49] Odd Arne Westad, *The Global Cold War: Third World Interventions and the Making of Our Times* (Cambridge: Cambridge University Press, 2005), 69.

[50] John K. Fairbank and Merle Goldman, *China: A New History, Second Enlarged Edition* (Cambridge, MA: Harvard University Press, 2006), 352; Xun Zhou, *Forgotten Voices of Mao's Great Famine, 1958–1962: An Oral History* (New Haven, CT: Yale University Press, 2013), 14.

[51] The PRC not only cut off relations with the Soviet Union, it also competed with it to become the leading model of economic development among countries in need of aid. See, e.g.: Jeremy Friedman, *Shadow Cold War: The Sino-Soviet Competition for the Third World* (Chapel Hill, NC: University of North Carolina Press, 2015).

[52] Wo Hongmei, "Zhongguo yixue tongjixue fazhan jianshi [Brief History of China's Medical Statistics, 1949–2012]," 152.

statistical reports. ... This is not only professional work, but also a political mission.[53]

During the Great Leap Forward, control of statistical collection passed from the State Statistical Bureau to local Party leadership.[54] Mao encouraged the local cadres of the people's communes to acquire statistical knowledge so that they could use statistics to communicate local realities to the Party leadership for centralized policy-making.[55] Valuing grass-roots mobilization, the Party trained local cadres to report statistics so that the central government could tackle problems objectively and without bias.[56] Each people's commune had its own statistics agency. Some communes also organized health survey teams with their leaders, who oversaw health statistics in the communes.[57] Nevertheless, the quality of the statistics collected remained questionable. In an oral history collected by Zhou Xun, Huang Manyi, a woman who was part of a people's commune in eastern Anhui, recalled life during the Great Famine that ravaged China a year after the Great Leap Forward began: "Our village used to be quite big, with a few hundred people. But in those days hardly anyone was left in our village. More than half of the villagers died during the famine, including quite a few entire families. But there were no official [death] statistics. Even now it's still forbidden to talk about what happened."[58]

The taboo on collecting death numbers dominated at the village level. The number of deaths as reported by the local cadres is therefore questionable, if not completely fabricated. The epidemiological reporting system also had limited capacity: Fang Xiaoping recounts how a disease outbreak took fifteen days to be confirmed by the central government, as the large size of the people's communes made epidemic reporting difficult. Fang also indicates that disease reporting became much faster when the size of the people's communes was reduced nationwide after 1962.[59]

The Great Leap Forward pushed the people's communes to make ever greater efforts to achieve the numbers needed. And as Mao announced new goals based on the statistics reported from the previous season, local production was caught in a vicious circle of impossibly high expectations.

[53] The Editor's Office, "Lizheng tongji nianbao gongzuo de dayuejin [Strive for a Great Leap Forward in Annual Statistical Reports]," *Tongji gongzuo [Statistical Work]*, no. 23 (1958): 5.
[54] Nai-Ruenn Chen, ed., *Chinese Economic Statistics in the Maoist Era: 1949–1965* (New Brunswick: Transaction Publishers, 2009), 56.
[55] Gross, *Farewell to the God of Plague*, 209.
[56] Ibid.
[57] Fang, "Diseases, Peasants, and Nation-Building in Rural China," 61.
[58] Zhou, *Forgotten Voices of Mao's Great Famine, 1958–1962*, 141.
[59] Fang, "Diseases, Peasants, and Nation-Building in Rural China," 61–2.

Scholars have also demonstrated that these inflated numbers were eventually crucially detrimental to Mao's governance, as he failed to grasp the true situation. Over-mobilization eventually resulted in widespread famine, leading to the deaths of between 11 million and 60 million people, according to various estimates.[60] Some scholars go further, arguing that it was the local leadership's exaggeration of economic statistics that caused the Great Famine.[61] There was no difference when it came to public health work: Zhou Xun's research chronicles the chaos on the ground with regard to statistical collection both before and during the Great Leap Forward. Without explicitly citing sociologists of quantification, Zhou describes a scene of "reactivity" toward the governance of statistics. That is, the collection of numbers was not only a way of reflecting the reality in the field, but also shaped how stakeholders conceived the subject matter, which changed how they reacted, with a view to obtaining the numbers they preferred.[62] Zhou writes that fieldworkers "came up with makeshift solutions," such as using government funds to buy snails to kill in order to meet the quota set by their superiors, or would simply "fabricate the numbers."[63]

Mass mobilization during the Great Leap Forward also impacted health statisticians at the Shanghai First Medical School. The school magazine meticulously documented how faculty members within the public health department were criticized by colleagues and students during the school's rectification movement. As early as March 1958, the magazine published criticism of the public health department for its lack of policy concern, thought education, or understanding of China and workers' lived experience.[64] Xu Shijin and his colleagues were sent to work in factories, epidemic prevention centers, and the Shanghai

---

[60] See, e.g.: Fu, *Autocratic Tradition and Chinese Politics*, 304; Xun Zhou, *The Great Famine in China, 1958–1962: A Documentary History* (New Haven, CT: Yale University Press, 2012), 43.

[61] Kenneth Walker's theory is the best known and stresses how the local leadership's exaggeration of grain production led to a high grain procurement rate, which led to local famine (Kenneth Walker, *Food Grain Procurement and Consumption in China* [Cambridge: Cambridge University Press, 1984]). Nevertheless, as Kimberley Ens Manning and Felix Wemheuer have indicated, some scholars argue that the Great Famine was actually due to other causes, such as bad weather (Kimberley Ens Manning and Felix Wemheuer, eds., *Eating Bitterness: New Perspectives on China's Great Leap Forward and Famine* [Vancouver: University of British Columbia Press, 2011], 9–10).

[62] Espeland and Sauder, *Engines of Anxiety*, 7, 196–8.

[63] Zhou, *The People's Health*, 60, 153.

[64] "Weishengxi jiaoxue gongzuo zhenggai fangan (Chugao) [Proposal to Reform the Public Health Department Following the Rectification Movement (First Draft)]," *The Magazine of the Shanghai First Medical School*, March 14, 1958.

Municipal Health Bureau for two hours per week.[65] Although thought reform impacted faculty members' weekly schedules, statistical practices became even more central to the department's curriculum. The course "Vital and Health Statistics" became a requirement for first-year students.[66] The teaching and research unit within the department asserted the importance of the principle of demonstration and statistical collection during the Rectification Movement, justifying the method as a way of customizing Soviet public health theories about water supply systems to rural China.[67] In terms of statistical discourse, members of the unit thus had aspirations similar to those of their interwar predecessors in Beijing and Ding Xian (see Chapters 2 and 4). Both generations had hoped to use statistical practices to import foreign theories and tailor health policies to the Chinese context. Experts occupying teaching positions, however, came under attack despite this continuity of thinking.

The events recounted above show that statistics remained a salient aspect of public health research and policy-making during the Great Leap Forward, possibly even more so than before, as statistics were needed to govern mass mobilization. Even though the academic statistician Xu became the target of criticism at the Shanghai First Medical School, vital and health statistics nonetheless became even more central to teaching and research.

## A Short-Lived Comeback for Mathematical Statistics

It is telling that mathematical statistics began to reappear in Chinese public health textbooks only a year after the Soviet Union canceled its technical assistance to China and repatriated its experts. In 1961, Xu published *Guidelines for Self-Learning Public Health Administration*, in which he detailed public health campaigns in China from the interwar period to the PRC years.[68] With a special focus on the PRC's public

[65] "Lai ge jiaoxue dafanshen bancheng yi ge Zhongguo de weishengxi – weishengxi zhaokai jiaoxue zhenggai cujin dahui [Let's Change Training and Organize a Chinese Public Health Department, Teaching Reform Meeting Convened by the Public Health Department]," *The Magazine of the Shanghai First Medical School*, April 4, 1958.
[66] Ibid.
[67] "Xiaomie san duo san shao, baozheng jiaoxue zhiliang tigao – huanjing weisheng jiaoyanzu tichu zhenggai jihua [Eliminating the Three Excesses and Three Lacks to Improve Teaching Quality: The Environmental Health Research and Teaching Unit Proposes Reforms]," *The Magazine of the Shanghai First Medical School*, March 28, 1958.
[68] Xu Shijin, *Baojian zuzhixue zixue zhidao [Guidelines for Self-Learning Public Health Administration]* (Shanghai: Shanghai First Medical School, 1961).

health organizations, from the Patriotic Health Campaign to the people's communes, Xu included statistical methods (covering mathematical statistics) ranging from survey design, data tabulation, and standard deviations to random sampling and the chi-squared test.[69] Though they were relegated to the annex, the fact that mathematical statistics were included at all can be considered part of their gradual reintegration, which was likely due to the departure of most Soviet experts after the Sino-Soviet split. Three years later, Guo and Xu published a second version of Guo's textbook with a new title, *Medical Mathematical Statistics Methodology*, in which the return of mathematical statistics was blatant. The textbook devotes only two chapters on descriptive statistics, and five others on deviations, secondary and Poisson distribution, normal distribution, statistical significance, and linear regression.[70]

This comeback for mathematical statistics was short-lived, as the Cultural Revolution led to the suppression of the statisticians' research venues. Xu's research and teaching activities were discontinued during the Cultural Revolution, when he was stigmatized as an anti-revolutionary academic authority. It was not until 1979 that Xu, in collaboration with his colleagues at the Shanghai First Medical School's public health statistics teaching and research unit, published another textbook, *Medical Statistical Methods*.[71] Guo and Xue, despite their positions within the military system, were also persecuted.

At the beginning of the Cultural Revolution, as during the Great Leap Forward, there was a reliance on vital and health statistics despite the criticisms of trained statistical experts.[72] For instance, during the first two years, the City of Shanghai undertook statistical collection reform and continued to collect vital and health statistics. The Ministry of Health informed its partners at the provincial and municipal levels that public health reporting forms had been simplified, but it continued to issue a monthly epidemic report and a biannual report on family planning. At the end of the decree, the Ministry of Health declared:

This year is the year that the proletariat's Cultural Revolution blooms. Collect actively, compile actively, and report actively, as this year's statistical data is

[69] Ibid.
[70] Guo Zuchao, *Yiyong shuli tongji fangfa [Medical Mathematical Statistics Methodology]*, eds. Xu Shijin and Li Guangyin (Beijing: Renmin weisheng chubanshe [People's Public Health Publishing House], 1963).
[71] Shanghai diyi yixueyuan weisheng tongjixue jiaoyanzu [Shanghai First Medical School Public Health Statistics Teaching and Research Unit], *Yixue tongji fangfa [Medical Statistical Methods]* (Shanghai: Shanghai kexue jishu chubanshe [Shanghai Science and Technology Publishing House], 1979).
[72] For example, Ghosh mentions that the State Statistical Bureau was particularly hard hit by the Cultural Revolution (Ghosh, *Making It Count*, 278).

meaningful. We hope that each province, self-governing region and municipal health bureau, based on the spirit of "grasp revolution and improve production," so as to secure the success of the proletariat's Cultural Revolution, will allocate appropriate resources to secure the public health statistical report for the year 1966.[73]

Like Mao's appeal during the Great Leap Forward, the quotation shows that statistical collection continued to be used in the PRC's public health administration at the outset of the Cultural Revolution. Even as experts were ousted and stigmatized, the administration tightened its grip on statistics for use in governance. A lack of access to archives makes it difficult to determine exactly how numbers were used during the Cultural Revolution. What is certain is that the administration's faith in statistics was not completely destroyed, as three important health statisticians – Xu, Guo, and Xue – regained their positions and resumed publishing in the 1970s.

\*

This chapter has shown that the PRC's decision to withdraw from the WHO was not a turn away from statistics. Despite refusing to share its numbers with the WHO, the regime carried on collecting vital and health statistics and shared them with other socialist countries.

Three threads of vital and health statistical practices intertwined with one another at one time or another during this period. First, there were the statistical practices employed at the national level, through which socialist statistics were imported to the PRC via Soviet experts and the State Statistics Bureau in the 1950s. But even when socialist statistics were at their most dominant, public health experts carrying out fieldwork – the second thread – had some independence in the ways they used numbers for their research and other activities, although mathematical statistics disappeared from textbooks. The fieldwork-based research of these experts involved demonstrations and test points that used the logic of sampling, a type of reasoning that socialist statisticians opposed. This in turn impacted the third thread – statistical collection for governmental health campaigns – as the same experts oversaw the training of officers in statistical collection at the beginning of the PRC. Statistical collection continued to have an important role in PRC health campaigns, despite statistical experts being persecuted during various periods. During the

---

[73] Translated from: Weisheng bu [Ministry of Health], "Ge sheng, zizhiqu, weisheng tingju [To the Departments and Health Bureaus of Provinces and Self-Governing Regions]," November 17, 1966, B242-1-1764, Shanghai Municipal Archives.

Great Leap Forward and the beginning of the Cultural Revolution, the PRC government repeatedly proclaimed the importance of statistical reporting for grasping local conditions and forming policies.

The events related here present an interesting case study in how statistical experts' authority and the authority of statistics interacted. The early years of the PRC indeed present a somewhat extreme example in that experts were constantly deprived of their authority during this period. Yet, even while public health statistical experts were losing their authority, the PRC administration was placing growing importance on the use of numbers for public health campaigns. PRC officers constantly emphasized and amended statistical reporting systems for their campaigns, as they were aware that collection on the ground was problematic. Indeed, statistical practices remained central within health campaigns, but the work was increasingly carried out by local cadres instead of public health experts. It is also likely that the comeback of public health statistical experts such as Xu Shijin, Guo Zuchao, and Xue Zhongsan following the Cultural Revolution was made possible by a continued faith in the power of statistics.

# Conclusion
## Numbers, Experts, and Policy-Making

The COVID-19 crisis and the resulting daily flood of models, graphs, and tables have shown how numbers – and the ways in which we visualize numbers – have grown ever more dominant since the period covered in this book. In many countries, political leaders and media outlets put forward the image of a COVID response "production line" in which statistics were automatically fed into policy-making via modeling: numbers fed into models, which produced prognostics, which then dictated policies. Some governments even cited the virus's basic reproduction number ($R_0$) when justifying their response policies. This reliance on models in policy-making has led many researchers to voice concerns about the necessarily simplistic nature of such models.[1]

And yet governments, despite experiencing similar transmission curves over time, undertook a large variety of different response measures: ordering the closure of different types of public establishments, for example, and enforcing different lengths of quarantine. This revealed the important role retained by policy-makers in interpreting the numbers. Policy-makers certainly continued to have leverage when it came to decision-making during the pandemic.[2] The French president, Emmanuel Macron, for example, went within a year from stressing the scientific nature of his decisions to calling the models – and hence the scientists – wrong. When facing increasing cases, policy-makers' discourse also differed: Donald Trump, then the United States president, more than once blamed the high number of cases in the country on increased testing. Is it really true that there was an over-reliance on models, and that numbers were fed directly into policy-making? Or was this reliance magnified in part by communication strategies aimed at making policy-making

---

[1] Warwick Anderson, "The Model Crisis, or How to Have Critical Promiscuity in the Time of Covid-19," *Social Studies of Science* 51, no. 2 (2021), 167–88.

[2] Sabina Leonelli, "Data Science in Times of Pan(Dem)ic," *Harvard Data Science Review*, no. 3.1 (2021), 3.

"conceivable" and at "depoliticizing" the debate, as Warwick Anderson has suggested?[3]

It will be up to future historians to assess how wide a gap existed between numbers and policies during the pandemic, and the true role played by experts in the policy-making process. The "number culture" in global health governance, made all the more evident by the COVID-19 crisis, did not arise in a vacuum; this book recounts the budding of that very culture by tracing the historical process by which public health actors at different levels and in different places learned to speak the language of statistics, a language they used to grasp health conditions in distant parts of the world, consolidate authority in matters of global health, and increase trust in their policies.

A historical, transnational network of public health experts laid the foundation for the trust in numbers that characterizes international health governance today. Underlying that network was a political context that has always been crucial to the success or failure of statistical collection. The League of Nations had to tread carefully when it sent an expert to tour Asian colonies; the United Nations Relief and Rehabilitation Administration depended on cooperation from the Allied countries; the young World Health Organization (WHO) collaborated with the United States, which aimed to make the organization an all-encompassing clearing house for statistics; and in China and Taiwan, public health statistics were driven in different directions as the two competing regimes sided with different camps in the Cold War.

Another hurdle faced by this global network of statisticians was the heterogeneity of the territories involved. Whereas interwar statisticians from North Atlantic countries were entrusted with standard-making, those from other regions were involved only at a later stage: learning pre-formulated standards and using them to collect numbers. The United Nations' ever-expanding membership eventually incited the WHO's statisticians to take local knowledge into account by including statisticians from different regions at an earlier stage of standard-making and by tailoring standards to local capacities. Nevertheless, the instructions for how to collect statistics in public health fieldwork were decided at the WHO headquarters in Geneva, while statisticians in the regional offices assumed the main responsibility to help countries to implement the decisions; in-country experts again found themselves relegated to a passive role, their contribution limited for the most part to reporting problems encountered in the field. Although local knowledge was integrated into

---

[3] Anderson, "The Model Crisis," 177.

the global statistical reporting system, once that system was established, quantification ended up sidelining local knowledge.[4]

This was not yet completely the case in the period studied here. Most of the actors discussed in this book boasted varied skill sets. They had mastered biostatistics in addition to having expertise in public health issues and the technologies and measures for tackling them, as well as on-the-ground knowledge of the field. This was true even of experts from outside the global health policy-making centers: they were skilled at adapting statistical practices using their local knowledge and the resources at hand. Interwar Chinese experts, for example, adapted statistical systems to the Chinese context and were fluent in reporting numbers when needed. Postwar Taiwanese experts, too, trained fieldworkers to understand the importance of numbers in directing policy decisions; they published the numbers they collected in academic journals, provided field data to support the WHO's policy statements, and took part in WHO meetings, bringing Taiwanese experiences to the table. Although statisticians in the People's Republic of China (PRC) turned away from the WHO and mathematical statistics during this period, the Communist regime nonetheless continued to rely on numbers. Public health experts in the PRC continued to conduct fieldwork-based research that used the logic of sampling from mathematical statistics, despite it being a form of reasoning that socialist statisticians opposed.

Given these diverse practices, to what extent did statistics really serve as a world language of public health that experts from different organizations used to communicate with one another? This book has explored the narrowing distance that separated statistics from policy-making, and the evolving roles of experts (and their knowledge of the field). During the period under study, statistics were gaining ground, and unquantifiable forms of knowledge were becoming marginalized in the process. Whereas interwar experts would use statistical practices at the start of their programs, their individual knowledge still had authority vis-à-vis their sponsors, regardless of the numbers collected. Their postwar colleagues, on the other hand, were forced to engage with and interpret statistics in their policy statements. Nevertheless, while statistics became indispensable in policy-making and communication, postwar experts continued to play an essential role in making sense of the numbers and turning them into policy. The distance between numbers and

---

[4] Merry, *The Seductions of Quantification*, 6–7. More recently, Seye Abimbola has written a poignant editorial calling for the inclusion of local-specific knowledge in knowledge production for global health (Seye Abimbola, "The Uses of Knowledge in Global Health," *BMJ Global Health* 6, no. 4 (2021): 1–7).

policy-making was narrowing, but experts (and their knowledge) were still the linchpins at both ends.

The quantification of health has accelerated on many fronts since 1960. The first and most significant change has been that health economists systematically factor the national economy into health policy-making, a calculation that still dictates most governments' allocation of resources. Two trends paved the way for this change. First, health economics emerged as a discipline, accelerating what historian Michelle Murphy calls "the economization of life."[5] Second, during the neoliberal turn in the 1980s, when countries cut government spending, the WHO experienced a budget crisis, and the World Bank gradually replaced it as the leading financer of health projects at the international level. The World Bank emphasized the need for public health projects to produce an economic return, contributing to what anthropologist Vincanne Adams calls "audit culture," in which quantification and numbers are crucial to devising, monitoring, and assessing health policies.[6]

The economization of life became even more pervasive in policy-making with the rise of indexes.[7] A case in point is the disability-adjusted life year (DALY) index, which was endorsed by the World Bank in 1993 to serve as the basic indicator of health policy design. Discussions of the DALY index have illustrated the dominance, and limits, of health indexes.[8] Devised by the Institute for Health Metrics and Evaluation at the University of Washington, the DALY makes commensurate years of life lost due to fatal disease or injury with years of life lived with a disability. The DALY index rates diseases based on statistical records of how much they reduce the number of disability-free lives as well as life expectancy within a population. Based on this approach, a disease's level of emergency is not based on the number of deaths it causes but on how many disability-free years of life it costs. Younger lives thus count more.[9] Over almost three decades of its existence, the DALY has become a predominant index for public health policy-makers at both the international and national levels. Tellingly, in 2020 alone, eighteen articles were published on PubMed that calculated the burden of COVID-19 using the DALY.

---

[5] Murphy, *The Economization of Life*.
[6] Adams, *Metrics: What Counts in Global Health*.
[7] Indicators involve yet another set of dynamics in policy-making, on which sociologists and anthropologists have conducted in-depth analysis. See, e.g.: Davis, Fisher, Kingsbury, and Merry, *Governance by Indicators*; Merry, *The Seductions of Quantification*.
[8] Jon Cohen, "A Controversial Close-Up of Humanity's Health," *Science* 338, no. 6113 (2012): 1414.
[9] Without citing the DALY, the same rationale was also used in Italian hospitals when deciding which COVID-19 patients should receive treatment using a ventilator.

Despite its sweeping influence, little attention has been paid to the fact that the creation of the DALY involved a number of experts and astute stakeholders. Since 1993, many have sought either to change the DALY's formulae or to include databases to draw attention to health problems in which they are interested.[10] The index has become central to public health policy-making despite raising considerable controversy. It is yet another case in which a deep trust in quantification has played an important role in today's global health goal-setting and policy-making. The controversy surrounding the DALY demonstrates the importance of studying the historical process by which health is quantified.[11] It is equally important to investigate how economic thinking and public health interact in real-life policy-making. Specifically, how did economics impact the ways in which health organizations perceived their programs when health affairs were integrated into the national economy? Are the numbers being collected directly linked to policy-making? What roles are played by experts in interpreting data? These are essential questions if we are to understand international health programming since the 1960s.

Recent growth in data-set size and computing capacity, producing what is known as Big Data, is another critical aspect that impacts our lives in numbers.[12] People have come to accept the collection and calculation of numbers in more and more areas of modern life. This includes epidemiology: as the number and types of communication devices and electronic medical equipment have exploded, data on the health conditions of their users are now stored digitally, ready for analysis.[13] "Infoveillance," epidemiological surveillance based on syndromic data posted online, has become an indispensable method for studying the recent epidemics of Zika virus disease and COVID-19, among others.[14] Apart from infoveillance, Big Data technologies have grown so pervasive that research on COVID-19 includes aspects that range from modeling to the identification of social and environmental needs, as Sabina Leonelli has

---

[10] Cohen, "A Controversial Close-Up of Humanity's Health," 1415–16.

[11] George Weisz and Noemi Tousignant have studied the historical context of the beginning of the DALY. See, e.g.: George Weisz and Noemi Tousignant, "International Health Research and the Emergence of Global Health in the Late Twentieth Century," *Bulletin of the History of Medicine* 93, no. 3 (2019): 365–400.

[12] For a historical investigation into the phenomena of Big Data, see: Elena Aronova, Christine von Oertzen, and David Sepkoski, "Introduction: Historicizing Big Data," *Osiris* 32, no. 1 (2017): 1–17.

[13] Marcel Salathé et al., "Digital Epidemiology," *PLoS Computational Biology* 8, no. 7 (2012): 1–5.

[14] On the Zika virus disease epidemic, see: Effy Vayena et al., "Policy Implications of Big Data in the Health Sector," *Bulletin of the World Health Organization* 96, no. 1 (2018): 66–8.

identified.[15] At the same time, the surveillance of health conditions has also drifted away from the holistic ideal of "complete physical, mental, and social well-being," as defined by the WHO,[16] and is increasingly based upon atomized bodily data, such as heart rate and blood pressure. And statistics are no longer just in the hands of experts; ordinary individuals can also monitor and adjust their lifestyles using quantified data.

As quantification has become pervasive, aspects that cannot be quantified have lost their visibility. To this day, geographical inequality in data has persisted, if not worsened. Data is being generated at an explosive rate in wealthy countries, but the WHO is still struggling to collect statistics in regions with weak public health services. The Ebola crisis in 2013 demonstrated the lack of reliable epidemic statistics reporting in some regions, a deficiency that delayed and hindered relief work.[17] The rise of an "audit culture" had created a blind spot in global health policy-making: territories that do not produce sufficient statistics are relegated to a secondary position, as they do not have the reliable quantified data required for putting forward a convincing argument for obtaining funding from international organizations.

As statistics penetrate all aspects of health policy-making, fully understanding the implications of public health numbers, indexes, and models has become an urgent issue. Only by disentangling the methodological presumptions behind statistical collection and examining reporting procedures in detail can global public health policies be decoupled from the rationale of economic returns, and the policy-making process be made truly transparent. And only by opening the black box of data can we use numbers in a well-informed way when devising global health policy.

---

[15]  Leonelli, "Data Science in Times of Pan(Dem)ic."
[16]  International Health Conference, "The Constitution of the World Health Organization," 1946. www.who.int/about/governance/constitution.
[17]  Suerie Moon et al., "Will Ebola Change the Game? Ten Essential Reforms before the next Pandemic. The Report of the Harvard-LSHTM Independent Panel on the Global Response to Ebola," *The Lancet* 386, no. 10009 (2015): 2204–21.

# Glossary of Chinese Key Terms

Bai Xiqing　白希清
Cai Fu　蔡福
Central Field Health Station (CFHS)　中央衛生實驗院
Central Statistics Bureau　國民政府主計處
Chaojhou (Chaozhou)　潮州(屏東)
Chen Wanyi (Ch'en Wan-I)　陳萬益
Chen Xixuan (Ch'en Hsi-Hsuan)　陳錫煊
Chen Zhengde (Ch'en Cheng Te, C. T. Ch'en)　陳政德
Chen Zhiqian (Ch'en Chih-Ch'ien, C. C. Ch'en)　陈志潜／陳志潛
Chinese National Association of the Mass Education Movement　中华平民教育促进会／中華平民教育促進會
Chishan　旗山
Chongqing (Chungking)　重慶
Ding Xian (Ting Hsien)　定县／定縣
Executive Yuan 行政院
Fang Yiji (Fang I-Chih, I. C. Fang)　方頤積
Gu Weilin　顾玮琳／顧瑋琳
Guo Zuchao　郭祖超
Guo Songgen (Quo Sung-Ken, S. K. Quo)　郭松根
Huang Zifang (Huang Tsefang, Tsefang F. Huang)　黃子方
Jiangning　江宁／江寧
Jin baoshan (King Pao-Zan, P. Z. King)　金宝善／金寶善
Jurong　句容
Li Jinghan (Lee Ching-Han)　李景汉／李景漢
Li Ting-An (Ting-An Lee)　李廷安
Liang Guangqi (Liang Kuang-Ch'i, K. C. Liang)　梁鑛琪
Lin Jingchen　林竟成
Liu Ruiheng (Jui-Heng Liu, J. Heng Liu)　劉瑞恆
Ministry of Health　卫生部／衛生部
Nanjing　南京
National Health Administration, Ministry of the Interior　內政部衛生署
Niuzhuang (Newchwang)　牛庄
Peiping Health Demonstration Station (Peking First Health Station, First Health Station Peiping)　北平市衛生局第一衛生區事務所
Rong Qirong (Winston Yung)　容啟榮

Taiwan Malaria Research Institute (TMRI) 臺灣省瘧疾研究所
Taiwan Provincial Health Administration 台灣省政府衛生處
Tangshan 汤山／湯山
Tao Rongjin (T'ao Jung-Chin, J. C. Tao) 陶榮錦
Tianjin (Tientsin) 天津
Wu Liande (Wu Lien-Teh) 伍连德／伍連德
Wusong (Woosung) 吳淞
Xu Shijing (Hsu Shih-Chin, S.C. Hsu) 许世瑾／許世瑾
Yan Yangchu (Y. C. James Yen) 晏阳初／晏陽初
Yang Guoliang 杨国亮／楊國亮
Yang Tingguang (Yang Ting-Kwong, Edward B. Young) 楊廷珖
Yuan Yijing (Yüan I-Chin, I. C. Yuan) 袁貽瑾
Zhou county 邹县／鄒縣

# Bibliography

## Primary Sources

### *Archives and Libraries*

Academia Historica, Taipei (國史館)
Alan Mason Chesney Medical Archives of the Johns Hopkins Medical Institutions, Baltimore (Johns Hopkins Medical Archives)
American Bureau for Medical Aid to China Records, Columbia University Libraries, New York
Archives of Ministry of Foreign Affairs of China, Beijing (中华人民共和国外交部档案馆)
Archives of Ministry of Foreign Affairs of the Republic of China (外交檔案), Institute of Modern History, Academia Sinica, Taipei (中央研究院近代史研究所)
Beijing Municipal Archives, Beijing (北京市档案馆)
League of Nations Archives, Geneva
Milbank Memorial Fund Archives, University of Yale, New Haven
National Archives and Records Administration, College Park
National Taiwan University Library, Taipei (台灣大學圖書館)
Peking Union Medical College Archives, Beijing (北京协和医学院档案馆)
Raymond Pearl's Papers, American Philosophical Society, Philadelphia
Rockefeller Archive Center, Tarrytown
Shanghai Library, Shanghai (上海图书馆)
Shanghai Municipal Archives, Shanghai (上海档案馆)
United Nations' Archives, New York
Welch Medical Library, Johns Hopkins University & Medicine, Baltimore
World Health Organization Archives, Geneva
World Health Organization Library, Geneva

### *Published Primary Sources*

Armstrong, Donald B. "The Framingham Health Tuberculosis Demonstration." *American Journal of Public Health* 7, no. 3 (1917): 318–22.
Balinska, Marta Aleksandra. "Ludwik Rajchman (1881–1965): Médecin polonais et citoyen du monde." *La Revue du Praticien* 55, no.4 (2005): 458–61.

Buck, Pearl S. "Tell the People: Mass Education in China." American Council Institute of Pacific Relations, 1945. Family/2.OMR/G/3/16. Rockefeller Archive Center.

Bi, Rugang 毕汝刚 and Guo Zuchao 郭祖超, eds. *Gonggong weisheng* 公共卫生 *[Public Health]*. Shanghai: Shangwu yinshuguan 商務印書館 [The Commercial Press], 1953.

Ch'en, C. C. "Scientific Medicine as Applied in Ting Hsien: Third Annual Report of the Rural Public Health Experiment in China." *The Milbank Memorial Fund Quarterly Bulletin* 11, no. 2 (1933): 97–129.

Ch'en, C. C. "Public Health in Rural Reconstruction at Ting Hsien: Fourth Annual Report of the Rural Public Health Experiment in China." *The Milbank Memorial Fund Quarterly* 12, no. 4 (1934): 370–78.

Ch'en, C. C. "The Rural Public Health Experiment in Ting Hsien, China." *The Milbank Memorial Fund Quarterly* 14, no. 1 (1936): 66–80.

Ch'en, C. C. "Ting Hsien and the Public Health Movement in China." *The Milbank Memorial Fund Quarterly* 15, no. 4 (1937): 380–90.

Ch'en, C. C., and Frederica M. Bunge. *Medicine in Rural China: A Personal Account*. Berkeley, CA: University of California Press, 1989.

Ch'en, C. T., and K. C. Liang. "Malaria Surveillance Programme in Taiwan." *Bulletin of the World Health Organization* 15, no. 3–5 (1956): 805–10.

Chen, Jinsheng 陳金生. "Taiwan weisheng xingzheng he yixue jiaoyu yibainian shi 台灣衛生行政和醫學教育一百年史 [One Hundred Years of Public Health Administration and Medical Education in Taiwan]," 2006. 410.3 7582. National Taiwan University Library.

Chen, Zhiqian 陳志潛. "Hebei Dingxian shiyan xiangcun weisheng 河北定縣實驗鄉村衛生 [Experimental Rural Health Program in Ding County, Hebei]." *Zhonghua yixue zazhi* 中華醫學雜誌（上海）*[National Medical Journal of China (Shanghai)]* 20, no. 9 (1934a): 1125–34.

Chen, Zhiqian 陳志潛. "Dingxian shehui gaizao shiye zhong zhi nongcun weisheng shiyan 定縣社會改造事業中之農村衛生實驗 [Reform of the Rural Health Experiment in Ding County]." *Weisheng yuekan* 衛生月刊 *[Health Monthly]* 4 (1934b): 4–13.

Chernow, Ron. *Titan: The Life of John D. Rockefeller, Sr.* New York: Knopf Doubleday Publishing Group, 2007.

Chow, C. Y., K. C. Liang, and Donald J. Pletsch. "Observations on Anopheline Populations in Human Dwellings in Southern Taiwan (Formosa)." *Indian Journal of Malariology* 5, no. 4 (1951): 569–77.

Chu, Chen-Yi 朱真一. "Nueji yanjiusuo ji zaoqi fuwu de qianbei – shang 瘧疾研究所及早期服務的前輩（上）[The Taiwan Malaria Research Institute and its Staff During its Founding Years. Part I]." *Taiwan Yijie* 台灣醫界 *[Taiwan Medical Journal]* 52, no. 3 (2009a): 58–61.

Chu, Chen-Yi 朱真一. "Nueji yanjiusuo ji zaoqi fuwu de qianbei – xia 瘧疾研究所及早期服務的前輩（下）[The Taiwan Malaria Research Institute and its Staff During its Founding Years. Part II]." *Taiwan Yijie* 台灣醫界 *[Taiwan Medical Journal]* 52, no. 5 (2009b): 53–6.

Committee on the Celebration of the Eightieth Birthday of Doctor William Henry Welch. *The Eightieth Birthday of William Henry Welch: The Addresses Delivered*. New York: Milbank Memorial Fund, 1930.

Department of Health. *Monthly Bulletin of the Department of Health of the City of New York*, October 1911. New York: The Department of Health, 1911. https://babel.hathitrust.org/cgi/pt?id=hvd.32044103093621;view=1up;seq=93.

Department of Health. *Malaria Eradication in Taiwan*. 2nd ed. Taipei: Centers for Disease Control, Department of Health, 2005.

Department of Health. *Taiwan punue jishi* 台灣撲瘧紀實 *[Malaria Eradication in Taiwan]*. 2nd ed. Taipei: 行政院衛生署疾病管制局 [Centers for Disease Control, Department of Health], 2005.

Eyler, John M. *Sir Arthur Newsholme and State Medicine, 1885–1935*. Cambridge: Cambridge University Press, 1997.

Farewell, Vern, and Tony Johnson. "Major Greenwood (1880–1949): A Biographical and Bibliographical Study." *Statistics in Medicine* 35, no. 5 (2016): 645–70.

Fine, Paul E. M. "A Commentary on the Mechanical Analogue to the Reed-Frost Epidemic Model." *American Journal of Epidemiology* 106, no. 2 (1977): 87–100.

Flexner, Simon and James Thomas Flexner. *William Henry Welch and the Heroic Age of American Medicine*. New York: The Viking Press, 1941.

Gamble, Sidney David. *Ting Hsien: A North China Rural Community*. New York: Institute of Pacific Relations, 1954.

Gear, Harry Sutherland, Yves Biraud, and Satya Swaroop. *International Work in Health Statistics, 1948–1958*. Geneva: WHO, 1961.

Grant, John B., T. F. Huang, and S. C. Hsu. "A Preliminary Note on Classification of Causes of Death in China." *National Medical Journal of China (Shanghai)* 13, no. 1 (1927): 1–23.

Gu, Weilin 顧瑋琳. "Wodui tingban shengming tongji shiban gongzuo de renshi 我對停辦生命統計試辦工作的認識 [My Knowledge of the End of Vital Statistics Demonstrations]." *Tongji gongzuo tongxun* 統計工作通訊 *[Statistical Work Bulletin]*, no.1 (1955): 38–9.

Guo, Zuchao 郭祖超. *Yixue yu shengwu tongji fangfa* 醫學與生物統計方法 *[Medical Science and Biological Statistical Methods]*. Shanghai: Zhengzhong shuju 正中書局 [Cheng Chung Book Company], 1948.

Guo, Zuchao 郭祖超. *Yiyong shuli tongji fangfa* 医用数理统计方法 *[Medical Mathematical Statistics Methodology]*, edited by Xu Shijin 许世瑾 and Li Guangyin 李光荫. Beijing: Renmin weisheng chubanshe 人民卫生出版社 [People's Public Health Publishing House], 1963.

Haas, William Joseph. *China Voyager: Gist Gee's Life in Science*. Armonk, NY: M.E. Sharpe, 1996.

"Hermann M. Biggs." *Science* 58, no. 1508 (1923): 413–15.

Howard-Jones, Norman. *The Scientific Background of the International Sanitary Conferences, 1851–1938*. Geneva: World Health Organization (WHO), 1974.

Hsieh, H. C., and K. C. Liang. "Residual Foci of Malarial Infection in the DDT-Sprayed Area of Taiwan." *Bulletin of the World Health Organization* 15, no. 3–5 (1956): 810–13.

International Health Conference. "The Constitution of the World Health Organization," 1946. www.who.int/about/governance/constitution.

Jennings, Herbert S. *"Biographical Memoir of Raymond Pearl (1879–1940),"* *National Academy of Sciences of the United States of America Biographical Memoirs Vol. XXII*, Washington, DC: National Academy of Sciences, 1942, 293–347.

Jin, Baoshan 金寶善. "Beijing zhi gonggong weisheng 北京之公共衛生 [Beijing's Public Health]." *Zhonghua yixue zazhi* 中華醫學雜誌 (上海) *[National Medical Journal of China (Shanghai)]* 12, no. 3 (1926): 253–61.

Jin, Baoshan 金寶善. "Xiwang yu Beijing weisheng dangju zhe 希望於北平衛生當局者 [Plea to the Peking Public Health Authority]." *Zhonghua yixue zazhi* 中華醫學雜誌 (上海) *[National Medical Journal of China (Shanghai)]* 14, no. 5 (1928): 1–4.

Jin, Baoshan 金寶善. "Weisheng yu jiuguo 衛生與救國 [Public Health and Saving Country]." *Weisheng yuekan* 衛生月刊 *[Health Monthly]* 4, no. 1 (1934): 2–3.

Jin, Baoshan 金寶善, and Xu Shijin 許世瑾. "Geshengshi xianyou gonggong weisheng sheshi zhi gaikuang 各省市現有公共衛生設施之概況 [The Current Conditions of Public Health Services in Provinces and Municipalities]." *Zhonghua yixue zazhi* 中華醫學雜誌 (上海) *[National Medical Journal of China (Shanghai)]* 23, no. 11 (1937): 1235–48.

Lin, Jingcheng 林竟成. "Zhongguo gonggong weisheng hangzheng zhi zhengjie 中國公共衛生行政之症結 [The Problems of Chinese Public Health Administrations]." *Zhonghua yixue zazhi* 中華醫學雜誌 (北京) *[National Medical Journal of China (Beijing)]* 22, no. 10 (1936): 951–72.

King, Willford I. "Edgar Sydenstricker." *Journal of the American Statistical Association* 31, no. 194 (1936): 411–14.

Kingsbury, John A. "The Effect of the Anti-Tuberculosis Campaign." *The World's Health Monthly Review of the League of Red Cross Society* 6, no. 2 (1925): 63–70.

Kopf, E. W., Otto R. Eichel, Raymond Pearl, and Edgar Sydenstricker. "Educational and Professional Standards for Vital Statisticians." *American Journal of Public Health* 15, no. 6 (1925): 518–20.

"Lai ge jiaoxue dafanshen bancheng yi ge Zhongguo de weishengxi – weishengxi zhaokai jiaoxue zhenggai cujin dahui 來個教學大翻身 辦成一個中國的衛生系 衛生系招開教學整改促進大會 [Let's Change Training and Organize a Chinese Public Health Department, Teaching Reform Meeting Convened by the Public Health Department]." 上海一医院刊 *[The Magazine of the Shanghai First Medical School]*, April 4, 1958.

*The League from Year to Year, October 1st, 1929–September 30th, 1930.* Geneva: League of Nations Information Section, 1931.

Liang, Fei-Yi 梁妃儀, and Tsai Duu-Jian 蔡篤堅. "Liang Kuangqi koushu lishi 梁鑛琪口述歷史 [Oral History of Liang Kuangqi]." *Taiwan fengwu* 台灣風物 *[The Taiwan Folkways]* 59 (2009): 9–39.

Liang, K. C. "The Priority of Malaria Eradication Programs." *Bulletin of the Pan American Health Organization* 9, no. 4 (1975a): 295–9.

Liang, K. C. "Priorities of the malaria eradication program." *Boletin de la Oficina Sanitaria Panamericana. Pan American Sanitary Bureau* 79, no. 6 (1975b): 508–13.

Liang, K. C. "Historical Review of Malaria Control Program in Taiwan." *The Kaohsiung Journal of Medical Sciences* 7, no. 5 (1991): 271–7.

Millard Publishing House. *The China Weekly Review 54.* Shanghai: Millard Publishing House, 1930.

Newsholme, Arthur. *The Elements of Vital Statistics in Their Bearing on Social and Public Health Problems.* London: George Allen & Unwin, 1923.

Parran, Thomas. "Proposals for the Establishment of An International Health Organization." In *Minutes of the Technical Preparatory Committee for the International Health Conference*, 46–50. WHO Official Records 1. Geneva: United Nations World Health Organization Interim Commission, 1947.

Paul, J. H., R. B. Watson, and K. C. Liang. "A Further Report on the Use of Chloroguanide (Paludrine) to Suppress Malaria Prevalence in Southern Formosan Villages." *Journal National Malaria Society (US)* 9, no. 4 (1950): 356–65.

Pearl, Raymond, and Lowell J. Reed. "On the Rate of Growth of the Population of the United States Since 1790 and its Mathematical Representation." *Proceedings of the National Academy of Sciences of the United States of America* 6, no. 6 (1920): 275–88.

Pletsch, Donald J., and C. T. Ch'en. "Economic and Social Effects on Malaria Control with Some Specific Instances from Taiwan," August 31, 1954. WHO Library. http://apps.who.int/iris/bitstream/10665/64287/1/WHO_Mal_108.pdf.

Pubmed Development Team. "Home – PubMed – NCBI." Accessed October 4, 2016. www.ncbi.nlm.nih.gov/pubmed.

Rajchman, Ludwik. "Report to the League of Nations." *National Medical Journal of China (Shanghai)* 13, no. 3 (1927): 288–92.

Riesman, David. "William Henry Welch, Scientist and Humanist." *The Scientific Monthly* 41, no. 3 (1935): 251–7.

Sawyer, Wilbur A. "Achievements of UNRRA as an International Health Organization." *American Journal of Public Health and the Nation's Health* 37, no. 1 (1947): 41–58.

Shalobaofu 沙洛保夫 [transliterated name]. *Sulian baojian, jiaoyu he wenhua tongji zuzhi* 蘇聯保健、教育和文化統計組織 *[The USSR's Public Health, Educational, and Cultural Statistical Organizations]*. Translated by Gu Weilin 顧瑋琳. Beijing: Caizheng jingji chubanshe 財政經濟出版社 [Financial and Economic Publishing House], 1955.

Shanghai diyi yixueyuan weisheng tongjixue jiaoyanzu 上海第一医学院卫生统计学教研组 [Shanghai First Medical School Public Health Statistics Teaching and Research Unit]. *Yixue tongji fangfa* 医学统计方法 *[Medical Statistical Methods]*. Shanghai: Shanghai kexue jishu chubanshe 上海科学技术出版社 [Shanghai Science and Technology Publishing House], 1979.

Shanghai yike daxue jishi bianzuan weiyuan hui 上海医科大学纪事编纂委员会 [Shanghai Medical College Chronicle Editorial Board]. *Shanghai yike daxue jishi* 上海医科大学纪事 *[Shanghai Medical College Chronicle (1927–2000)]*. Shanghai: Fudan University Press, 2000.

Song, Zhiai 宋志愛 and Jin Naiyi 金乃逸. "Woguo haigang jianyi shiwu yange 我國海港檢疫事務沿革 [History of Our Country's Maritime Quarantine Affairs]," *Zhonghua yixue zazhi* 中華醫學雜誌 （上海） *[National Medical Journal of China (Shanghai)]* 25, no. 12 (1939): 1068–74.

Štampar, Andrija. "Suggestions Relating to the Constitution of an International Health Organization." In *Minutes of the Technical Preparatory Committee for the International Health Conference*, 54–61. WHO Official Records 1. Geneva: United Nations World Health Organization Interim Commission, 1947.

Swaroop, Satya, and WHO. *Statistical Notes for Malaria Workers*. Geneva: WHO, 1956. http://apps.who.int/iris/handle/10665/64526.

Swaroop, Satya, and WHO. *Statistical Methodology in Malaria Work*. Geneva: WHO, 1957. https://apps.who.int/iris/handle/10665/64527.

Swaroop, Satya, and WHO. "Statistical Considerations and Methodology in Malaria Eradication." Geneva: WHO, 1959. https://apps.who.int/iris/handle/10665/64660.

Swaroop, Satya, Alan Brownlie Gilroy, Kazuo Uemura, and WHO. *Statistical Methods in Malaria Eradication*. Geneva: WHO, 1966. https://apps.who.int/iris/handle/10665/41775.

Sydenstricker, Edgar. "The Statistical Evaluation of the Results of Social Experiments in Public Health." *Journal of the American Statistical Association* 23, no. 161 (1928a): 155–65.

Sydenstricker, Edgar. "The Statistician's Place in Public Health Work." *Journal of the American Statistical Association* 23, no. 162 (1928b): 115.

Sydenstricker, Edgar. *The Proposed Public Health Program for Ting Hsien, China, of the Chinese National Association of the Mass Education Movement in Collaboration with the Milbank Memorial Fund*. New York: Milbank Memorial Fund, 1930.

Sydenstricker, Edgar. "The Decline in the Tuberculosis Death Rate in Cattaraugus County." In *The Challenge of Facts: Selected Public Health Papers of Edgar Sydenstricker*, edited by Richard V. Kasius, 370–78. New York: Prodist, 1974a.

Sydenstricker, Edgar. "The Measurement of Results of Public Health Work: An Introductory Discussion." In *The Challenge of Facts: Selected Public Health Papers of Edgar Sydenstricker*, edited by Richard V. Kasius, 39–64. New York: Prodist, 1974b.

Sze, Szeming. "The Birth of WHO: Interview [with] Dr Szeming Sze." World Health, May 1989. http://apps.who.int//iris/handle/10665/45224.

Tao, Jung-Chin. "Pulmonary Tuberculosis in Chinese Students." *American Review of Tuberculosis* 56, no. 1 (1947): 22–6.

Tao, Jung-Chin. "Community Approach to Tuberculosis." *Journal of the American Medical Women's Association* 14, no. 12 (1959a): 1077–83.

Tao, Jung-Chin. "Tuberculosis in Taiwan (Formosa)." *American Review of Respiratory Disease* 80, no. 3 (1959b): 359–70.

Tao, Jung-Chin. "Organizing a Simplified Case-Finding Service for Developing Countries. People with Little Formal Education Can Be Trained to Examine the Sputum." *Bulletin – National Tuberculosis and Respiratory Disease Association* 56, no. 2 (1970a): 9–11.

Tao, Jung-Chin. "Tuberculosis. Training, Supervision and Motivation of Personnel." *Bulletin of the International Union Against Tuberculosis* 43, no. 6 (1970b): 87–92.

Tao, Jung-Chin. "The Fight Against Tuberculosis. A Cheap and Efficient Case-Finding Method." *Journal of the West Australian Nurses* 37, no. 1 (1971): 20–22.

Tao, Jung-Chin. "Tuberculosis Control in the Western Pacific Region of WHO 1951–1970." *WHO Chronicle* 27, no. 12 (1973): 507–15.

Tao, Jung-Chin. "BCG Vaccination in the Control of Tuberculosis and the Organisation of a National BCG Vaccination Programme." *Bulletin of the International Union Against Tuberculosis* 49, suppl. 1 (1974a): 154–60.

Tao, Jung-Chin. "Tuberculosis in the Western Pacific Region." *Bulletin of the International Union Against Tuberculosis* 49, suppl. 1 (1974b): 18–23.

The American Journal of Hygiene. *The School of Hygiene and Public Health of the Johns Hopkins University*. The American Journal of Hygiene Monographic Series 6. Baltimore, MD: The American Journal of Hygiene, 1926.

The China Weekly Review. "Chinese Take Over Shanghai Quarantine Service," September 20, 1930. Millard Publishing House.

The Editor's Office. "Lizheng tongji nianbao gongzuo de dayuejin 力争统计年报工作的大跃进 [Strive for a Great Leap Forward in Annual Statistical Reports]." *Tongji gongzuo* 统计工作 *[Statistical Work]*, no. 23 (1958): 5–6.

The Rockefeller Foundation. "The Rockefeller Foundation Annual Report 1913–1914," 1914. www.rockefellerfoundation.org/wp-content/uploads/Annual-Report-1913-1914-1.pdf.

"Tuberculosis Chemotherapy Centre, Madras." *Tubercle* 49, no. 1 (1968): 114–21.

Tsai, Duu-Jian 蔡篤堅, and Yu Yumei 余玉梅, eds. *Taiwan yiliao daode zhi yanbian — ruogan licheng ji gean tantao* 台灣醫療道德之演變—若干歷程及個案探討 *[The Evolution of Medical Ethics in Taiwan: Selected Histories and Case Studies]*. Taipei: National Health Research Institutes, 2003.

Velu, S., R. H. Andrews, S. Devadatta, et al. "Progress in the Second Year of Patients with Quiescent Pulmonary Tuberculosis after a Year of Chemotherapy at Home or in Sanatorium, and Influence of Further Chemotherapy on the Relapse Rate." *Bulletin of the World Health Organization* 23, no. 4–5 (1960): 511–33.

Watson, R. B., and K. C. Liang. "Seasonal Prevalence of Malaria in Southern Formosa." *Indian Journal of Malariology* 4, no. 4 (1950): 471–86.

Weisheng bu 中央人民政府衛生部 [Ministry of Health]. "jiancha tongji gongzuo de jianyao baogao 關於檢查統計工作的簡要報告 [Brief Report on the Examination of Statistical Work]." *Tongji gongzuo tongxun* 統計工作通訊 *[Statistical Work Bulletin]*, 11 (July 3, 1953).

Weisheng bu 中華民國衛生部 [Ministry of Health]. *Taiwan diqu gonggong weisheng fazhan shi (er)* 台灣地區公共衛生發展史（二） *[The History of Public Health Development in Taiwan Vol. II]*. Taipei: Weisheng bu 衛生部 [Ministry of Health], 1995.

"Weishengxi jiaoxue gongzuo zhenggai fangan (Chugao) 卫生系教学工作整改方案（初稿） [Proposal to Reform the Public Health Department Following the Rectification Movement (First Draft)]." 上海一医院刊 *[The Magazine of the Shanghai First Medical School]*, March 14, 1958.

Weisheng Yuekan 衛生月刊, "Wei qing xing wen kangyi Meiguo zhengfu weipai yiguan zai hu jianyi bing ken sushe haigang jianyi jiguan chen gaijin weisheng jianshe yi du jiekou you 為請行文抗議美國政府委派醫官在滬檢疫並懇速設海港檢疫機關、陳改進衛生建設以杜藉口由 [Plea for Protest Against the US Government's Appointment of Medical Officers in Shanghai for Quarantine and for the Prompt Establishment of a Maritime Quarantine Authority to Improve Public Health Infrastructure so as to Eliminate Justifications]." *Weisheng yuekan* 衛生月刊 *[Health Monthly]* 2, no.7 (1929): 32–4.

Whipple, George C. Review of *The Biology of Death*, by Raymond Pearl. *Journal of the American Statistical Association* 18, no. 143 (1923): 926–8.

WHO. "Minutes of the First Session of the Interim Commission," July 1946. Official Record 03. WHO Library.

WHO. "Expert Committee on Health Statistics: Report on the First Session," Geneva: WHO, 1950a.

WHO. "Expert Committee on Health Statistics: Report on the Second Session," Geneva: WHO, 1950b.

WHO. "Bureau de Recherches sur la Tuberculose (Copenhague)," November 10, 1952a. EB11/12. WHO Library.

WHO. "Expert Committee on Health Statistics Third Report," Geneva: WHO, 1952b.

WHO. "Expert Committee on Malaria Fifth Report," WHO Technical Report Series 80. Geneva: WHO, 1954.

WHO. "Expert Committee on Health Statistics Fifth Report," Geneva: WHO, 1957a.

WHO. "Expert Committee on Health Statistics Sixth Report," Geneva: WHO, 1957b.

WHO. "Expert Committee on Malaria Sixth Report," Geneva: WHO, 1957c.

WHO. "Expert Committee on Health Statistics Seventh Report," Geneva: WHO, 1961.

WHO. "Expert Committee on Malaria Thirteenth Report," WHO Technical Report Series 357. Geneva: WHO, 1967.

WHO. "Expert Committee on Health Statistics Fifteenth Report," Geneva: WHO, 1972.

WHO. "The Organizational Structure of the World Health Organization (1948–1974) Vol. II," 1974. WHO Library.

WHOIC. *Minutes of the Technical Preparatory Committee for the International Health Conference.* WHO Official Records 1. Geneva: World Health Organization Interim Commission, 1947.

Wiehl, Dorothy G. "Edgar Sydenstricker: A Memoir." In *The Challenge of Facts: Selected Public Health Papers of Edgar Sydenstricker,* edited by Richard V. Kasius, 3–17. New York: Prodist, 1974.

Winslow, C. E. A. *Health on the Farm and in the Village: A Review and Evaluation of the Cattaraugus County Health Demonstration.* New York: The Macmillan Company, 1931.

Winslow, C. E. A., and Myrdal, Gunnar. "The Economic Values of Preventive Medicine (Fifth World Health Assembly Technical Discussion)." Geneva: WHO, 1952. apps.who.int/iris/handle/10665/101988.

Wu, Liande 伍連德. "Haigang jianyi guanlichu di si nian zhi gongzuo 海港檢疫管理處第四年之工作 [The Fourth Year of Work of the National Quarantine Service]," *Zhonghua yixue zazhi* 中華醫學雜誌 （上海） *[National Medical Journal of China (Shanghai)]* 20, no. 1 (1934): 130–35.

Wu, Zhengji 伍正己. "Dao min jian qu! Banli xiangcun weisheng de kunnan 到民間去！ 辦理鄉村衛生的困難 [Go to the People! The Difficulties in Implementing Rural Health Programs]." *Weisheng yuekan* 衛生月刊 *[Health Monthly],* no. 1–2 (1935): 108–11.

"Xiaomie san duo san shao, baozheng jiaoxue zhiliang tigao – huanjing weisheng jiaoyanzu tichu zhenggai jihua 消灭三多三少 保证教学质量提高 环境卫生教研组提出整改计划 [Eliminating the Three Excesses and Three Lacks to Improve

Teaching Quality: The Environmental Health Research and Teaching Unit Proposes Reforms]." 上海一医院刊 *[The Magazine of the Shanghai First Medical School]*, March 28, 1958.

Xu, Shijin 許世瑾. "Wo ruhe banli weisheng tongji 我如何辦理衛生統計 [How I Implemented Public Health Statistics Collection]," *Fuwu yuekan* 服務月刊 *[Service Monthly]* 2, no. 3–4 (1929): 18–20.

Xu, Shijin 許世瑾. "Shiban Jurong xian Shengming tongji ernian lai gaikuang 試辦句容縣生命統計二年來概況 [Two Years after Implementing Vital Statistics Collection System in Jurong]," *Gonggong weisheng yuekan* 公共衛生月刊 *[Public Health Monthly]* 1–6 (1936): 153.

Xu, Shijin 許世瑾. "Nanjing shi shengming tongji lianhe banshichu diernian gongzuo baogao 南京市生命統計辦事處第二年工作報告 [The Second Annual Report of the United Vital Statistical Office of Nanjing City]," October 1936, 10, Shanghai Library.

Xu, Shijin 許世瑾 and Wang Zuxiang 王祖祥. "Nanjing shi yinger siwanglu diaocha 南京市嬰兒死亡率調查 [Infantile Mortality Investigation in Nanjing City]," *Gonggong weisheng yuekan* 公共衛生月刊 *[Public Health Monthly]*, no. 4 (1935): 23–27.

Xu, Shijin 许世瑾. *Baojian zuzhixue zixue zhidao* 保健组织学自学指导 *[Guidelines for Self-Learning Public Health Administration]* (Shanghai: Shanghai First Medical School, 1961).

Yang, Guoliang 杨国亮. "Qu Subei diaocha yasi gongzuo de jingguo qingkuang he yixie tihui 去苏北调查亚斯工作的经过情况和一些体会 [My Field Survey on Yaws Work in Subei]." 上海一医院刊 *[The Magazine of the Shanghai First Medical School]*, October 16, 1956a.

Yang, Guoliang 杨国亮. "Qu Subei diaocha yasi gongzuo de jingguo qingkuang he yixie tihui 去苏北调查亚斯工作的经过情况和一些体会 [My Field Survey on Yaws Work in Subei]." 上海一医院刊 *[The Magazine of the Shanghai First Medical School]*, November 1, 1956b.

Zhongguo kexueyuan Hebeisheng fenyuan jingji yanjiusuo zichanjieji tongjixue pipan xiaozu 中国科学院河北省分院经济研究所资产阶级统计学批判小组 [China Science Council's Critic Group Against Bourgeois Statistical Research] and Nankai daxue jingjixi zichanjieji tongjixue pipan xiaozu 南开大学经济系资产阶级统计学批判小组 [Nankai University's Critic Group Against Bourgeois Statistical Research]. *Suqing zichan jieji tongji xueshu sixiang de liudu* 肃清资产阶级统计学术思想的流毒 *[Cleaning the Remaining Poison of Bourgeois Statistical Research]*. Shanghai: Shanghai renmin chubanshe 上海人民出版社 [Shanghai People's Publishing House], 1958.

## Secondary Sources

Abimbola, Seye. "The Uses of Knowledge in Global Health." *BMJ Global Health* 6, no. 4 (2021): 1–7.

Adams, Vincanne, ed. *Metrics: What Counts in Global Health*. Durham, NC: Duke University Press, 2016.

Adler, Richard. *Robert Koch and American Bacteriology*. Jefferson, NC: McFarland, 2016.

Akami, Tomoko. "A Quest to be Global: The League of Nations Health Organization and Inter-Colonial Regional Governing Agendas of the Far Eastern Association of Tropical Medicine 1910–25." *The International History Review* 38, no. 1 (2016): 1–23.

Akami, Tomoko. "Imperial Polities, Intercolonialism, and the Shaping of Global Governing Norms: Public Health Expert Networks in Asia and the League of Nations Health Organization, 1908–37." *Journal of Global History* 12, no. 1 (2017): 4–25.

Amrith, Sunil. "In Search of a 'Magic Bullet' for Tuberculosis: South India and Beyond, 1955–1965." *Social History of Medicine* 17, no. 1 (2004): 113–30.

Amrith, Sunil. *Decolonizing International Health: India and Southeast Asia, 1930–65.* New York: Palgrave Macmillan, 2006.

Anderson, Benedict. *Imagined Communities: Reflections on the Origin and Spread of Nationalism.* London: Verso, 2006.

Anderson, Warwick. *Colonial Pathologies: American Tropical Medicine, Race, and Hygiene in the Philippines.* Durham, NC: Duke University Press, 2006.

Anderson, Warwick. "The Model Crisis, or How to Have Critical Promiscuity in the Time of Covid-19." *Social Studies of Science* 51, no. 2 (2021): 167–88.

Andreas, Joel. *Rise of the Red Engineers: The Cultural Revolution and the Origins of China's New Class.* Stanford, CA: Stanford University Press, 2009.

Arnold, David. *Colonizing the Body: State Medicine and Epidemic Disease in Nineteenth-Century India.* Berkeley, CA: University of California Press, 1993.

Aronova, Elena, Christine von Oertzen, and David Sepkoski. "Introduction: Historicizing Big Data." *Osiris* 32, no. 1 (2017): 1–17.

Barry, Andrew, Thomas Osborne, and Nikolas Rose, eds. *Foucault and Political Reason: Liberalism, Neo-Liberalism and the Rationalities of Government.* Chicago, IL: Chicago University Press, 1996.

Bashford, Alison, and Philippa Levine, eds. *The Oxford Handbook of the History of Eugenics.* Oxford: Oxford University Press, 2010.

Bernstein, Thomas P., and Hua-Yu Li, eds. *China Learns from the Soviet Union, 1949–Present.* The Harvard Cold War Studies Book Series. Lanham, MD: Lexington Books, 2010.

Bhattacharya, Sanjoy. "International Health and the Limits of its Global Influence: Bhutan and the Worldwide Smallpox Eradication Programme." *Medical History* 57, no. 4 (2013): 461–86.

Birn, Anne-Emanuelle. *Marriage of Convenience: Rockefeller International Health and Revolutionary Mexico.* Rochester, NY: University of Rochester Press, 2006.

Birn, Anne-Emanuelle. "The Stages of International (Global) Health: Histories of Success or Successes of History?" *Global Public Health* 4, no. 1 (2009): 50–68.

Birn, Anne-Emanuelle. "Backstage: The Relationship between the Rockefeller Foundation and the World Health Organization, Part I: 1940s–1960s." *Public Health* 128, no. 2 (2014): 129–40.

Birn, Anne-Emanuelle, and Nikolai Krementsov. "'Socialising' Primary Care? The Soviet Union, WHO and the 1978 Alma-Ata Conference." *BMJ Global Health* 3, suppl. 3 (2018): 1–15.

Birn, Anne-Emanuelle, and Raùl Necochea López, eds. *Peripheral Nerve: Health and Medicine in Cold War Latin America.* Durham, NC: Duke University Press, 2020.

Birn, Anne-Emanuelle, Yogan Pillay, and Timothy H. Holtz. *Textbook of Global Health*. Oxford: Oxford University Press, 2017.

Boecking, Felix. *No Great Wall: Trade, Tariffs and Nationalism in Republican China, 1927–1945*. Cambridge, MA: Harvard University Asia Center, 2017.

Borowy, Iris. "Counting Death and Disease: Classification of Death and Disease in the Interwar Years, 1919–1939." *Continuity and Change* 18, no. 3 (2003): 457–81.

Borowy, Iris. "Maneuvering for Space: International Health Work of the League of Nations During World War II." In *Shifting Boundaries of Public Health: Europe in the Twentieth Century*, edited by Susan Gross Solomon, Lion Murard, and Patrick Zylberman, 87–113. Rochester Studies in Medical History. Rochester, NY: University of Rochester Press, 2008.

Borowy, Iris. *Coming to Terms with World Health: The League of Nations Health Organisation 1921–1946*. Bern: Peter Lang, 2009a.

Borowy, Iris. "Thinking Big – League of Nations Efforts Towards a Reformed National Health System in China." In *Uneasy Encounters: The Politics of Medicine and Health in China 1900–1937*, edited by Iris Borowy, 205–28. Frankfurt am Main: Peter Lang, 2009b.

Bouk, Dan. *How Our Days Became Numbered: Risk and the Rise of the Statistical Individual*. Chicago, IL: University of Chicago Press, 2015.

Brazelton, Mary Augusta. "Western Medical Education on Trial: The Endurance of Peking Union Medical College, 1949–1985." *Twentieth-Century China* 40, no. 2 (2015): 126–45.

Brazelton, Mary Augusta. *Mass Vaccination: Citizens' Bodies and State Power in Modern China*. Ithaca, NY: Cornell University Press, 2019.

Bréard, Andrea. "Robert Hart and China's Statistical Revolution." *Modern Asian Studies* 40, no. 3 (2006): 605–29.

Breckenridge, Keith, and Simon Szreter. *Registration and Recognition: Documenting the Person in World History*. Oxford: Oxford University Press/ British Academy, 2012.

Brian, Éric. "Statistique administrative et internationalisme statistique pendant la seconde moitié du XIXe siècle." *Histoire & Mesure* 4, no. 3 (1989): 201–24.

Brimnes, Niels. "BCG Vaccination and WHO's Global Strategy for Tuberculosis Control 1948–1983." *Social Science & Medicine* 67, no. 5 (2008): 863–73.

Brown, Theodore M., Marcos Cueto, and Elizabeth Fee. "The World Health Organization and the Transition from 'International' to 'Global' Public Health." *American Journal of Public Health* 96, no. 1 (2006): 62–72.

Bu, Liping. *Public Health and the Modernization of China, 1865–2015*. London: Routledge, 2017.

Bu, Liping, and Elizabeth Fee. "John B. Grant International Statesman of Public Health." *American Journal of Public Health* 98, no. 4 (2008): 628–9.

Bu, Liping, and Ka-Che Yip, eds. *Public Health and National Reconstruction in Post-War Asia: International Influences, Local Transformations*. London: Routledge, 2015.

Bullock, Mary Brown. *An American Transplant: The Rockefeller Foundation and Peking Union Medical College*. Berkeley, CA: University of California Press, 1980.

Bullock, Mary Brown, and Bridie Andrews, eds. *Medical Transitions in Twentieth-Century China.* Bloomington, IN: Indiana University Press, 2014.

Burchell, Graham, Colin Gorden, and Peter Miller, eds. *The Foucault Effect: Studies in Governmentality.* Chicago, IL: University of Chicago Press, 1991.

Burkman, Thomas W. *Japan and the League of Nations.* Honolulu, HI: University of Hawai'i Press, 2008.

Cao, Cong. *China's Scientific Elite.* London: Routledge, 2004.

Carrillo, Ana María, and Anne-Emanuelle Birn. "Neighbours on Notice: National and Imperialist Interests in the American Public Health Association, 1872–1921." *Canadian Bulletin of Medical History* 25, no. 1 (2008): 225–54.

Chang, Shu-Ching 張淑卿. "Fanglao tixi yu jiankong jishu: Taiwan jiehebing shi yanjiu (1945–1970s) 防癆體系與監控技術:台灣結核病史研究（1945–1970s）[The System of Tuberculosis Control and the Techniques of Surveillance: The History of Tuberculosis in Taiwan (1945–1970s)]." Hsinchu: National Tsing Hua University, 2004.

Chang, Shu-Ching 張淑卿. "Zhanhou Taiwan de fanglao baojianyuan 戰後台灣的防癆保健員 [Lay Home Visitors in Tuberculosis Control after World War II in Taiwan]." *Jindai zhongguo funushi yanjiu* 近代中國婦女史研究 *[Research on Women in Modern Chinese History]*, no. 14 (2006): 89–123.

Chang, Shu-Ching 張淑卿. "1950 & 60 niandai Taiwan de kajiemiao yufang jiezhong jihua 1950、60 年代台灣的卡介苗預防接種計畫 [The BCG Vaccination Program in Taiwan in the 1950s and 1960s]." *Keji, yiliao yu shehui* 科技醫療與社會 *[Taiwanese Journal for Studies of Science, Technology and Medicine]*, no. 8 (2009): 121–72.

Chang, Li 張力. *Guoji hezuo zai Zhongguo: Guoji Lianmeng jiaose de kaocha* 國際合作在中國: 國際聯盟角色的考察 *[International Collaboration in China: A Study of the Role of the League of Nations (1919–1946)].* Taipei: Academia Sinica, 1999.

Cheek, Timothy. *The Intellectual in Modern Chinese History.* Cambridge: Cambridge University Press, 2015.

Chen, Nai-Ruenn, ed. *Chinese Economic Statistics in the Maoist Era: 1949–1965.* New Brunswick: Transaction Publishers, 2009.

Chiffoleau, Sylvia. *Genèse de la santé publique internationale: de la peste d'Orient à l'OMS.* Rennes: Presses universitaires de Rennes, 2012.

Cohen, Jon. "A Controversial Close-Up of Humanity's Health." *Science* 338, no. 6113 (2012): 1414–16.

Connelly, Matthew. *Fatal Misconception: The Struggle to Control World Population.* Cambridge, MA: Harvard University Press, 2008.

Conrad, Sebastian. *What Is Global History?* Princeton, NJ: Princeton University Press, 2016.

Cueto, Marcos. "The ORIGINS of Primary Health Care and SELECTIVE Primary Health Care." *American Journal of Public Health* 94, no. 11 (2004): 1864–74.

Cueto, Marcos. *Cold War, Deadly Fevers: Malaria Eradication in Mexico, 1955–1975.* Washington, DC: Woodrow Wilson Center Press, 2007a.

Cueto, Marcos. *The Value of Health: A History of the Pan American Health Organization.* Rochester, NY: University of Rochester Press, 2007b.

Cueto, Marcos. "International Health, the Early Cold War and Latin America." *Canadian Bulletin of Medical History* 25, no. 1 (2008): 17–41.

Cueto, Marcos, Theodore M. Brown, and Elizabeth Fee. *The World Health Organization: A History*. Cambridge: Cambridge University Press, 2019.

Cullather, Nick. *The Hungry World*: America's Cold War Battle against Poverty in Asia. Cambridge, MA: Harvard University Press, 2010.

David, Thomas, and Ludovic Tournès. "Introduction. Les philanthropies: un objet d'histoire transnationale." *Monde(s)*, no. 6.2 (2014): 7–22.

Davis, Kevin, Angelina Fisher, Benedict Kingsbury, and Sally Engle Merry, eds. *Governance by Indicators: Global Power Through Quantification and Rankings*. Oxford: Oxford University Press, 2012.

Desrosières, Alain. *La politique des grands nombres: histoire de la raison statistique*. Paris: Éditions La Découverte, 1993.

Desrosières, Alain. *Gouverner par les nombres*. Paris: Presses de l'Ecole des mines, 2008a.

Desrosières, Alain. *Pour une sociologie historique de la quantification*. Paris: Presses de l'Ecole des mines, 2008b.

Didier, Emmanuel. "Globalization of Quantitative Policing: Between Management and Statactivism." *Annual Review of Sociology* 44, no. 1 (2018): 515–34.

Donnelly, Michael. "William Farr and Quantification in Nineteenth-Century English Public Health." In *Body Counts: Medical Quantification in Historical and Sociological Perspectives/La Quantification Médicale, Perspectives Historiques et Sociologiques*, edited by George Weisz, Annick Opinel, Gérard Jorland, and Fondation Mérieux, 251–65. Montreal: McGill-Queens, 2005.

Douki, Caroline, and Philippe Minard. "Histoire globale, histoires connectées: un changement d'échelle historiographique?" *Revue d'histoire moderne et contemporaine* 5, no. 54–4, no. 5 (2007): 7–21.

Du, Lihong 杜丽红. "Zhidu kuosan yu zaidihua: Lan Ansheng zai Beijing de gonggong weisheng shiyan, 1921–1925 制度擴散與在地化: 蘭安生 (John B. Grant) 在北京的公共衛生試驗, 1920–1925 [Institutional Diffusion and Localization: John B. Grant's Public Health Experiments in Beijing, 1921–1925]." *Zhongyang Yanjiuyuan jindaishi yanjiusuo jikan* 中央研究院近代史研究所集刊 *[Bulletin of the Institute of Modern History Academia Sinica]*, no.86 (2014): 1–47.

Duffy, John. *The Sanitarians: A History of American Public Health*. Urbana: University of Illinois Press, 1992.

Ekbladh, David. *The Great American Mission: Modernization and the Construction of an American World Order*. Princeton, NJ: Princeton University Press, 2011.

Endicott, Stephen Lyon, and Edward Hagerman. *The United States and Biological Warfare: Secrets from the Early Cold War and Korea*. Bloomington, IN: Indiana University Press, 1998.

Engel, Jonathan. *Doctors and Reformers: Discussion and Debate over Health Policy, 1925–1950*. Social Problems and Social Issues. Columbia, SC: University of South Carolina Press, 2002.

Escobar, Arturo. *Encountering Development: The Making and Unmaking of the Third World*. Princeton, NJ: Princeton University Press, 1995.

Espeland, Wendy Nelson, and Mitchell L. Stevens. "Commensuration as a Social Process." *Annual Review of Sociology* 24, no. 1 (1998): 313–43.

Espeland, Wendy Nelson, and Mitchell L. Stevens. "A Sociology of Quantification." *European Journal of Sociology* 49, no. 3 (2008): 401–36.

Espeland, Wendy Nelson, and Michael Sauder. *Engines of Anxiety: Academic Rankings, Reputation, and Accountability*. New York: Russell Sage Foundation, 2016.

Fairbank, John K., and Mary C. Wright. "Introduction." *The Journal of Asian Studies* 17, no. 1 (1957): 55–60.

Fairbank, John K., and Merle Goldman. *China: A New History, Second Enlarged Edition*. Cambridge, MA: Harvard University Press, 2006.

Fang, Xiaoping. *Barefoot Doctors and Western Medicine in China*. Rochester, NY: University of Rochester Press, 2012.

Fang, Xiaoping. "Diseases, Peasants, and Nation-Building in Rural China. Social Conformity, Institutional Strengthening, and Political Indoctrination." In *Public Health and National Reconstruction in Post-War Asia: International Influences, Local Transformations*, edited by Liping Bu and Ka-Che Yip, 52–71. New York: Routledge, 2015.

Fang, Xiaoping. *China and the Cholera Pandemic: Restructuring Society under Mao*. Pittsburgh, PA: University of Pittsburgh Press, 2021.

Farley, John. *To Cast Out Disease: A History of the International Health Division of Rockefeller Foundation*. Oxford: Oxford University Press, 2004.

Farley, John. *Brock Chisholm, the World Health Organization, and the Cold War*. Vancouver: University of British Columbia Press, 2009.

Fee, Elizabeth. *Disease and Discovery: A History of the Johns Hopkins School of Hygiene and Public Health, 1916–1939*. Baltimore, MD: Johns Hopkins University Press, 1987.

Feng-Yuan, Hsu 許峰源. "Shijie weisheng zuzhi yu Taiwan nueji de fangzhi (1950–1972) 世界衛生組織與台灣瘧疾的防治（1950–1972） [Taiwan–World Health Organization Malaria Control Measures (1950–1972)]." Taipei: National Chengchi University, 2013.

Fox, Daniel M. "The Significance of the Milbank Memorial Fund for Policy: An Assessment at its Centennial." *The Milbank Quarterly* 84, no. 1 (2006): 5–36.

Fox, Daniel M. "Foundations and Health: Innovation, Marginalization, and Relevance since 1900." In *American Foundations: Roles and Contributions*, edited by Helmut K. Anheier and David C. Hammack. Washington, DC: Brookings Institution Press, 2010.

Fu, Zhengyung. *Autocratic Tradition and Chinese Politics*. Cambridge: Cambridge University Press, 1993.

Friedman, Jeremy. *Shadow Cold War: The Sino-Soviet Competition for the Third World*. Chapel Hill: University of North Carolina Press, 2015.

Gao, Xi. "Foreign Models of Medicine in Twentieth-Century China." In *Medical Transitions in Twentieth-Century China*, edited by Mary Brown Bullock and Bridie Andrews, 173–211. Bloomington, IN: Indiana University Press, 2014.

Gardey, Delphine. *Écrire, calculer, classer: comment une révolution de papier a transformé les sociétés contemporaines, 1800–1940*. Paris: Éditions La Découverte, 2008.

Ghosh, Arunabh. "Accepting Difference, Seeking Common Ground: Sino-Indian Statistical Exchanges 1951–1959." *BJHS Themes* 1 (2016): 61–82.

Ghosh, Arunabh. *Making It Count: Statistics and Statecraft in the Early People's Republic of China*. Princeton, NJ: Princeton University Press, 2020.

Gorsky, Martin, and Christopher Sirrs. "World Health by Place: The Politics of International Health System Metrics, 1924–c. 2010." *Journal of Global History* 12, no. 3 (2017): 361–85.

Gross, Miriam. *Farewell to the God of Plague: Chairman Mao's Campaign to Deworm China*. Berkeley, CA: University of California Press, 2016.

Hacking, Ian. *The Taming of Chance*. Cambridge: Cambridge University Press, 1990.

Hardy, Anne, and M. Eileen Magnello. "Statistical Methods in Epidemiology: Karl Pearson, Ronald Ross, Major Greenwood and Austin Bradford Hill, 1900–1945." *Sozial- und Präventivmedizin* 47, no. 2 (2002): 80–89.

Harrison, Mark. *Contagion: How Commerce Has Spread Disease*. New Haven, CT: Yale University Press, 2013.

Hayford, Charles Wishart. *To the People: James Yen and Village China*. New York: Columbia University Press, 1990.

Herren, Madeleine, Martin Rüesch, and Christiane Sibille. *Transcultural History: Theories, Methods, Sources*. Berlin: Springer, 2012.

Higgs, Edward. *The Information State in England: The Central Collection of Information on Citizens Since 1500*. New York: Palgrave Macmillan, 2004.

Hoffman, Beatrix. *The Wages of Sickness: The Politics of Health Insurance in Progressive America*. Chapel Hill, NC: University of North Carolina Press, 2001.

Huber, Valeska. "The Unification of the Globe by Disease? The International Sanitary Conferences on Cholera, 1851–1894." *The Historical Journal* 49, no. 2 (2006): 453–76.

Hsu, Sheng-Kai 徐聖凱. *Rizhi shiqi Taipei gaodeng xuexiao yu jingying yangcheng* 日治時期臺北高等學校與菁英養成 *[Higher Education and Elite Formation in Taipei During the Japanese Rule Period]*. Taipei: Airiti Press, 2012.

Iriye, Akira. *Global Community: The Role of International Organizations in the Making of the Contemporary World*. Berkeley, CA: University of California Press, 2004.

Iriye, Akira. *Global and Transnational History: The Past, Present, and Future*. New York: Palgrave Macmillan, 2013.

Iriye, Akira, and Pierre-Yves Saunier. *The Palgrave Dictionary of Transnational History: From the Mid-19th Century to the Present Day*. New York: Palgrave Macmillan, 2009.

Joseph, Jonathan. *The Social in the Global: Social Theory, Governmentality and Global Politics*. Cambridge: Cambridge University Press, 2012.

Keenan, Barry. *The Dewey Experiment in China: Educational Reform and Political Power in the Early Republic*. Cambridge, MA: Council on East Asian Studies, Harvard University, 1977.

Kiersey, Nicholas J., and Doug Stokes, eds. *Foucault and International Relations: New Critical Engagements*. London: Routledge, 2011.

Kirby, Maurice W. *Operational Research in War and Peace: The British Experience from the 1930s to 1970*. London: Imperial College Press, 2003.

Kirby, William C. "The Internationalization of China: Foreign Relations at Home and Abroad in the Republican Era." *The China Quarterly*, no. 150 (1997): 433–58.

Kuo, Wen-Hua 郭文華. "Yijiuwuling zhi qiling niandai Taiwan jiating jihua: Yiliao zhengce yu nuxing shi de tantao 一九五零至七零年代台灣家庭計畫: 醫療政策與女性史的探討 [Family Planning in Taiwan from 1950 to 1970: An Exploration of Medical Policy and Women's History]." Hsinchu: Institute of History, National Tsing Hua University, 1997.

Kuo, Wen-Hua 郭文華. "Meiyuan xia de weisheng zhengce: 1960 niandai Taiwan jiating jihua de tantao 美援下的衛生政策: 1960 年代台灣家庭計劃的探討 [Public Health Policy with US Aid: Discussions of Taiwan's Family Planning in the 1960s]." In *Diguo yu xiandai yixue* 帝國與現代醫學 *[Empires and Modern Medicine]*, edited by Shang-jen Li, 325–65. Taipei: Linking Publishing, 2008.

Kuo, Wen-Hua 郭文華. "Ruhe kandai Meiyuan xia de weisheng? Yi ge lishi shuxie de fanxing yu zhanwang 如何看待美援下的衛生? 一個歷史書寫的反省與展望 [How to Write a History of Public Health under US Aid in Taiwan: A Critical Review]." *Taiwan shi yanjiu* 台灣史研究 *[Taiwan Historical Research]* 17, no. 1 (2010): 175–210.

Lam, Tong. *A Passion for Facts: Social Surveys and the Construction of the Chinese Nation-State, 1900–1949*. Berkeley, CA: University of California Press, 2011.

Lampland, Martha, and Susan Leigh Star. *Standards and Their Stories: How Quantifying, Classifying, and Formalizing Practices Shape Everyday Life*. Ithaca, NY: Cornell University Press, 2009.

Lei, Hsiang-Lin 雷祥麟. "Weisheng weihe bushi baowei shengming? Minguo shiqi linglei de weisheng, ziwo, yu jibing 衛生爲何不是保衛生命? 民國時期另類的衛生、自我、與疾病 [Why Weisheng Is Not About Guarding Life? Alternative Conceptions of Hygiene, Self, and Illness in the Republican China]." *Taiwan shehui yanjiu jikan* 台灣社會研究季刊 *[Taiwan: A Radical Quarterly in Social Studies]*, no. 54 (2004): 17–59.

Lei, Sean Hsiang-Lin. "Habituating Individuality: The Framing of Tuberculosis and its Material Solutions in Republican China." *Bulletin of the History of Medicine* 84, no. 2 (2010): 248–79.

Lei, Sean Hsiang-Lin. *Neither Donkey nor Horse: Medicine in the Struggle Over China's Modernity*. Chicago, IL: University of Chicago Press, 2014.

Leitenberg, Milton. "A Chinese Admission of False Korean War Allegations of Biological Weapon Use by the United States." *Asian Perspective* 40, no. 1 (2016): 131–46.

Leonelli, Sabina. "Data Science in Times of Pan(Dem)ic." *Harvard Data Science Review*, no. 3.1 (2021): 3.

Li, Tania Murray. *The Will to Improve: Governmentality, Development, and the Practice of Politics*. Durham, NC: Duke University Press Books, 2007.

Li, Shang-Jen 李尚仁. "Shijiu shiji Zhongguo tongshang gangbu de weisheng zhuangkuang: haiguan yiguan de guandian 十九世紀通商港埠的衛生狀況: 海關醫官的觀點 [Health Conditions of Treaty Ports in China during 19th Century: From the Perspective of Customs Medical Officer]." In *Jiankang yu shehui: Huaren weisheng xinshi* 健康與社會: 華人衛生新史 *[Health and Society: The New History of Chinese Hygiene]*, edited by Chu Ping-Yi, 69–93. Taipei: Linking Books, 2013.

Lin, Yi-Ping, and Shiyung Liu. "A Forgotten War: Malaria Eradication in Taiwan 1905–1965." In *Health and Hygiene in Chinese East Asia: Policies and Publics in the Long Twentieth Century*, edited by Angela Ki Che Leung and Charlotte Furth, 183–203. Durham and London: Duke University Press, 2010.

Lin, Yi-Tang 林意唐. "Waiguo weisheng zuzhi yu Minguo huangjin shinian de gonggong weisheng shiyan: Dingxian xiangcun baojian xi tong yu zhongyang weisheng sheshi shiyanchu de Jiangning shiyanxian (1928–1937) 外国卫生组织与民国黄金十年的公共卫生实验：定县乡村保健系统与中央卫生设施实验处的江宁实验县(1928–1937) [Foreign Health Organizations and Public Health Experiments during the Nanjing Decade: Ting Hsien Rural Health Experiment System and the Central Field Health Station's Jiangning County Experiment (1928–1937)]." *Yiliao shehuishi yanjiu* 医疗社会史研究 *[Journal of Social History of Medicine]* 3, no. 1 (2017a): 156–75.

Lin, Yi-Tang. "Making Standards to Quantify All Health Matters: The World Health Organization's Statistical Practices (1946–1960)." *Monde(s)*, no. 11(2017b): 247–66.

Litsios, Socrates. "Selskar Gunn and China: The Rockefeller Foundation's 'Other' Approach to Public Health." *Bulletin of the History of Medicine* 79, no. 2 (2005): 295–318.

Liu, Michael Shiyung. "The Theory and Practices of Malariology in Colonial Taiwan." In *Disease, Colonialism, and the State: Malaria in Modern East Asian History*, edited by Ka-Che Yip, 49–60. Hong Kong: Hong Kong University Press, 2009.

Liu, Michael Shiyung. "From Japanese Colonial Medicine to American-Standard Medicine in Taiwan: A Case Study of the Transition in the Medical Profession and Practices in East Asia." In *Science, Public Health and the State in Modern Asia*, edited by Liping Bu, Darwin H. Stapleton, and Ka-Che Yip, 161–76. London: Routledge, 2012.

Löhr, Isabella, and Roland Wenzlhuemer, eds. *The Nation State and Beyond: Governing Globalization Processes in the Nineteenth and Early Twentieth Centuries*. Heidelberg: Springer, 2013.

Lu, Li 李璐 and Zhang Daqing 张大庆. "Lan Ansheng de gongxian: Zhongguo gonggong weisheng jingyan zai yindu de zhuanyi" 兰安生的贡献:中国公共卫生经验在印度的转移 [John Black Grant's Contribution: Chinese Public Health Experiences' Transplant in India]. *Yixue yu Zhexue* 医学与哲学 *[Medicine and Philosophy]* 36, no. 09A (2015): 81–4.

Luesink, David, William H. Schneider, and Zhang Daqing. *China and the Globalization of Biomedicine*. Rochester, NY: University of Rochester Press, 2019.

Magnello, Eileen. "The Introduction of Mathematical Statistics into Medical Research: The Roles of Karl Pearson, Major Greenwood and Austin Bradford Hill." In *The Road to Medical Statistics*, edited by Eileen Magnello and Anne Hardy, 95–123. Amsterdam; New York: Rodopi, 2002.

Magnello, Eileen, and Anne Hardy, eds. *The Road to Medical Statistics* (Amsterdam; New York: Rodopi, 2002)

Manderson, Lenore. "Wireless War in the Eastern Arena: Epidemiological Surveillance, Disease Prevention and the Work of the Eastern Bureau of the League of Nations Health Organisation." In *International Health Organisations and Movements, 1918–1939*, edited by Paul Weindling, 109–33. Cambridge: Cambridge University Press, 1995.

Manela, Erez. "A Pox on Your Narrative: Writing Disease Control into Cold War History." *Diplomatic History* 34, no. 2 (2010): 299–323.

Manning, Kimberley Ens, and Felix Wemheuer, eds. *Eating Bitterness: New Perspectives on China's Great Leap Forward and Famine*. Vancouver: University of British Columbia Press, 2011.

Marks, Shula. "What is Colonial About Colonial Medicine? And What has Happened to Imperialism and Health?" *Social History of Medicine* 10, no. 2 (1997): 205–19.

Matthews, J. Rosser. *Quantification and the Quest for Medical Certainty*. Princeton, NJ: Princeton University Press, 1995.

McMillen, Christian W. *Discovering Tuberculosis – A Global History, 1900 to the Present*. New Haven, CT: Yale University Press, 2015.

Mennicken, Andrea, and Wendy Nelson Espeland. "What's New with Numbers? Sociological Approaches to the Study of Quantification." *Annual Review of Sociology* 45, no. 1 (2019): 223–45.

Meng-Hui, Wu 鄔孟慧. "Zhanhou Taiwan de feijiehebing fangzhi (1950– 1966) 戰後台灣的肺結核病防治 (1950–1966) [Prevention of Pulmonary Tuberculosis in Taiwan after the Second World War (1950–1966)]." Master's dissertation, Nantou: National Chi-Nan University, 2004.

Merry, Sally Engle. *The Seductions of Quantification: Measuring Human Rights, Gender Violence, and Sex Trafficking*. Chicago, IL: University of Chicago Press, 2016.

Mitter, Rana. "Imperialism, Transnationalism, and the Reconstruction of Post-War China: UNRRA in China, 1944–7." *Past & Present* 218, suppl. 8 (2013): 51–69.

Moon, Suerie, Devi Sridhar, Muhammad A. Pate, et al. "Will Ebola Change the Game? Ten Essential Reforms Before the Next Pandemic. The Report of the Harvard-LSHTM Independent Panel on the Global Response to Ebola." *The Lancet* 386, no. 10009 (2015): 2204–21.

Morabia, Alfredo. *A History of Epidemiologic Methods and Concepts*. Basel: Birkhäuser, 2004.

Moriyama, Iwao, Ruth M. Loy, Alastair H. T. Robb-Smith, et al. *History of the Statistical Classification of Diseases and Causes of Death*. Hyattsville, MD: National Center of Health Statistics, 2011.

Murard, Lion. "Atlantic Crossings in the Measurement of Health: From US Appraisal Forms to the League of Nations' Health Indices." In *Medicine, the Market and the Mass Media: Producing Health in the Twentieth Century*, edited by Virginia Berridge and Kelly Loughlin, 19–54. London: Routledge, 2004.

Murard, Lion. "La santé publique et ses instruments de mesure: des barèmes évaluatifs américains aux indices numériques." In *Body Counts: Medical Quantification in Historical and Sociological Perspectives/La Quantification*

*Médicale, Perspectives Historiques et Sociologiques*, edited by Gérard Jorland, Annick Opinel, and George Weisz, 266–93. Montreal: McGill-Queens University Press, 2005.

Murard, Lion. "Designs within Disorder: International Conferences on Rural Health Care and the Art of the Local, 1931–1939." In *Shifting Boundaries of Public Health: Europe in the Twentieth Century*, edited by Susan Gross Solomon, Lion Murard, and Patrick Zylberman, 141–174, Rochester Studies in Medical History. Rochester, NY: University of Rochester Press, 2008.

Murphy, Michelle. *The Economization of Life*. Durham, NC: Duke University Press, 2017.

Nield, Robert. *China's Foreign Places: The Foreign Presence in China in the Treaty Port Era, 1840–1943*. Hong Kong: Hong Kong University Press, 2015.

Ninkovich, Frank. "The Rockefeller Foundation, China, and Cultural Change." *The Journal of American History* 70, no. 4 (1984): 799–820.

Packard, Randall M. "Malaria Dreams: Postwar Visions of Health and Development in the Third World." *Medical Anthropology* 17, no. 3 (1997): 279–96.

Packard, Randall M. "'Roll Back Malaria, Roll in Development'? Reassessing the Economic Burden of Malaria." *Population and Development Review* 35, no. 1 (2009): 53–87.

Packard, Randall M. *The Making of a Tropical Disease: A Short History of Malaria*. Baltimore, MD: Johns Hopkins University Press, 2007.

Packard, Randall M. *A History of Global Health: Interventions into the Lives of Other Peoples*. Baltimore, MD: Johns Hopkins University Press, 2016.

Paillette, Céline. "Épidémies, santé et ordre mondial. Le rôle des organisations sanitaires internationales, 1903–1923." *Monde(s)*, no. 2 (2012): 235–56.

Parmar, Inderjeet. *Foundations of the American Century: The Ford, Carnegie, and Rockefeller Foundations in the Rise of American Power*. New York: Columbia University Press, 2012.

Pearson, Jessica Lynne. *The Colonial Politics of Global Health: France and the United Nations in Postwar Africa*. Cambridge, MA: Harvard University Press, 2018.

Porter, Theodore M. *The Rise of Statistical Thinking: 1820–1900*. Princeton, NJ: Princeton University Press, 1986.

Porter, Theodore M. *Trust in Numbers: In Pursuit of Objectivity in Science and Public Life*. Princeton, NJ: Princeton University Press, 1995.

Porter, Theodore M. *Karl Pearson: The Scientific Life in a Statistical Age*. Princeton, NJ: Princeton University Press, 2004.

Raj, Kapil. "Colonial Encounters and the Forging of Knowledge and National Identities: Great Britain and India, 1760–1850." In *Social History of Science in Colonial India*, edited by S. Irfan Habib and Dhruv Raina, 83–101. Oxford: Oxford University Press, 2007.

Ramsden, Edmund. "Carving up Population Science Eugenics, Demography and the Controversy over the 'Biological Law' of Population Growth." *Social Studies of Science* 32, no. 5–6 (2002): 857–99.

Rasmussen, Anne. "L'hygiène en congrès (1852–1912): circulation et configuration internationales." In *Les Hygiénistes: Enjeux, modèles et pratiques (XVIIIe-XXe Siècles)*, edited by Patrice Bourdelais, 213–39. Paris: Belin, 2011.

Reinisch, Jessica. "Introduction: Relief in the Aftermath of War." *Journal of Contemporary History* 43, no. 3 (2008): 371–404.

Reinisch, Jessica. "'Auntie UNRRA' at the Crossroads." *Past & Present* 218, suppl. 8 (2013): 70–97.

Reubi, David. "A Genealogy of Epidemiological Reason: Saving Lives, Social Surveys and Global Population." *BioSocieties* 13, no. 1 (2017): 1–22.

Revel, Jacques, ed. *Jeux d'échelles. La micro-analyse à l'expérience*. Paris: Seuil, 1996.

Rogaski, Ruth. *Hygienic Modernity: Meanings of Health and Disease in Treaty-Port China*. Berkeley, CA: University of California Press, 2004.

Rosen, George. *A History of Public Health*. Baltimore, MD: Johns Hopkins University Press, 2015.

Rosenberg, Clifford. "The International Politics of Vaccine Testing in Interwar Algiers." *The American Historical Review* 117, no. 3 (2012): 671–97.

Salathé, Marcel, Linus Bengtsson, Todd J. Bodnar, et al. "Digital Epidemiology." *PLoS Computational Biology* 8, no. 7 (2012): 1–5.

Sauder, Michael, and Wendy Nelson Espeland. "The Discipline of Rankings: Tight Coupling and Organizational Change." *American Sociological Review* 74, no. 1 (2009): 63–82.

Saunier, Pierre-Yves. "Circulations, connexions et espaces transnationaux." *Genèses* 57, no. 4 (2004): 110–26.

Saunier, Pierre-Yves. *Transnational History*. New York: Palgrave Macmillan, 2013.

Scott, James C. *Seeing Like a State: How Certain Schemes to Improve the Human Condition Have Failed*. New Haven, CT: Yale University Press, 1998.

Sealander, Judith. *Private Wealth and Public Life: Foundation Philanthropy and the Reshaping of American Social Policy from the Progressive Era to the New Deal*. Baltimore, MD: Johns Hopkins University Press, 1997.

Singaravélou, Pierre. *Tianjin Cosmopolis. Une histoire de la mondialisation en 1900*. Paris: Le Seuil, 2017.

Sluga, Glenda. *Internationalism in the Age of Nationalism*. Philadelphia: University of Pennsylvania Press, 2013.

Soon, Wayne. *Global Medicine in China: A Diasporic History*. Stanford, CA: Stanford University Press, 2020.

Stapleton, Darwin H. *Creating a Tradition of Biomedical Research: Contributions to the History of the Rockefeller University*. New York: Rockefeller University Press, 2004.

Stapleton, Darwin H. "Malaria Eradication and the Technological Model: The Rockefeller Foundation and Public Health in East Asia." In *Disease, Colonialism, and the State: Malaria in Modern East Asian History*, edited by Ka-Che Yip, 71–84. Hong Kong: Hong Kong University Press, 2009.

Starr, Paul. *The Social Transformation of American Medicine*. New York: Basic Books, 1982.

Stromquist, Shelton. *Reinventing "The People": The Progressive Movement, the Class Problem, and the Origins of Modern Liberalism*. Urbana and Chicago, IL: University of Illinois Press, 2006.

Susser, Mervyn, and Zena Stein. *Eras in Epidemiology: The Evolution of Ideas*. Oxford and New York: Oxford University Press, 2009.

Szreter, Simon. "The Idea of Demographic Transition and the Study of Fertility Change: A Critical Intellectual History." *Population and Development Review* 19, no. 4 (1993): 659–701.

Taylor, Kim. *Chinese Medicine in Early Communist China, 1945–63: A Medicine of Revolution.* London: Routledge, 2004.

Teller, Michael E. *The Tuberculosis Movement: A Public Health Campaign in the Progressive Era.* Contributions in Medical Studies 22. New York: Greenwood Press, 1988.

Thomas, Karen Kruse. *Health and Humanity: A History of the Johns Hopkins Bloomberg School of Public Health, 1935–1985.* Baltimore, MD: Johns Hopkins University Press, 2016.

Toon, Elizabeth. "Selling the Public on Public Health: The Commonwealth and Milbank Health Demonstrations and the Meaning of Community Health Education." In *Philanthropic Foundations: New Scholarship, New Possibilities,* edited by Ellen Condliffe Lagemann, 119–30. Bloomington and Indianapolis, IN: Indiana University Press, 1999.

Tournès, Ludovic. *Les États-Unis et la Société des Nations (1914–1946): le système international face à l'émergence d'une superpuissance.* Bern: Peter Lang, 2016.

Tworek, Heidi J. S. "Communicable Disease: Information, Health, and Globalization in the Interwar Period." *American Historical Review* 124, no. 3 (2019): 813–42.

Tyrrell, Ian. *Reforming the World: The Creation of America's Moral Empire.* Princeton, NJ: Princeton University Press, 2010.

Van de Ven, Hans. *Breaking with the Past: The Maritime Customs Service and the Global Origins of Modernity in China.* New York: Columbia University Press, 2014.

Vargha, Dóra. *Polio Across the Iron Curtain: Hungary's Cold War with an Epidemic.* Cambridge: Cambridge University Press, 2018.

Vayena, Effy, Joan Dzenowagis, John S. Brownstein, and Aziz Sheikh. "Policy Implications of Big Data in the Health Sector." *Bulletin of the World Health Organization* 96, no. 1 (2018): 66–8.

Walker, Kenneth. *Food Grain Procurement and Consumption in China.* Cambridge: Cambridge University Press, 1984.

Watt, John R. *Saving Lives in Wartime China: How Medical Reformers Built Modern Healthcare Systems Amid War and Epidemics, 1928–1945.* Leiden: Brill, 2014.

Weathersby, Kathryn. "New Evidence on the Korean War." *Cold War International History Project Bulletin* 11 (1998): 176–99.

Weindling, Paul. "German Overtures to Russia, 1919–1925: Between Racial Expansion and National Coexistence." In *Doing Medicine Together: Germany and Russia Between the Wars,* edited by Susan Gross Solomon, 35–60. German and European Studies 4. Toronto: University of Toronto Press, 2006.

Weindling, Paul. "American Foundations and the Internationalizing of Public Health." In *Shifting Boundaries of Public Health: Europe in the Twentieth Century,* edited by Susan Gross Solomon, Lion Murard, and Patrick Zylberman, 63–86. Rochester Studies in Medical History. Rochester, NY: University of Rochester Press, 2008.

Weisz, George, and Noemi Tousignant. "International Health Research and the Emergence of Global Health in the Late Twentieth Century." *Bulletin of the History of Medicine* 93, no. 3 (2019): 365–400.

Westad, Odd Arne. *The Global Cold War: Third World Interventions and the Making of Our Times.* Cambridge and New York: Cambridge University Press, 2005.

Wheatley, Steven. "The Partnerships of Foundations and Research Universities." In *American Foundations: Roles and Contributions*, edited by Helmut K. Anheier and David C. Hammack, 73–97. Washington, DC: Brookings Institution Press, 2010.

Wo, Hongmei 沃紅梅. "Zhongguo yixue tongjixue fazhan jianshi 中国医学统计学发展简史 [Brief History of China's Medical Statistics, 1949–2012]." Master's dissertation, Nanjing Medical College, 2013.

Wu, Harry Yi-Jui. "World Citizenship and the Emergence of the Social Psychiatry Project of the World Health Organization, 1948–c.1965." *History of Psychiatry* 26, no. 2 (2015): 166–81.

Wu, Harry Yi-Jui. *Mad by the Millions: Mental Disorders and the Early Years of the World Health Organization.* Cambridge, MA: MIT Press, 2021.

Xu, Guoqi. *China and the Great War: China's Pursuit of a New National Identity and Internationalization.* Cambridge: Cambridge University Press, 2005.

Yang, Xiangyin 杨祥银 and Wang Pong 王鹏. "Minzu zhuyi yu xiandaihua: Wu Liande dui shouhui haigang jianyiquan de hunhe lunshu 民族主义与现代化: 伍连德对收回海港检疫权的混合论述 [Nationalism and Modernization: The Mixed Discourse of Wu Liande Regarding the Takeover of Maritime Quarantine]." *Huaren huaqiao lishi yanjiu [Journal of Overseas Chinese History Studies]*, no. 1 (2014): 51–60.

Yang, Nianqun 杨念群. "Beijing 'weisheng shifanqu' de jianli yu chengshi kongjian gongneng de zhuanhuan 北京'卫生示范区'的建立与城市空间功能的转换 [The Establishment of Beijing Health Demonstration and the Transformation of Urban Space Functions]." *Beijing dangan shiliao* 北京档案史料 *[Beijing Archives Series]*, no. 1 (2000): 205–31.

Yang, Nianqun 杨念群. "'Lan Ansheng moshi' yu Minguo chunian Beijing shengsi kongzhi kongjian de zhuanhuan '兰安生模式'与民国初年北京生死控制空间的转换 [The John B. Grant Model and the Transfer of Spaces of Birth and Death Control in the Early Years of the Republic of China]." *Shehuixue yanjiu* 社会学研究 *[Sociological Studies]*, no.4 (1999): 98–133.

Yang, Nianqun 杨念群. "Minguo chunian Beijing de shengsi kongzhi yu kongjian zhuanhuan 民国初年北京的生死控制与空间转换 [Birth and Death Control and the Transformation of Space at the Beginning Years of the Republic of China]." In *kongjian jiyi shehui zhuanxing*: "xin shehui shi" yanjiu lunwen jingxuan ji 空间·记忆·社会转型: 「新社会史」研究论文精选集 *[Space, Memory, Transformation of Society: Compilation of New Social History Papers]*, edited by Nianqun Yang. Shanghai: Shanghai People's Publishing House, 2001.

Yang, Nianqun 杨念群. *Zaizao "bingren": Zhongxiyi chongtu xia de kongjian zhengzhi (1832–1985)* 再造"病人": 中西医冲突下的空间政治 (1832–1985) *[Remaking "Patients": Space Politics under the Conflict Between Chinese and Western Medicine (1832–1985)].* Beijing: China Renmin University Press, 2006.

Yip, Ka-Che. *Health and National Reconstruction in Nationalist China: The Development of Modern Health Services, 1928–1937.* Ann Arbor, MI: Association for Asian Studies Incorporated, 1995.

Youde, Jeremy. *Biopolitical Surveillance and Public Health in International Politics.* New York: Palgrave Macmillan, 2010.

Yu, Xinzhong 余新忠. "Fuza xing yu xiandaixing: wan Qing jianyi jizhi yin-jianzhong de shehui fanying 复杂性与现代性：晚清检疫机制引建中的社会反应 [Complexity and Modernity: Social Reactions Toward the Establishment of Quarantine Measures in the Late Qing Dynasty]." *Jindaishi Yanjiu* 近代史研究 *[Modern Chinese History Studies]* 188, no. 2 (2012): 47–64.

Zanasi, Margherita. "Exporting Development: The League of Nations and Republican China." *Comparative Studies in Society and History* 49, no. 1 (2007): 143–69.

Zhou, Xun. *The Great Famine in China, 1958–1962: A Documentary History.* New Haven, CT: Yale University Press, 2012.

Zhou, Xun. *Forgotten Voices of Mao's Great Famine, 1958–1962: An Oral History.* New Haven, CT: Yale University Press, 2013.

Zhou, Xun. "From China's 'Barefoot Doctor' to Alma Ata: The Primary Health Care Movement in the Long 1970s." In *China, Hong Kong, and the Long 1970s: Global Perspectives,* edited by Priscilla Roberts and Odd Arne Westad, 135–57. New York: Palgrave Macmillan, 2017.

Zhou, Xun. *The People's Health: Health Intervention and Delivery in Mao's China 1949–1983.* Montreal: McGill-Queen's University Press, 2020.

Zunz, Olivier. *Philanthropy in America: A History.* Princeton, NJ: Princeton University Press, 2014.

# Index

Please note that page numbers in italics direct the reader to tables, photographs or other images.

www.ingramcontent.com/pod-product-compliance
Ingram Content Group UK Ltd.
Pitfield, Milton Keynes, MK11 3LW, UK
UKHW022001190125
453752UK00007B/53

9 781108 845922